C. D. Claussen · E. K. Fishman · B. Marincek · M. Reiser (Eds.)

Multislice CT · A Practical Guide

Springer-Verlag Berlin Heidelberg GmbH

C. D. Claussen · E. K. Fishman
B. Marincek · M. Reiser (Eds.)

With the Collaboration of A. Kopp

Multislice CT

A Practical Guide

Proceedings of the 6th International SOMATOM CT
Scientific User Conference
Tuebingen, September 2002

With 115 Figures, 29 in colours
and 17 Tables

Springer

Prof. Dr. med. C.C. Claussen
Radiologische Universitätsklinik Tübingen
Abt. Radiologische Diagnostik
Hoppe-Seyler-Str. 3
D-72076 Tübingen

Prof. Dr. med. Borut Marincek
UniversitätsSpital Zürich
Institut für Diagnostische Radiologie
Rämistr. 100
CH-8091 Zürich

Elliot K. Fishman M.D.
Professor of Radiology and Oncology
Director, Diagnostic Radiology and Body CT
Department of Radiology and
Radiological Science
The Johns Hopkins Hospital
600 North Wolfe Street Baltimore
Maryland 21287
USA

Prof. Dr. med. M. Reiser
Institut für Klinische Radiologie
Universitätsklinik München
Standort Großhadern
Marchioninistr. 15
D-81377 München

ISBN 978-3-642-62279-3

Cataloging-in-Publication Data applied for Bibliographic information published by Die Deutsche Bibliothek. Die Deutsche Bibliothek lists this publication in the Deutsche Nationalbibliografie; detailed ibliographic data is abailable in the Internet at http://dnb.ddb.de.

ISBN 978-3-642-62279-3 ISBN 978-3-642-18758-2 (eBook)
DOI 10.1007/978-3-642-18758-2

springeronline.com

Originally published by Springer-Verlag Berlin Heidelberg New York in 2004
Softcover reprint of the hardcover 1st edition 2004

Cover-Design: design & production, Heidelberg
Typesetting: Goldener Schnitt, Sinzheim

Printed on acid-free paper 18/3130 – 5 4 3 2 1 0

Contents

I Technical Aspects, Workflow, Dose

II Neuro, Head and Neck

III Abdomen and Chest

IV Contrast/CT-Angiography

V Cardio CT

VI Screening

Preface

The 6th International SOMATOM CT Scientific User Conference was held in Tübingen on September 27 and 28, 2002, under the auspices of the Eberhard Karls University Tübingen, the University Hospital Zurich, the Ludwig Maximilians University, Munich, and the Johns Hopkins University, Baltimore. Siemens AG Medical Solutions, Forchheim, was again very gracious in sponsoring the course and the associated events.

There have been remarkable achievements in CT technology, workflow management and applications since the last SOMATOM user conference in Zurich in June 2000. The next generation of multidetector-row CT, now capable of acquiring 16 slices during a single rotation has been introduced. The meeting in Tübingen was the very first conference where research groups from all over the world were presenting their very first results with this new technology in the various fields of CT imaging. It became obvious that these new technical possibilities will again have significant impact on the clinical use of CT.

Tübingen offered a special and inspiring atmosphere for the meeting, an atmosphere which has been preserved throughout time. For more than 500 years the university – one of the oldest in Germany – has been a source for new ideas being pursued by famous philosophers, poets and scientists such as Hölderlin, Mörike, Hegel, Schelling, Kepler, Butenandt and many more.

The experiences presented at the meeting are collected in this book. The chapters will facilitate a thorough understanding of 4- and 16-slice multidetector-row CT and its clinical applications. This will help to fully exploit the diagnostic potential of this technology. We would like to thank all authors for their enthusiasm and superb work. The excellent work of the editorial team at Springer Verlag is also greatly acknowledged.

Claus D. Claussen, M.D.
Professor and Chairman
Department of Diagnostic Radiology
University Hospital Tübingen

Elliot Fishman, M.D.
Professor
Department of Radiology
Johns Hopkins Hospital, Baltimore

Borut Marincek, M.D.
Professor and Chairman
Institute of Diagnostic Radiology
University Hospital Zurich

Maximilian Reiser, M.D.
Professor and Chairman
Department of Radiology
Klinikum Großhadern, Munich

Authors

Editors

C.D. Claussen
Radiologische Universitätsklinik Tübingen, Abt. Radiologische Diagnostik, Hoppe-Seyler-Straße 3, 72076 Tübingen, Germany

Borut Marincek
Universitäts-Spital Zürich, Institut für Diagnostische Radiologie, Rämistraße 100, 8091 Zürich, Schweiz

M. Reiser
Institut für Klinische Radiologie, Universitätsklinik München – Standort Großhadern, Marchioninistraße 15, 81377 München, Germany

Elliot K. Fishman
Professor of Radiology and Oncology, Diagnostic Radiology and Body CT, Department of Radiology and Radiological Science, The Johns Hopkins Hospital
600 North Wolfe Street Baltimore, Maryland 21287, USA

List of Corresponding Authors

K. Ty Bae
Assistant Professor of Radiology, Mallinckrodt Institute of Radiology, Washington Univ. Sch. Med., 510 S Kingshighway Blvd, Box 8131, St. Louis, MO, USA

Christoph Becker
Institut für Klinische Radiologie, Universitätsklinik München – Standort Großhadern, Marchioninistraße 15, 81377 München, Germany

Roman Fischbach
Institut für Klinische Radiologie, Albert-Schweitzer-Straße 33, 48129 Münster, Germany

ELLIOT K. FISHMAN
Professor of Radiology and Oncology, Director Diagnostic Radiology and Body CT, Department of Radiology and Radiological Science, The Johns Hopkins Hospital, 600 North Wolfe Street Baltimore, Maryland 21287, USA

THOMAS FLOHR
Siemens Computertomographie, Siemensstraße 1, 91301 Forchheim, Germany

ANDREAS F. KOPP
Radiologische Universitätsklinik Tübingen, Abt. Radiologische Diagnostik, Hoppe-Seyler-Straße 3, 72076 Tübingen, Germany

GABRIEL P. KRESTIN
Professor and Chairman, Department of Radiology, University Hospital Rotterdam, Dr. Molewaterplein 40, 3015 GD Rotterdam, The Netherlands

MICHAEL LELL
Institut für Diagnostische Radiologie, Universität Erlangen-Nürnberg, Maximiliansplatz 1, 91054 Erlangen, Germany

MICHAEL MACARI
Assistant Professor of Clinical, Department of Radiology, New York University Medical Center, 560 First Avenue, New York, NY, 10016, USA

ALEC MEGIBOW
Professor of Radiology, Department of Radiology, New York University Medical Center, 560 First Avenue, New York, NY, 10016, USA

DAVID NAIDICH
Professor of Radiology, Department of Radiology, New York University School of Medicine, 560 First Avenue, New York, NY 10016, USA

BERND OHNESORGE
Siemens Computertomographie, Siemensstraße 1, 91301 Forchheim, Germany

ROBERTO PASSARIELLO
Professor and Chairman Department of Radiology, University of Rome »La Sapienza«, Viale Regina Elena, 324, 00161, Rome, Italy

MARTINE REMY-JARDIN
Department of Radiology, Hospital Calmette, University Center of Lille, Blvd Jules Leclerq, 59037 Lille cedex, France

PABLO R. ROS
Brigham and Women's Hospital, Harvard Medical School, Boston, Massachusetts
75 Francis Street, Boston, MA 02115, USA

Stefan Schaller
Siemens Computertomographie, Siemensstraße 1, 91301 Forchheim, Germany

U. Joseph Schoepf
Department of Radiology, Brigham and Women's Hospital, Harvard Medical School, 75 Francis Street, Boston, MA 02115, USA

Bernhard Schuknecht
Universitäts-Spital Zürich, Institut für Neuroradiologie, Frauenklinikstrasse 10, 8091 Zürich, Schweiz

Marilyn J. Siegel
Professor of Radiology and Pediatrics, Washington University School of Medicine, Department of Radiology, 660 South Euclid Avenue, Campus Box 8131, St. Louis, MO 63110, USA

I Technical Aspects, Workflow, Dose

1 Computed Tomography – Past, Present and Future

S. Schaller, T. Flohr

Historical Development of CT

The basic principles of computed tomography go back to the work of J.H. Radon, a Bohemian mathematician, who in 1917 published the mathematical framework for reconstruction of an object from its line integrals [1]. First experiments on medical applications of tomography were conducted by A.M. Cormack [2], a hospital physicist at Groote Schuur Hospital in Kapstadt, who without knowledge of Radon's prior work, set out to improve radiation therapy planning. Cormack developed a method for reconstructing the absorption coefficient of a slice of the human body from transmission measurements but was not able to prove the medical significance of this invention. Only later, in the 1970s, did Cormack learn about the prior work of Radon and first applications of his theory in radioastronomy [3]. G.N. Hounsfield, who today is widely recognized as the inventor of computed tomography, independently discovered the method in 1972, and was the first to develop a successful practical implementation [4]. He began his experiments using radioisotopes as sources for his transmission measurements, with measurement times on the order of 9 days. Using more powerful X-ray tubes, it still took about 9 h to complete a measurement. Nevertheless, Hounsfield was able to install a first prototype of his CT system at Atkinson Morley's Hospital in London, and, working closely with neuroradiologist J. Ambrose, successfully scanned the first patient in 1972. A photograph of the early system is shown in Fig. 1. This development sparked a wave of excitement in the medical community. For the first time it was possible to obtain cross-sectional images of the head free of superposition with dramatically improved low-contrast resolution capabilities. In 1979 Hounsfield and Cormack were awarded the Nobel Prize for their invention.

Maybe as surprising as the invention itself was the fact that it originated not from one of the large manufacturers of medical imaging equipment, but from the company EMI, known to many only as the record label of the Beatles. By 1974, EMI had a total of 60 scanners installed and other vendors, including Siemens, quickly followed suit. In 1974 Siemens introduced their first CT scanner, the SIRETOM. Figure 2 shows a photograph of the system and the head image in Fig. 3 illustrates the level of image quality that could be obtained. Rather than using the time-consuming algebraic reconstruction technique employed by the EMI scanners, the SIRETOM used the so-called filtered backprojection reconstruction, a method essentially still in use today.

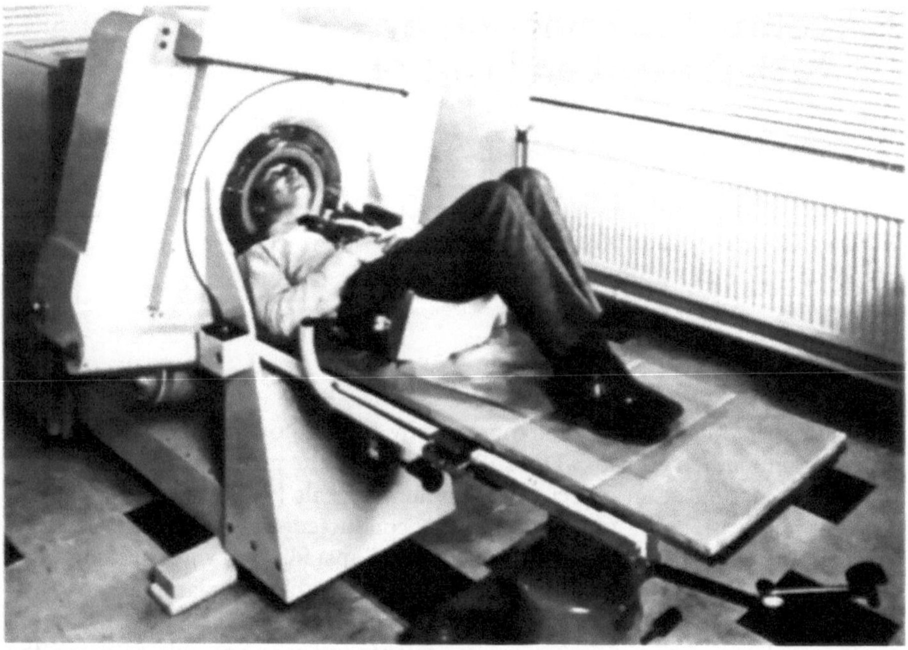

Fig. 1. Early prototype installation of Godfrey N. Hounsfield's first CT scanner. The scanner acquired a total of 28 800 measurements per scan (160 positions at 180 angles) in 5 min. Thus, six times two images could be acquired in about 35 min

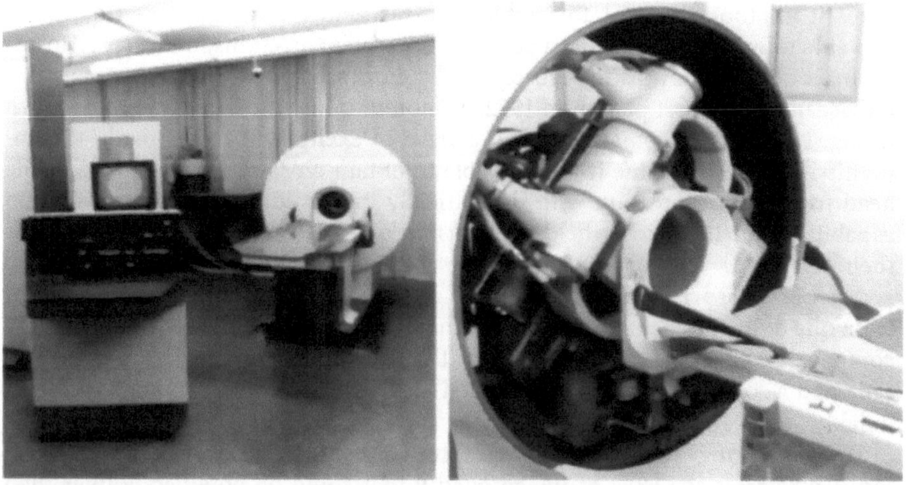

Fig. 2. The Siemens SIRETOM, Siemens' first CT scanner, introduced in 1974. The acquisition time was 5 min for an 80 x 80 image in a 25-cm measurement field of view. The slicewidth was 10 mm and the in-plane spatial resolution was 4 lp/cm

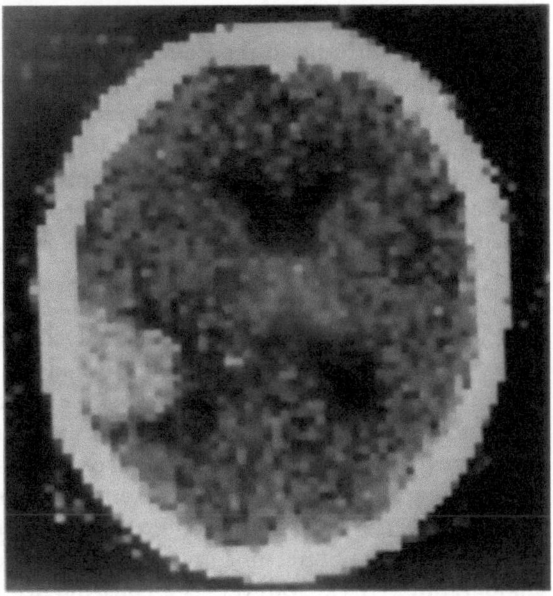

Fig. 3. Early head image in an 80 x 80 image matrix. Although the individual pixels are very coarse, the low-contrast lesion can be clearly depicted

While these early scanners were limited to scanning the head, R.S. Ledley at Georgetown University in Washington worked on developing the first body CT scanner. The decisive step here was to be able to do away with the water bag that was previously required to avoid beam-hardening artefacts. This scanner was introduced at the RSNA 1974 as ACTA scanner (Automatic Computerized Transverse Axial scanner). The scanner with measurement times of 5 min was later commercially distributed by Pfizer. At the same meeting. Ohio Nuclear also introduced their full-body CT scanner DELTA Scan 50, which went into production in 1975 [5].

In general, the years 1973 to 1976 can be regarded as the gold-rush years in CT. As early as in 1974, three generations of CT scanners were known: first, second, and third generation scanners. First generation scanners worked according to the so-called translation-rotation principle [6]. A pencil beam was measured and traversed across the object. After acquisition of a full set of parallel rays, the setup was rotated by an angular increment and the measurement was repeated until a half rotation was acquired. In the second generation, multiple rays were measured concurrently, cutting down the measurement times. In the third generation, a tube and a detector arc on the opposite side rotated without translation. A full fan of rays was acquired at any point in time, cutting down measurement times from minutes to seconds. However, in 1975 and 1976 the performance of today's third-generation design was not fully anticipated and it appeared as if the translation-rotation design with measurement times on the order of 20 s could survive for a longer while. Two years later, yet another system design was introduced, the so-called fourth generation, using a stationary full detector ring.

All vendors introduced new systems in rapid succession [6]. In spring 1977, Ohio Nuclear introduced their new system DELTA-Scan 2000, effectively stalling order income for their DELTA-Scan 50 FS. Other companies felt a pressure to react, resulting in three vendors prematurely exhibiting systems at the RSNA 1977 without any clinical images. This was a remarkable year in many respects, with a total of 18 vendors in tough competition, offering a total of 25 different systems. With a market volume of 750 systems, this resulted in an average of 30 systems per model per year. Some vendors even had to face much smaller numbers and some soon had to give up, resulting in a drastic consolidation of vendors during the following years. The 1980s focused on further reducing scanning times and brought only incremental technical improvements.

Continuously rotating CT systems, based on slip-ring technology, were first introduced in 1987 and were the basis for the introduction of spiral CT in the early nineties by W.A. Kalender, which resulted in a fundamental and far-reaching improvement of CT imaging [7,8]. For the first time, entire scan ranges could be acquired in a single breath-hold, effectively avoiding misregistration caused by breathing. Overlapping image reconstruction greatly benefited many kinds of 3-D applications. Spiral imaging also paved the way for applications like CT angiography (CTA). However, as a consequence of increasing clinical demands, single-slice spiral CT with 1-s gantry rotation time soon encountered its limitations. The goal of acquiring image data of a scan range covering e.g., the thorax or the abdomen at isotropic resolution within a single breath-hold could not be met. In clinical practice, compromises had to be made with regard to either scan range or longitudinal resolution, or the scan range could not be covered within a single breath-hold [9].

Larger volume coverage and improved transverse resolution can be achieved by simultaneous acquisition of more than one slice and by a shorter gantry rotation time. The first step towards multislice acquisition was a two-slice CT scanner introduced in 1993, the Elscint TWIN. In 1998, all major CT manufacturers introduced four-slice CT systems, typically with rotation times of 0.5 s. The corresponding increase in performance clinically translates into

1. increased scan speed, important for trauma, uncooperative patients or very long scan ranges, or
2. increased longitudinal resolution, which for the first time makes it possible to obtain nearly isotropic volume data.

As a consequence, volumetric viewing and diagnosis in a volumetric mode have become integrated elements of the routine workflow [10–12].

Furthermore, new applications have been introduced in clinical practice, the most important application being cardiac CT. With a gantry rotation time of 0.5 s and dedicated image reconstruction approaches, the temporal resolution of an image could be reduced to 250 ms and below [13, 14], which proved to be sufficient for motion-free imaging of the heart in the mid- to end-diastolic phase at low to moderate heart rates. The improved transverse resolution in combination with the excellent low-contrast detectability of modern CT systems allowed for high-resolution CTAs of the coronary arteries [15–18]. In the meantime, first clinical studies have demonstrated the potential of multislice CT to not only detect but also classify lipid, fibrous and calcified plaques in the coronary arteries based on their CT density [19].

Despite all promising advances, clinical challenges and limitations remain for four-slice CT systems. True isotropic resolution for routine applications has not yet been reached, since the transverse resolution of about 1 mm does not fully match the in-plane resolution of about 0.5 mm. For long-range studies, such as peripheral CTAs, even thicker slices (2.5-mm collimated slice width) have to be chosen for acceptable scan times. Scan times are often still too long to allow for CTAs in the purely arterial phase. For a CTA of the circle of Willis, for instance, a scan range of about 100 mm has to be covered. With four-slice scanning at 1-mm collimated slice width using a pitch of 1.5 and 0.5 s gantry rotation time this takes about 9 s; considering the brain circulation time, it should be less than 5 s to avoid venous overlay. In cardiac examinations, stents or severely calcified arteries cannot yet be adequately visualized and suffer from »blooming«, mainly due to partial volume artefacts as a consequence of the still not fully sufficient transverse resolution [18]. For patients with higher heart rates, careful selection of separate reconstruction intervals for left and right coronary artery becomes mandatory [20], yet a diagnostic outcome cannot be guaranteed in this case. The scan time of about 40 s required to cover the entire heart volume (~12 cm) with 4 x 1-mm collimation is at the limit for a single breath-hold scan, it may be problematic for patients who cannot adequately cooperate.

Current State of the Art

Consequently, more than four simultaneously acquired slices combined with submillimeter collimation for routine clinical applications were the next step on the way towards true isotropic scanning with multislice CT, leading to the introduction of a 16-slice CT system in 2001, the SOMATOM Sensation 16 [21]. To improve the temporal resolution of cardiac imaging in a clinically stable way, gantry rotation times have been further reduced to 0.42 s [22].

When looking at the number of slices of multislice CT systems versus the year of their market introduction (see Fig. 4), it can be observed that it approximately follows an exponential law, roughly doubling every 2.5 years. This is an interesting parallel to Moore's law in the microelectronics sector. Table 1 gives an overview of the development of other performance parameters and Fig. 5 shows the resulting improvement in resolution over the last 30 years, illustrated as the corresponding reduction in size of a voxel element.

All recently introduced 16-slice CT systems employ Adaptive Array Detectors. The Siemens SOMATOM Sensation 16 uses 24 detector rows [21]. The 16 central rows define 0.75 mm collimated slice width at iso-center, the 4 outer rows on both sides define 1.5-mm collimated slice width (see Fig. 6). The total coverage in the transverse direction is 24 mm at the iso-center. By appropriate combination of the signals of the individual detector rows, either 12 or 16 slices with 0.75 or 1.5-mm collimated slice width can be acquired simultaneously.

For multislice CT scanning a certain dose increase compared to single-slice CT is unavoidable due to the underlying physical principles. The collimated dose

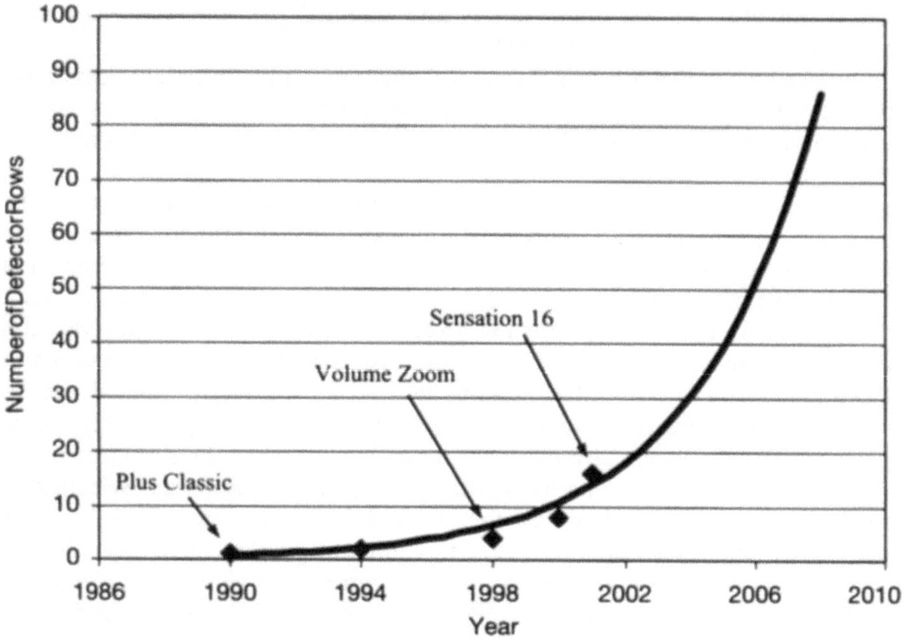

Fig. 4. Number of available slices in multislice CT scanners plotted vs. the year of their market introduction. The number of slices doubles approximately every 2.5 years

Table 1. Overview of the development of different performance parameters

	1972	1980	1990	1998	2002
Min. scan time	300 s	5 s	1 s	0.5 s	0.42s
Data per 360 scan	58 kb	1 mB	2 MB	12 MB	50 MB
Data per spiral scan	-	-	< 50 mB	< 500 MB	< 1 GB
Image matrix	80 x 80	256 x 256	512 x 512	512 x 512	512 x 512
Power	2 kW	10 kW	40 kW	60 kW	60 kW
Collimation	13 mm	2–10 mm	1–10 mm	0.5–5 mm	0.75–1.5 mm
Spatial resolution	3 lp cm^{-1}	12 lp cm^{-1}	15 lp cm^{-1}	24 lp cm^{-1}	24 lp cm^{-1}
Contrast resolution	5 mm/5 HU/ 50 mGy	3 mm/3 HU/ 30 mGy	3 mm/3 HU/ 30 mGy	3 mm/3 HU/ 30 mGy	3 mm/3 HU/ 30 mGy

profile is a trapezoid in the transverse direction. This is a consequence of the finite length of the focal spot and the prepatient collimation. In the plateau region of the trapezoid, X-rays emitted from the entire area of the focal spot illuminate the detector. In the penumbra regions only a part of the focal spot illuminates the detector while other parts are blocked off by the prepatient collimator. With single-slice CT, the entire trapezoidal dose profile can contribute to

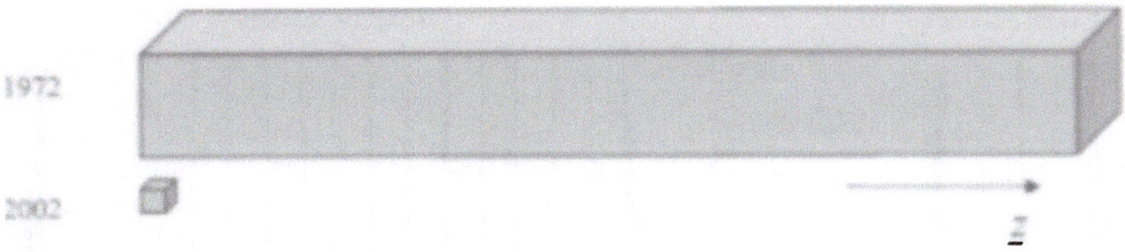

Fig. 5. Change in size of a voxel element over 30 years

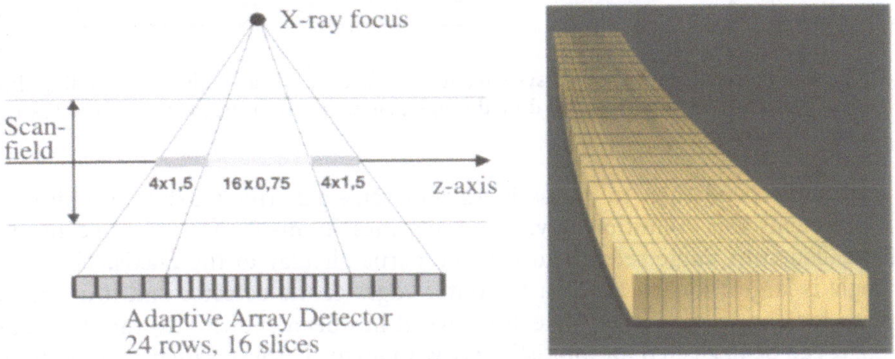

Fig. 6. Detector configuration of the Siemens SOMATOM Sensation 16

the detector signal and the collimated slice width is determined as the full width at half maximum (FWHM) of this trapezoid. With multislice CT, only the plateau region of the dose profile may be used to ensure equal signal level for all detector slices. The penumbra region has to be discarded, either by a postpatient collimator or by the intrinsic self-collimation of the multislice detector, and represents »wasted« dose. The relative contribution of the penumbra region increases with decreasing slice width, and it decreases with increasing number of simultaneously acquired slices. This is demonstrated by Fig. 7, which compares the »minimum width« dose profiles for a 4-slice CT system and a corresponding 16-slice CT system with equal collimated width of one detector slice. Correspondingly, the relative dose utilization of a representative 4-slice CT scanner (SOMATOM Sensation 4, Siemens AG, Forchheim, Germany) is 70% for 4 x 1-mm collimation and 85% for 4 x 2.5-mm collimation. A comparable 16-slice CT system (SOMATOM Sensation 16) has an improved dose utilization of 76 or 82% for 16 x 0.75-mm collimation and 85 or 89% for 16 x 1.5-mm collimation, depending on the size of the focal spot (large or small).

An important parameter to characterize a spiral scan is the pitch, defined as p = tablefeed per rotation/total width of the collimated beam [1].

Two-dimensional image reconstruction approaches used in commercially available single-slice CT scanners, such as the standard filtered-backprojection reconstruction, require all measurement rays contributing to an image to run in

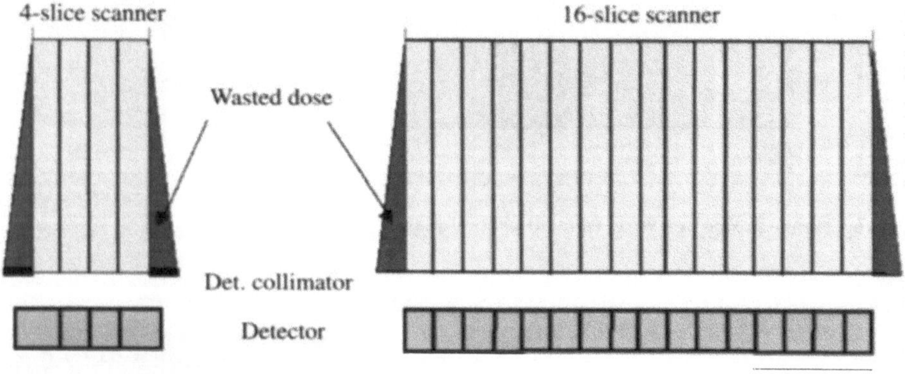

Fig. 7. Dose profiles for a 4-slice CT system and a 16-slice CT system with corresponding slice widths. The relative effect of wasted dose through penumbra effects decreases with increasing number of slices

a plane perpendicular to the patient's transverse axis (the **z**-axis). In multislice CT systems this condition is violated, the measurement rays are tilted by the so-called cone angle relative to a plane perpendicular to the **z**-axis. The cone angle is largest for the slices at the outer edges of the detector and it increases with increasing number of detector rows. It has been shown [10] that the cone angle can be neglected for multislice CT with up to six slices. When a larger number of slices is acquired, however, cone-beam artefacts appear at a level that cannot be tolerated, hence the effect needs to be taken into account by the image reconstruction algorithm.

Two different types of cone-beam reconstruction algorithms are currently implemented in state-of-the art 16-slice CT systems. The first one uses 3-D back-projection and generalizes the Feldkamp algorithm [25], which was originally introduced for sequential cone-beam scanning, to spiral scanning. The second reconstruction approach is based on nutating-slice algorithms, which split up the 3-D reconstruction into a series of 2-D reconstructions on tilted intermediate image planes individually adapted to the local curvature of the spiral path [23]. An example is the Adaptive Multiple Plane Reconstruction (AMPR; Fig. 8) implemented in the SOMATOM Sensation 16 [24]. AMPR is characterized by the following properties:

- The cone-beam geometry of the measurement rays is taken into account, cone-beam artefacts are effectively suppressed. The currently implemented AMPR can be expanded to medical CT systems with up to 64 slices, a modified version (SMPR – Segmented Multiple Plane Reconstruction) is compatible with up to 256 slices.
- The effective slicewidth *d* (FWHM of the spiral SSP) is independent of the spiral pitch, which is freely selectable in the range 0.5 to 2.0. For each collimation (e.g., 16 x 0.75 mm or 16 x 1.5 mm) a wide range of different slice-widths is available for retrospective reconstruction.
- The image noise for fixed effective mAs is independent of the spiral pitch.
- The dose for fixed effective mAs is independent of the spiral pitch and equals the dose of a sequential scan with the same mAs.

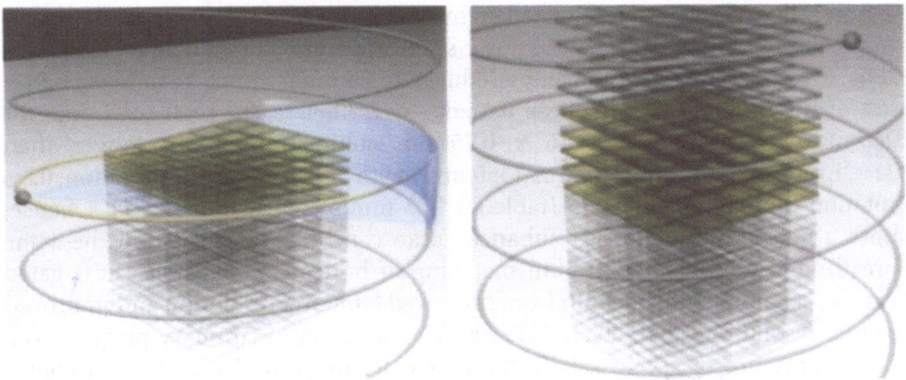

Fig. 8. Illustration of the AMPR approach. As a first step the multislice spiral data are used to reconstruct several images on double oblique image planes, which are individually adapted to the slope of the spiral path. As a second step the final images are calculated by a z-interpolation between the tilted image planes

One of the most exciting new applications of multislice CT is the ability to image the heart and the cardio-thoracic anatomy without motion artefacts. For ECG-synchronized examinations of the cardio-thoracic anatomy, either ECG-triggered axial scanning or ECG-gated spiral scanning can be used. In ECG-triggered axial scanning, the heart volume is covered by axial scans in a »step-and-shoot« technique. With retrospective ECG gating, the heart volume is covered continuously by a spiral scan. The patient's ECG signal is recorded simultaneously to allow for a retrospective selection of the data segments used for image reconstruction. Only scan data acquired in a predefined cardiac phase, usually the diastolic phase, is used for image reconstruction [13, 14, 22]. The data segments contributing to an image start with a user-defined offset relative to the onset of the R waves. The temporal resolution of an image can be improved up to $T_{rot}/(2N)$ by using scan data of N subsequent heart cycles for image reconstruction. T_{rot} is the gantry rotation time of the CT scanner. Image reconstruction during different heart phases is feasible by shifting the start points of the data segments used for image reconstruction relative to the R waves.

The latest generation of 16-slice CT systems allows for truly isotropic imaging in virtually any application. As a consequence, the distinction between transverse and in-plane resolution is gradually becoming a historical remnant, and the traditional axial slice is losing its clinical predominance. It is replaced by interactive viewing and manipulation of isotropic volume images, with only the key slices or views in arbitrary directions used for filming or stored for a demonstration of the diagnosis. Improved transverse resolution goes hand in hand with considerably reduced scan times, facilitating the examination of uncooperative patients and reducing the amount of contrast agent needed, but also requiring optimized contrast agent protocols. New clinical applications are evolving as a result of the tremendously increased volume scan speed, such as CT angiographic examinations in the pure arterial phase. A CTA of the circle of Willis with 16 x 0.75-mm collimation, 0.5 s rotation time and pitch 1.5 requires only 3.5 s for a scan range of 100 mm (table feed 36 mm/s). A thorax-abdomen scan with sub-mm collimation takes about 17 s for a scan range of 600 mm. For a CTA of the renal arteries, the table feed can be reduced to 24 mm/s (pitch 1) to make better use of the tube output for obese patients; nevertheless, the total scan time for 250-mm scan range with 16 x 0.75-mm collimation is not longer than 11 s. Examining the entire thorax (350 mm) with 16 x 0.75 mm-collimation, 0.5 s rotation time and pitch 1.375 (table feed 33 mm/s) can be done in 11 s, hence, both a native and a contrast-enhanced scan can be obtained within the same breath-hold period for optimum matching of both image volumes. ECG-gated cardiac scanning benefits both from improved temporal resolution and improved spatial resolution. Characterization and classification of coronary plaques even in the presence of severe calcifications is entering clinical routine as a consequence of the increased clinical robustness of the method. A recent study for

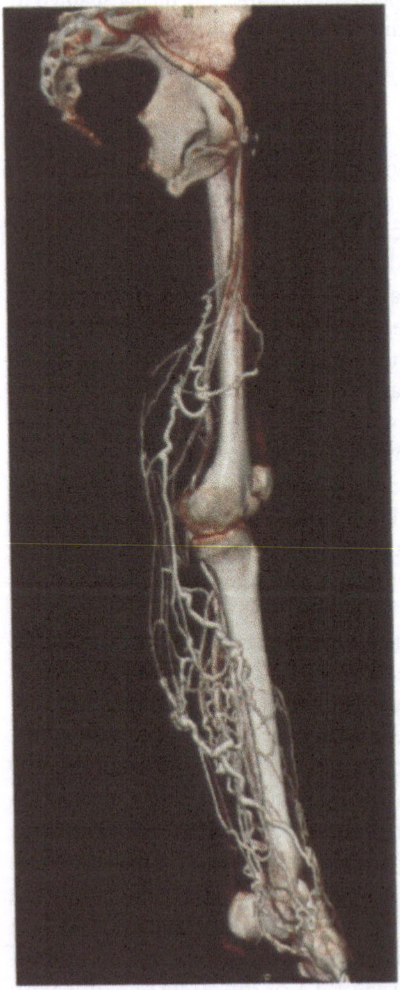

Fig. 9. CT angiogram of the lower peripheral vasculature scanned with 1.5-mm collimation at a table feed of 24 mm per rotation, 120 kV, 150 mAs, 0.5 s rotation, 2 mm reconstructed slice width, scan range 91 cm, total scan time 19 s

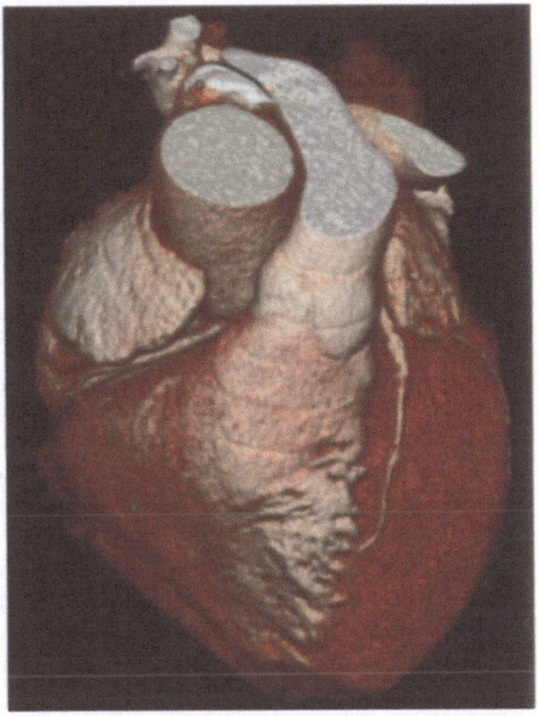

Fig. 10. Coronary angiography scanned with 0.75-mm collimation at a table feed of 2.8 mm per rotation, 120 kV, 500 mAs, 0.42 s rotation, 1 mm reconstructed slice width, scan range 13 cm, total scan time 19 s. Gating parameters were –500 ms

coronary CTA with a 16-slice system on 59 patients demonstrated 86% specificity and 95% sensitivity. None of the patients had to be excluded [27].

Typical image quality obtained with 16-slice CT is illustrated in Fig. 9, an example of a CT angiography of the peripheral vasculature and in Fig. 10, an example of a coronary CTA examination.

Future Developments

With a spatial resolution of 0.5 x 0.5 x 0.6 mm^3 16-slice CT sets today's benchmark in spatial resolution for non-invasive coronary artery imaging. Motion artefacts in patients with higher heart rates remain the most important challenge for multislice coronary CTA, although diagnostic image quality can be achieved in most cases by administration of beta-blockers. Improved temporal resolution is desirable in the future to avoid patient preparation, requiring increased gantry rotation speed rather than multisegment reconstruction approaches for robust clinical performance. Obviously, significant development efforts will be needed to handle the substantial increase of mechanical forces (~ 17 G for 0.42 s rotation time, >33 G for 0.3 s rotation time) and increased data transmission rates. Rotation times of less than 0.2 s (mechanical forces >75 G) required to provide a temporal resolution of less than 100 ms independent of the heart rate appear to be beyond today's mechanical limits. An alternative to further increased rotation speed is the reconsideration of a scanner concept with multiple tubes and multiple detectors that was described for the first time in 1975. For general-purpose CT, we will see a further increase in the number of simultaneously acquired slices; the resulting clinical benefits, however, may not be substantial and have to be carefully considered in the light of the necessary technical efforts. Potential further improvement of the spatial resolution will have to be reserved to special applications due to the inevitable increase of dose that has to be applied for adequate signal-to-noise ratio. It will have to go along with the development of more powerful X-ray tubes and generators. Instead of a mere quantitative enhancement of scan parameters with doubtful clinical relevance the introduction of area detectors large enough to cover the entire heart or the entire brain in one axial scan (~120 mm scan range) could bring a new quality to medical CT.

With these systems dynamic volume scanning would become possible, and a whole spectrum of new applications, such as functional or volume perfusion studies, could arise. Area detector technology is currently under development, yet no commercially available solution so far fulfills the high requirements of medical CT concerning dynamic range of the acquisition system and fast data readout. Initial experience with today's CsJ-aSi flat-panel detector technology originally used for conventional catheter angiography is limited in low-contrast resolution and scan speed. Due to the intrinsic slow signal decay of flat-panel detectors, rotation times of at least 20 s are needed to acquire a sufficient number

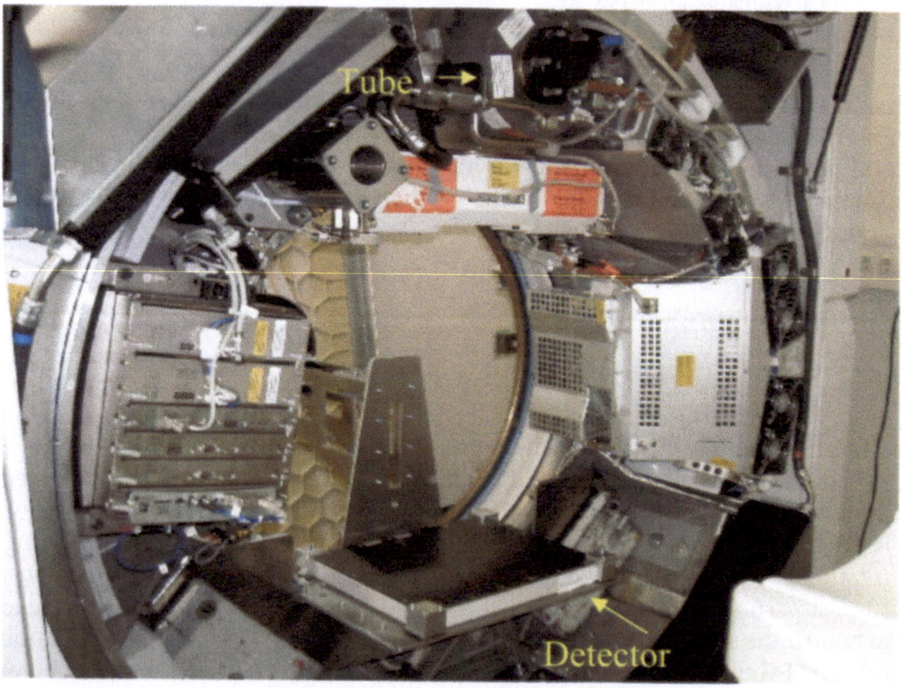

Fig. 11. Volume CT prototype setup, incorporating a flat panel detector into a standard CT gantry (SOMATOM Sensation 16)

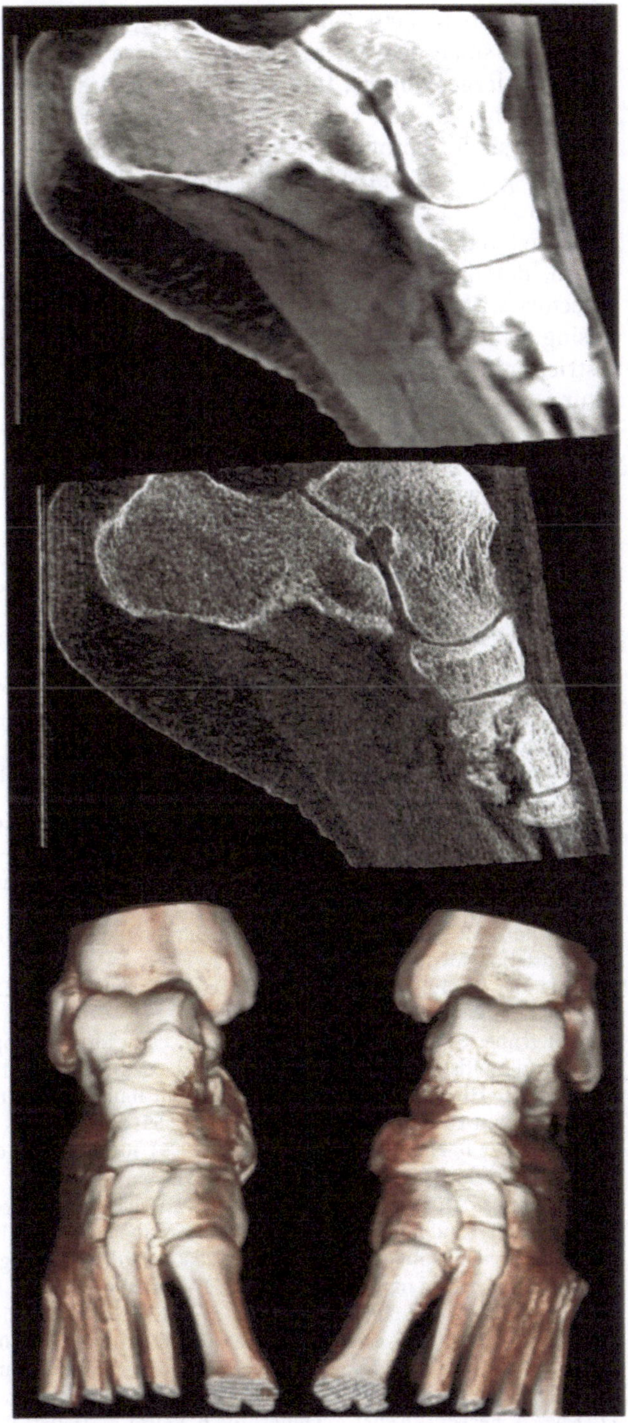

Fig. 12. MPRs and VRTs of a foot specimen, scanned with the volume CT prototype. *Top* soft tissue reconstruction; *middle* high resolution reconstruction; *bottom* VRT

of projections (= 600). On the other hand, high-contrast resolution is excellent due to the small detector pixel size, yet dose requirements preclude the examination of larger objects. Initial experimental results are limited to small high-contrast objects such as joints, inner ear or contrast-filled vessel specimens. Figure 11 shows a prototype setup incorporating a flat-panel detector into a standard CT gantry (SOMATOM Sensation 16, Forchheim, Germany). The detector covers a 25 x 25 x 18 cm^3 scan field of view, the pixel size is 250 x 250 μm^2, both measured in the center of rotation. Figure 12 shows MPRs and VRTs of a foot specimen, demonstrating excellent spatial resolution. The combination of area detectors with sufficient quality with fast gantry rotation speeds will be a promising technical concept for medical CT systems. Due to the present technical restrictions, however, these systems will probably not be available in the near future.

References

1. Radon JH (1917) Über die Bestimmung von Funktionen durch ihre Integralwerte längs gewisser Mannigfaltigkeiten. Berichte über die Verhandlungen der Königlich Sächsischen Gesellschaft der Wissenschaften zu Leipzig 69, 262
2. Cormack AM (1963) Representation of a function by its line integrals, with some radiological applications. J. Appl Phys 34: 2722
3. Bracewell RN (1956) Strip integration in radioastronomy. J. Phys 9: 198–217
4. Hounsfield GN (1973) Computerized transverse axial scanning (tomography), Part I. Description of the system. Br J Radiol 46: 1016.
5. Dümmling K (1984) 10 Jahre Computertomographie – ein Rückblick. Electromedica 52: 13–28
6. Kalender WA (2000) Computed tomography. Publicis MCD Munich
7. Kalender W, Seissler W, Klotz E, Vock P (1990) Spiral volumetric CT with single-breath-hold technique, continuous transport and continuous scanner rotation. Radiology 176: 181–183
8. Crawford CR, King KF (1990) Computed tomography scanning with simultaneous patient translation. Med Phys 17: 967–982
9. Kalender W (1995) Thin-section three-dimensional spiral CT: is isotropic imaging possible? Radiology 197: 578–580
10. Klingenbeck-Regn K, Schaller S, Flohr T, Ohnesorge B, Kopp AF, Baum U (1999) Subsecond multislice computed tomography: basics and applications. EJR 31:110–124
11. Hu H, He HD, Foley WD, Fox SH (2000) Four multidetector-row helical CT: image quality and volume coverage speed. Radiology 215: 55–62
12. Ohnesorge B, Flohr T, Schaller S et al. (1999) Technische Grundlagen und Anwendungen der Mehrschicht-CT. Radiologe 39:923–931
13. Kachelriess M, Ulzheimer S, Kalender W (2000) ECG-correlated image reconstruction from subsecond multislice spiral CT scans of the heart. Med Phys 27: 1881–1902
14. Ohnesorge B, Flohr T, Becker C et al. (2000) Cardiac imaging by means of electro-cardiographically gated multisection spiral CT – initial experience. Radiology 217:564–571
15. Achenbach S, Ulzheimer S, Baum U et al. (2000) Noninvasive coronary angiography by retrospectively ECG-gated multislice spiral CT. Circulation 102:2823–2828
16. Becker C, Knez A, Ohnesorge B, Schöpf U, Reiser M (2000) Imaging of non calcified coronary plaques using helical CT with retrospective EKG gating. AJR 175:423–424
17. Knez A, Becker C, Leber A, Ohnesorge B, Reiser M, Haberl R (2000) Non-Invasive Assessment of Coronary Artery Stenoses with Multidetector Helical Computed Tomography. Circulation 101:e221–e222

18. Nieman K, Oudkerk M, Rensing B et al. (2001) Coronary angiography with multislice computed tomography. Lancet 357: 599–603
19. Schroeder S, Kopp A, Baumbach A et al. (2001) Noninvasive detection and evaluation of atherosclerotic coronary plaques with multislice computed tomography. JACC 37(5): 1430–1435
20. Kopp A, Schröder S, Küttner A et al. (2001) Coronary arteries: retrospectively ECG-gated multi-detector row CT angiography with selective optimization of the image reconstruction window. Radiology 221(3): 683–688
21. Flohr T, Stierstorfer K, Bruder H, Simon J, Schaller S (2002) New technical developments in multislice CT, part 1. Approaching isotropic resolution with sub-mm 16-slice scanning. Fortschr Röntgenstr 174: 839–845
22. Flohr T, Bruder H, Stierstorfer K, Simon J, Schaller S, Ohnesorge B (2002) New technical developments in multislice CT, part 2. Sub-millimeter 16-slice scanning and increased gantry rotation speed for cardiac imaging. Fortschr Röntgenstr 174: 1022–1027
23. Kachelrieß M, Schaller S, Kalender WA (2000) Advanced single-slice rebinning in cone-beam spiral CT. Med Phys 27(4): 754–772
24. Schaller S, Stierstorfer K, Bruder H, Kachelrieß M, Flohr T (2001) Novel approximate approach for high-quality image reconstruction in helical cone beam CT at arbitrary pitch. Ed: SPIE (The International Society for Optical Engineering) San Diego. In: proceeding SPIE international symposium medical imaging 4322: 113–127
25. Feldkamp LA, Davis LC, and Kress JW (1984) Practical cone-beam algorithm. J. Opt Soc Am. A1: 612–619
26. Kudo H, Noo F, Defrise M (1998) Cone-beam filtered-backprojection algorithm for truncated helical data. Phys Med Biol 43: 2885–2909
27. Nieman K, Cademartiri F, Lemos PA, Raaijmakers R, Pattynama PMT, de Feyter PJ (2002) Reliable non-invasive coronary angiography with fast submillimeter multislice spiral computed tomography. Circulation 106:2051–2054

2 Multidetector CT and the Future of CT Scanning – The Coming Revolution in Workflow and Process Design

E. K. Fishman

Introduction

The medical headlines on CNN were most impressive on that early fall morning in September 2003. The announcer described a new non-invasive imaging technique developed at the same English company that in the past had brought us such musical superstars as Britney Spears and Eminem (note: I had to update singers for relevance as the Beatles are so yesterday) just introduced a scanning device that goes by the acronym of a CT scanner, short for computed tomography. Using the latest hardware and computer technology, the scanner is in constant motion and rotates around the patient every 500 milliseconds. The scanner allows 16 individual scans or slices to be obtained per scanner rotation or 32 scans per second. The system can acquire isotropic data where the x, y, and z resolution is equal. Typical scanning parameters used are 0.75 mm slice thickness, 0.5 mm interscan spacing, and post processing of data which allows reconstruction of 6 slices per second. The speed of acquisition means that a pancreas, liver or kidney can be evaluated with isotropic datasets in under 10 seconds. Depending on the study between 500 and 1200 individual slices are obtained for review with some studies such as vascular run-off studies generating 1500–2000 slices. The manufacturer noted that future generations of the scanner will have 32–256 detectors before the next wave of technology goes to flat panel detectors.

The story continues and the announcer then goes to a leading medical institution and shows the images to a startled and awed home-viewing public. Now for my question. Does anyone actually believe that the images demonstrated would be axial CT scans or are they more likely to be images from a volumetric 3D display? Does anyone believe that an axial display would even be a consideration if this new system were indeed introduced today? I doubt it. Yet, most of us still look at our shiny new 16-slice scanner and review axial images. However, the times are changing.

As we approach the 30th anniversary of the introduction of computed tomography (CT) into clinical practice, CT technology continues to evolve and it is thriving. In the early years of CT, technical advancements were typically measured by decreasing scan times and increasing speed of data reconstruction. Individual study times decreased from 90 min in the early 1980s to less than 20 min by the end of that decade. Although this increased speed definitely represented progress, the first truly revolutionary concept change in CT occurred in the late 1980s with the introduction of helical or spiral CT. This technology along with significant advancements in image post-processing software revitalized CT and allowed the development of new CT applications such as CT angiography and virtual imaging [1–3]. The era of true volume imaging had begun in earnest.

Next, the transition from single-detector to multi-detector-row CT represented another pivotal event in the evolution of CT imaging. Initially 4-, then 8-detector scanners were developed. But it was the introduction of 16-detector scanners, which has really revolutionized CT scanning and requires changes in our core operative structure. 16-slice MDCT represents what Andrew Grove, Ph.D. (co-founder and former CEO of Intel Inc.) called a strategic inflection point. It is defined as a change, which is not a 5–10% improvement over previous capabilities, but one that strategically changes the whole landscape. It can also be defined as a disruptive technology. 16-slice CT is not just simply four times faster than 4-slice scanning. It is far more than an incremental improvement. 16-slice MDCT, with true isotropic datasets, promises to further advance volume-imaging and all its resultant advantages. Volume-imaging will no longer be considered as a supplement to traditional axial imaging in select cases, but instead, may now be utilized for primary display and analysis. This paradigm shift will require a rethinking of many of the core processes in CT ranging from image transfer and data storage to redefining the role of CT across a wide spectrum of clinical applications. For example, the coronary arteries or peripheral runoff studies were once considered possible but impractical with 4-slice technology. These applications are now a reality (4–7). Workstations like the 3D Virtuoso, which worked so well with single slice or even 4-slice MDCT, can not handle these new volume datasets and provide real-time interactivity. Workstations are no longer a simple accessory to the CT scanner but the central core of processing and display.

CT continues to prosper in the medical imaging marketplace today with a growth rate of 10–15% in yearly CT volume. The new scanners have increased throughput capabilities to at least 3–4 patients an hour with the limitations being the time it takes to place the patient in the scanner and prepare them for a study. The problems of tube heating or slow data processing are for the most part a thing of the past. Many of these cases are more complex and require multiphase acquisitions. These increased capabilities coupled with increased experience can result in 3000–5000 images (or more) being generated per hour. A specific example is the 4D cardiac studies that require reconstruction at 9 intervals (10–90% of the cardiac cycle) which represents about 3000 images in a single exam. This total volume of data is in the 30–50 gigabyte range per day and the challenges presented by this have been the subject of many articles in imaging journals and in radiology web chat rooms.

Volume Visualization

The solution to the problem of large volume visualization with 4- and now 16-slice MDCT is not simply a modification of standard techniques such as faster scrolling with a computer mouse or roller ball or novel filming protocols (i.e. film every 5th or 10th image). Rather, it focuses on the data volume itself with the understanding that volume acquisition requires true volume visualization. The introduction of programs such as InSpace on the Siemens Sensation-16 scanners and on the Leonardo workstation addresses this paradigm shift from axial images to volume images. The study volumes can be presented in a range of formats including volume rendering, maximum intensity projection, minimum intensity projection and multiplanar visualization (coronal, sagittal, axial; Figs. 1 and 2).

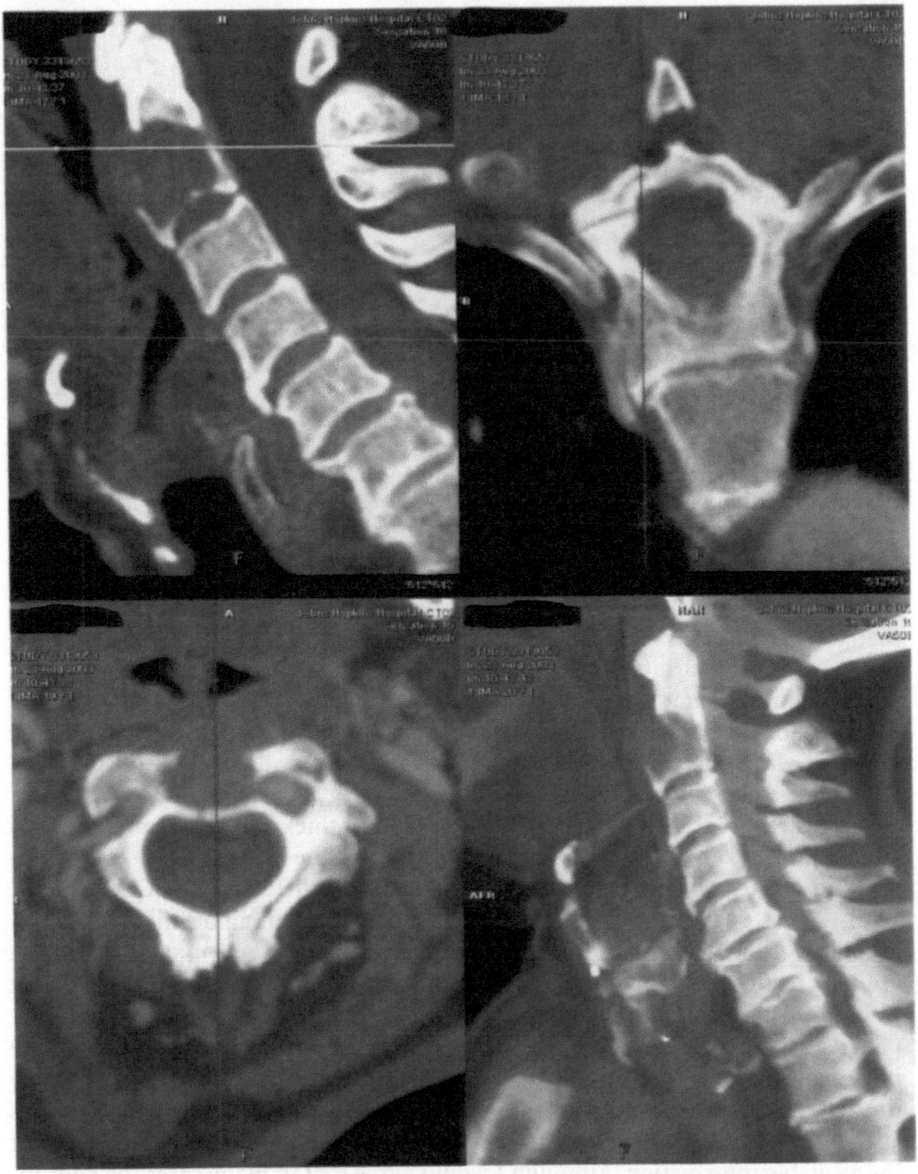

Fig. 1. Metastatic thyroid cancer to bone. (a) Composite image demonstrates the lytic lesion in the C-2 vertebral body. The true extent of the lesion is shown in a composite image of axial, sagittal, coronal and 3D volume rendering views. (Clockwise from bottom left image)

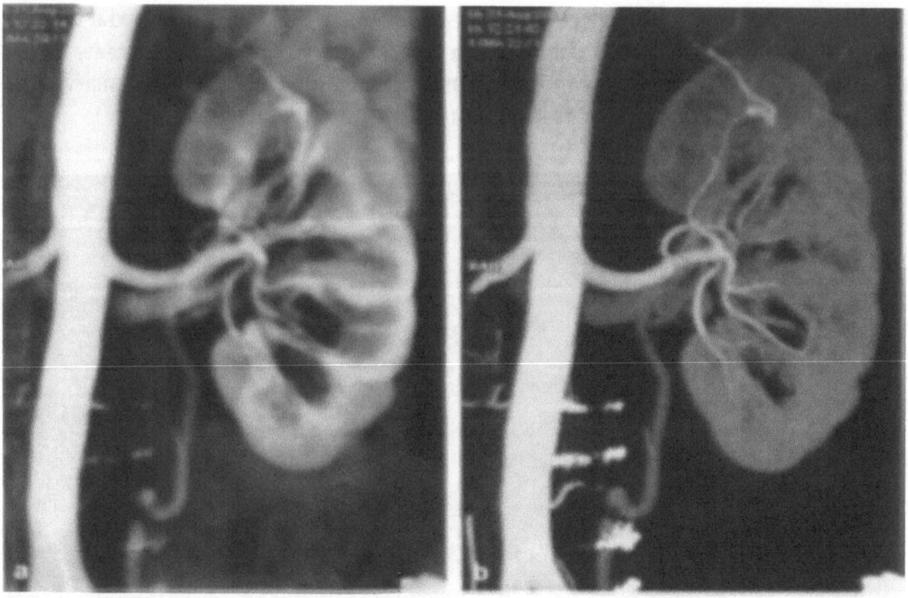

Fig. 2a, b. Normal CT angiogram of a kidney. **a** Volume rendered view defines cortical medullary differentiation as well as defining arterial and venous anatomy. **b** Maximum intensity projection view shows lack of differentiation of cortex and medulla but better detail of the branching renal arteries

InSpace allows primary analysis of the data volume in real time which is a necessity given that it is no longer practical to review CT slices on film or even using a film surrogate, the PAC's workstation or review station. For instance, with a 4-slice MDCT a dual phase dataset using 1.25 mm thick sections of the liver or pancreas was composed of 400–500 sections. At that point, it was still possible, although cumbersome, to scroll through these images on standard workstations. Yet, in fact, most centers reviewed images at 5-mm thickness and 5-mm intervals and at best looked at the 1-mm sections as part of the 3D examination. Regardless, this strategy of image review is not possible with 16-slice MDCT scanners. With the use of the Sensation-16 scanner we are performing detailed CT angiographic work with 0.75 mm thick sections reconstructed at 0.5 mm intervals. The optimal reconstruction interval overlap is 0.25 mm, which provides a dataset ideal for 3D reconstruction and multiplanar imaging. If we scan an area like the pancreas we are typically doing arterial phase images followed by venous phase imaging. This results in 400–500 individual slices per acquisition. If you view this dataset on a workstation or film, it is likely that you only reconstructed data at 3- or 5-mm intervals which means you are looking at between 10 and 16% of the available information. Although I would agree that in many cases the additional slices do not change the specific diagnosis, they may change the staging of disease especially in regards to vascular invasion. The concept that must be understood is the ability to use a 16-slice scanner in the optimum mode which requires a new workflow strategy. This shift to volume display not only affects the radiologist at time of interpretation of the study but also the referring physician at the time when they review the study.

The impact of the changes due to 16-slice MDCT has not taken the referring physician needs into the equation. Imagine their frustration looking at X-ray jackets with 20–100 CT sheets of film trying to find the key image. In many ways for our colleagues more is simply less. I would conclude that unless handled correctly more information (i.e. more slices per study) might provide less diagnostic information due to a breakdown in information transfer. This is a critical problem our colleagues are becoming frustrated with and that can be addressed with new visualization strategies.

Image Storage and Transfer

This paradigm shift to volume visualization has some challenges to overcome. Although a solution for volume image viewing has been addressed with InSpace, the ability to move images through the radiology department as well as the hospital or health care enterprise remains a challenge. Similarly, the amount of data generated provides perplexing problems for data storage and retrieval. Studies that range in size from 600 megabytes to 1 gigabyte are truly a challenge that must be addressed. New solutions must be identified and implemented. The size of the datasets per case make it no longer possible to use 5.2 gigabyte Sony MO storage devices (Sony Inc. NY, NY) as these hold but a handful of cases (usually 3–8 depending on use of image compression). This process as currently defined is the worst case scenario: it is expensive, time-consuming, and inefficient. Yet, most 16-slice scanners still ship with 5.2 G MO storage devices. A new workflow design with massive storage is necessary either as part of the hospital or clinic master plan (institutional PAC's system) or as a freestanding enterprise solution within the CT environment.

Even with a central archive not all issues are resolved. We require rapid data retrieval which may be limited by network transfer times with limited bandwidth which can paralyze the entire operation. Although this is commonly felt to be a problem for the radiology department, it is, in truth, a problem for the scanner vendors. Simply supplying »data acquisition devices« like a CT scanner is no longer enough as it is neither a solution or a system alone. Scanner manufacturers need to address workflow and process design. Siemens Medical Systems seems to have recognized the future by changing its name to Siemens Medical Solutions, but now comes the hard part. Name changes are easy, but providing those solutions that live up to your name is the challenge. Similarly, GE Medical is focusing their operations as providing system solutions rather than hardware solutions. Time will tell if they are successful. We can only hope they are. Recently, GE Medical has teamed up with EMC, the leader in enterprise storage solutions. We look forward to seeing any novel solution this may bring to our clinical environment.

Another issue that relates to workstations like the Leonardo is the amount of system storage available. These systems typically have hard drives in the 60 gigabytes range (55 G to be exact). This is insufficient in an environment where 20–30 cases per day are in need of analysis, whether it be CT angiography, 3D imaging, virtual colonoscopy or whole body screening [8–10]. I recently purchased from Apple Computer a 400-gigabyte hard drive for 700 dollars. This should be the bare minimum on a workstation although 1–3 terabytes probably as better number. More sophisticated storage strategies should also be made available for sites like ours where we typically keep months or years of CT angiographic and 3D studies online. I would guess a system with 10–40 terabytes storage is not undoable and would be cost-effective. This need for massive local storage should come as no surprise to anyone. The problem is that most of the major vendors are operated that the people who design the system do not have an understanding of what the user needs or wants. I have been told several times by major vendors that the problem of limited storage is not the manufacturer's lack of understanding of the clinical environment but mine (!).

Another problem with some current workstations is that they have not taken the clinical environment into their planning process for their database design. The databases are not flexible enough to allow user-selected partitions such that case studies could be divided by topic (i.e. pancreas, liver) as well as being limited in how many absolute cases can be stored within the database. Although some might be tempted to suggest that a workstation was never meant to store cases, this is again not a real-world analysis or solution. As a user I need a minimum of 4–6 weeks of 3D cases, and ideally at least 3 months on line. Clinicians will commonly want to review studies done in the past 4–6 weeks or longer (especially for renal donors) and they must be available. The limitations currently provided are real and not theoretical. As of March 2003, we had three 16-slice MDCTs feeding a workstation in our 3D imaging lab. The volume of data results in a purging of the database as least twice a week. This is both time-consuming and interfering with delivery of services. The concept of a strategic inflection point could have predicted problems of this scale and magnitude. Disrupture technologies have a habit of creating new challenges and opportunities.

Another issue common in many institutions is the need to minimize the time from data acquisition to when the radiologist is able to read the case. This problem may vary and will be different depending on the scanner and its configuration. If a Siemens Wizard (satellite console) or Leonardo workstation is used as the second console and is dedicated to physician review then the shared database with the main scanner provides easy access to current scan data. This is very efficient for throughput and consultation with the referring physician. However, if it is not available, other solutions including a PAC's workstation can be used, but there will be no shared database. Sufficient network bandwidth is needed to prevent any bottlenecks in this scenario as the information is sent across the network. Radiology, like many other businesses, is becoming ever more dependent on the quality and reliability of our network backbone. It is critical to our ability to efficiently practice radiology in the 21st century.

Referring Physicians

An area that is commonly overlooked with 16-slice MDCT is the impact these changes in technology are having on our referring physicians. The referring physician is not interested in stacks of images on film or on a workstation. Clinicians demand rapid access to critical information and images displayed in a user-friendly environment. Hundreds or thousands of images per patient on film or on a computer screen or computer disc are not acceptable. In contrast, an interactive volume display may be the answer. The combination of a limited number of selected volume visualizations coupled with the capability of real-time 3D rendering should prove ideal for a wide range of applications. If our personal experience is any guide, the acceptance of volume displays is immediate and complete (Figs. 3 to 7). The physicians come down to the scanner to view the 3D volume displays and several of them have even taken the time to learn how to use the software.

The concept of InSpace or a similar system when available on multiple workstations or PAC's systems across the enterprise moves us one step closer to the true »virtual« radiology department. That is, it matters little where the information is acquired, as it is available for a primary read or review anywhere throughout the enterprise. This enterprise-wide solution is critical to the radiologist and the referring physicians who would also have access to the volume datasets. The quality of a volume dataset is of little value unless the information can be used.

Our experience is that nearly all referring physicians, but especially surgeons have an increased need for access to our data files. The details provided by 16-slice MDCT are being used for detailed surgical mapping and planning. The need for more interactive tools in the clinic and the operating room are two of the common requests that I am currently seeing. Companies like TeraRecon (San Mateo, CA) have addressed this issue with a thin client environment solution that decreases the cost per seat on the network by 50–75%. It will be interesting to see

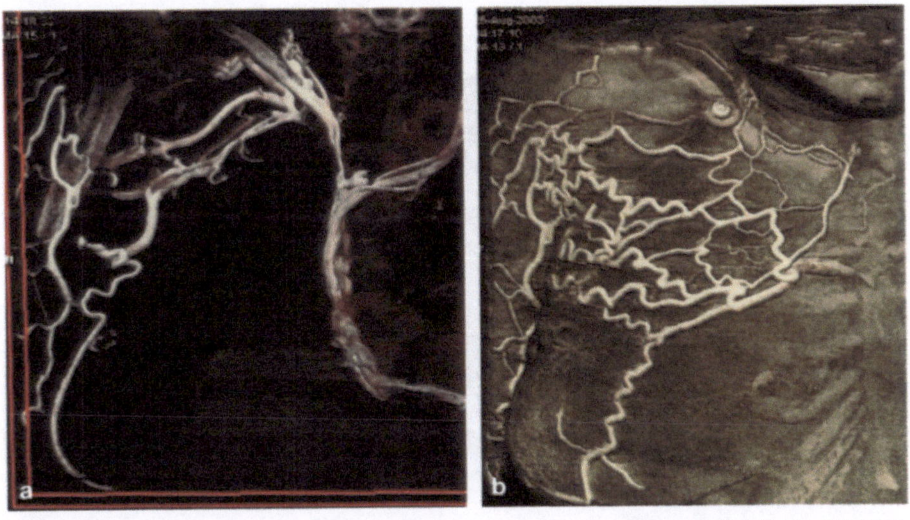

Fig. 3a, b. Occlusion of right brachiocephalic vein with chest wall collaterals. **(a–b)** a volume display is ideal for defining the site of obstruction as well as the chest wall collaterals that develop as a consequence

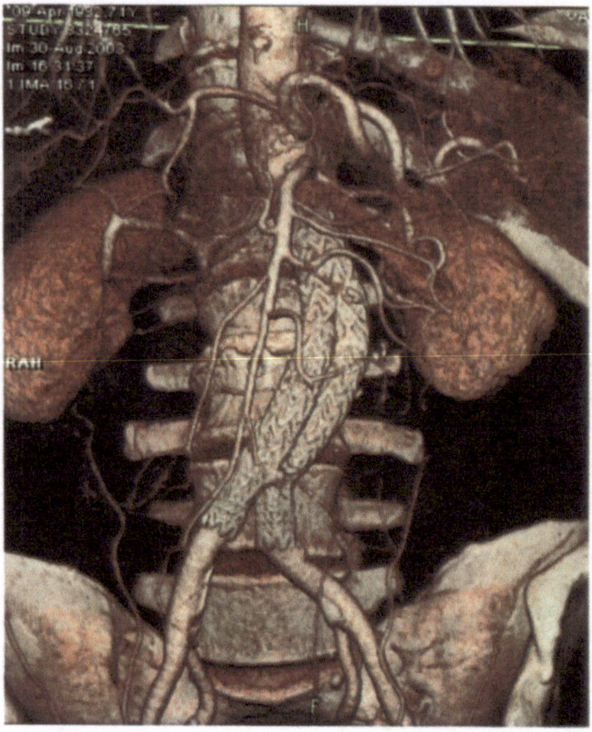

Fig. 4. Endovascular stent study as part of a routine exam follow-up. Volume rendered view defines the graft in good position without any complications such as endoleak or graft failure. This single view was constructed from over 800 individual .75 mm CT slices

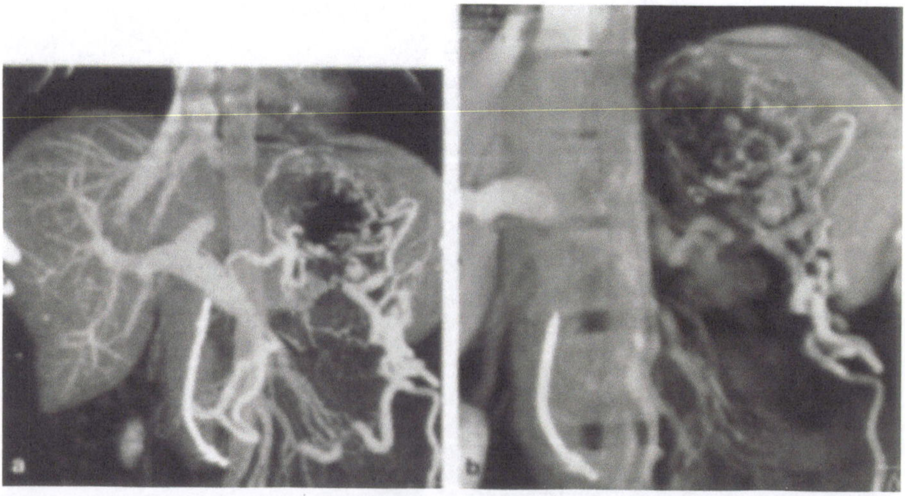

Fig. 5a, b. Occluded splenic vein with gastric varices. **(a–b)** a pancreatic mass occluded the splenic vein resulting in a classic collateral pathway through gastroepiploic vessels. The gastric varices were especially prominent.

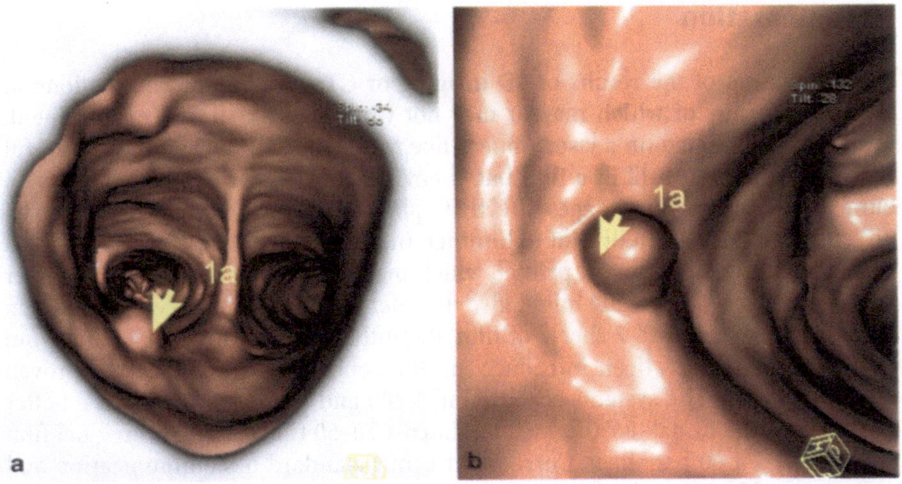

Fig. 6a, b. Endoluminal view of a mass in the trachea just above the bifurcation in a patient with tracheal papillomatosis. **(a–b)** volume display in an endoluminal view is valuable in guiding biopsy and/or removal of the papilloma.

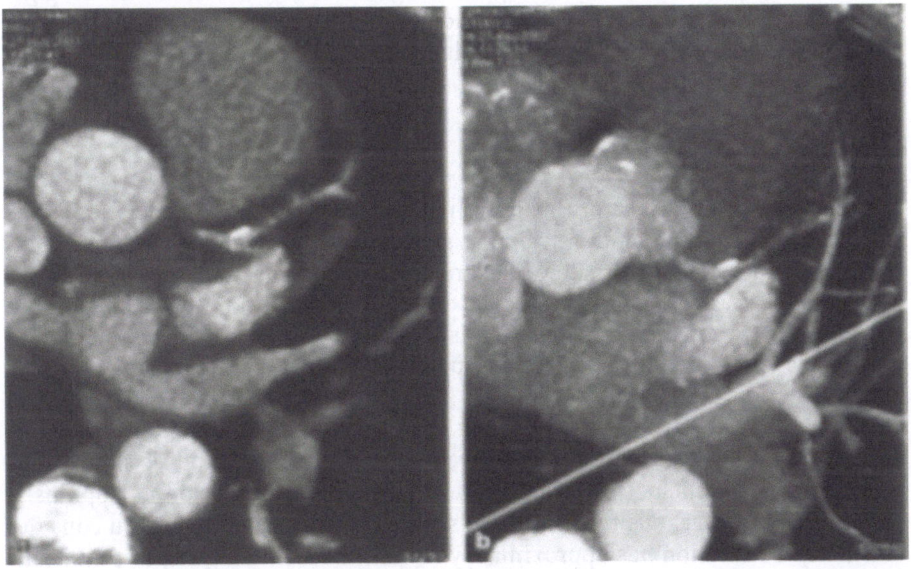

Fig. 7a, b. CT coronary angiogram detects calcified plaque on left anterior descending coronary artery without significant vessel narrowing. **(a–b)** 3D mapping defines the calcified plaque but is able to define the patent lumen as well.

how well this model catches on. Some radiologists are concerned that sharing data may decrease the radiologist's control of the information. Although this is in part correct, I believe that if radiology leads this new work paradigm we will remain the central player even in a distributed information environment.

Documentation

Documentation of the results of 3D imaging or CT angiography can be done in several ways, any of which may or may not work in your clinical environment. Images can be filmed on a laser camera like routine CT scans. This can be useful especially if you are still in a film-based environment. What is perhaps better in our experience is to film images directly to photographic film, which is then given directly to the physician or sent to him/her. In the past, we have done this using a Kodak 8650 dye sublimation printer, which makes good quality images at under $ 3.00 per page. We typically might give the referring physician anywhere between 6 and 14 images or 3 to 7 sheets of film. Recently, a new lower-cost camera from Olympus (p-400) has been introduced in the consumer market, but has proven ideal for our lab. The systems cost around $ 400 and produces images of a better quality than the Kodak 8650, which might cost 20–50 times more. Individual film cost is only $ 1.60 per sheet. Currently it is our standard of communication and well accepted by our referring physicians. Other elegant methods of image transfer to the referring physician are via the web as TIFF or PICT files or via CDs or DVD s. CDs are especially useful when studies that incorporate motion such as virtual colonoscopy are done. CDs are limited to 700 megabytes and may not hold an entire study without compressing the images. DVDs can hold around 4.7 gigabytes, and therefore seem to be a better solution in these cases. An analysis of your own environment is critical in determining the optimal delivery system.

Training

Another important aspect of this brave new world of volume visualization is the challenge of training and retraining staff radiologists and radiologic technologists and perhaps ultimately select referring clinicians. Whether this training is on the CT scanner, a workstation, or on a piece of software that runs on both systems, the training process needs revisiting and redesign. The usual method of training is for an imaging specialist to spend 2–5 days at the site of a new scanner or workstation installation. Additional training may be provided at a central location where the training is typically didactic with some hands-on available. This scenario has worked reasonably well for nearly 20 years, but is showing its age. A simple mathematical calculation at an institution like Johns Hopkins is that even a one-week visit for training is grossly inadequate. When you consider our Body CT division has approximately 20 fulltime technologists, 11 physicians who read CT, and 10 fellows and 24 residents who want to learn CT you can see the dilemma. Hands-on training typically helps but a privileged few. The majority of users rely on second-hand training. The same is true with the 3D workstations where much of the training may be combined with the scanner training. It is not surprising that over 95% of radiologists and technologists surveyed by the author over the past 3 years have been unsatisfied with their training or workstation expertise.

The problem then requires new solutions and a new teaching paradigm. E-based teaching has proven successful in other fields and will need to be adapted for radiology. The introduction of www.InsideInspace.com in March 2003 attempts to solve some of these problems. Developed as a website dedicated exclusively to using the real-time 3D program InSpace, the site combines technical information, »how to do it« information, and case studies for use by the users or potential users of InSpace. There is a question and answer section for which answers to the most common questions are provided, as well as an »ask the expert« section which puts the user in direct contact with program developers, support staff and radiologists knowledgeable in system performance and clinical applications. The site also provides lectures and allows downloadable presets for 3D rendering developed at leading academic and research centers for users to improve their practice. We believe this represents the first attempt to create a true users community within a medical imaging product. It will be interesting to see how successful the site becomes and whether it becomes the prototype for other products and applications. The site is free to the medical community. Whether this paradigm shift catches on and becomes a standard or »crashes and burns« will be of interest to us all. Our personal experience with our own website suggests that radiologists and technologists are ready to learn via the web and that this area will be an exciting one in the next decade [11–13].

Conclusion

CT continues to make amazing technical advancements and is currently enjoying unprecedented popularity based on its ever-changing capabilities. These capabilities provide unique opportunities to improve patient care while at the same time pose unique challenges to maximize the capabilities provided by these new technologies. The workflow that has worked so well for nearly 30 years will need to be revisited and redesigned as we move more fully into this world of volume imaging. The opportunity for change is there, we must just embrace it.

References

1. Horton KM, Fishman EK (2003) The current status of multidetector row CT and three-dimensional imaging of the small bowel. Radiol Clin North Am 41: 199–212
2. Macari M, Bini EJ, Xue X et al. (2002) Colorectal neoplasms: prospective comparison of thin-section low-dose multi-detector row CT colonography and conventional colonoscopy for detection. Radiology 224: 383–392
3. Lawler LP, Corl FM, Haponik EF, Fishman EK (2002) Multidetector row computed tomography and 3-dimensional volume rendering for adult airway imaging. Curr Probl Diagn Radiol 31: 115–133
4. Klingenbeck-Regn K, Flohr T, Ohnesorge B, Regn J, Schaller S (2001) Strategies for cardiac CT imaging. Int J Cardiovasc Imaging 18: 143–145
5. Flohr T, Ohnesorge B (2001) Heart rate adaptive optimization of spatial and temporal resolution for electrocardiogram-gated multislice spiral CT of the heart. J Comput Assist Tomogr 25: 907–902
6. Funabashi N, Kobayashi Y, Perlroth M, Rubin GD (2003) Coronary artery: quantitative evaluation of normal diameter determined with electron-beam CT compared with cine coronary angiography initial experience. Radiology 226: 263–271

7. Rubin GD, Schmidt AJ, Logan LJ, Sofilos MC (2001) Multi-detector row CT angiography of lower extremity arterial inflow and runoff: initial experience. Radiology 221: 146–158
8. Lawler LP, Pannu HK, Corl FM, Fishman EK (2002) Multidetector row computed tomography with volume rendering-an aid. Curr Probl Diagn Radiol 31: 230–243
9. Lawler LP, Corl FM, Fishman EK (2002) Multi-detector row and volume-rendered CT of the normal and accessory flow pathways of the thoracic systemic and pulmonary veins. RadioGraphics 22: S45–60
10. Fishman EK, Horton KM (2001) Imaging pancreatic cancer: the role of multidetector CT with three-dimensional CT angiography. Pancreatology 1: 610–624
11. Scatarige JC, Garland MR, Corl FM, O'Keefe CF, Fishman EK (2002) Visitors and content preferences on an educational web site dedicated to clinical body computed tomography: results of a 2001 audit and online survey. Invest Radiol 37: 53–59
12. Corl FM, Kuszyk BS, Garland MR, Fishman EK (1999) 3-D volume rendering as an anatomical reference for medical illustration. J Biocommun 26: 2–7
13. Horton KM, Garland MR, Fishman EK (2000) The Internet as a potential source of information about radiological procedures for patients. J Digit Imaging 13: 46–47

3 Pediatric Multidetector CT: Practice Guidelines

M. J. Siegel

Introduction

Multidetector CT has further advanced the imaging capabilities of CT in children. The rapid acquisition times have improved scan quality by reducing motion artifacts and decreasing the need for sedation. The ability to cover large volumes faster with thin slices improves the evaluation of small lesions and small vessels, and allows high-quality reconstructions and three-dimensional (3-D) renderings. However, unlike for adults, standard protocols cannot be used for pediatric patients because of their varying body size. Adjustments must be made for the technical parameters used for the CT examinations and for methods and rates of administering intravenous contrast agents [1–3]. This chapter addresses techniques that are helpful for optimizing the use of multidetector CT in pediatric patients and reviews the common clinical applications for performing CT in children. The role of multiplanar and 3-D reconstructions is emphasized.

Patient Preparation

Pediatric patients have some inherent problems that are not present in adults, including patient motion, small body size, and lack of perivisceral fat. The introduction of multidetector CT has substantially reduced patient motion and also reduced the need for sedation [4, 5]. In one study, sedation was necessary in only about 3% children undergoing CT examination with a 4-row detector scanner [5]. With the introduction of 16-row detector scanners, it is reasonable to assume that sedation requirements will diminish even further.

Bowel Opacification

The problems of small body size and lack of perivisceral fat can be minimized or eliminated by appropriate use of oral and intravenous contrast medium. Oral contrast agents are needed for most examinations of the abdomen, because unopacified bowel loops can simulate a mass or abnormal fluid collection. The exceptions to the use of oral contrast medium are patients with depressed mental status who are at risk of aspiration and those with acute blunt abdominal trauma where there may be insufficient time for contrast administration. A water-soluble

Table 1. Amount of oral contrast versus patient age

Patient Age	Minimum amount given at least 45 min prior to scanning	Additional volume given 15 min prior to scanning
Less than 1 month	2–3 ounces (60–90 ml)	1–1.5 ounces (30–45 ml)
1 month–1 year	4–8 ounces (120–240 ml)	2–4 ounces (60–120 ml)
1–5 years	8–16 ounces (240–480 ml)	4–8 ounces (120–180 ml)
6–12 years	16–36 ounces (480–1000 ml)	8–18 ounces (180–540 ml)
13 years and older	36 ounces (1000 ml)	18 ounces (500 ml)

contrast agent is used most often for bowel opacification. This can be given by mouth or through a nasogastric tube. If administered orally, the unpleasant taste of the contrast agent can be masked by mixing with a fruit-flavored drink or fruit juice.

Enteric contrast medium is given 45 min to 1 h prior to scanning. This initial volume should approximate an average feeding. The remaining contrast (about one-half the initial volume) is given about 15 min prior to scanning. If distal bowel opacification is inadequate, additional contrast can be given orally, and scanning can be repeated after a delay to allow the contrast medium to pass distally. The volumes of oral contrast material versus patient's age are given in Table 1. Rectal contrast material may be administered if necessary to opacify the distal colon, which can help delineate pelvic pathology.

Techniques

Intravenous Contrast Medium Administration

With the use of multidetector CT, examinations can be performed with high level of contrast enhancement, which allows the ability to perform CT angiography and multiphase scanning. These options were more difficult or impossible to achieve on single-detector row scanners. Scanning can also be performed using lower doses of contrast medium.

When intravenous contrast material is to be administered, an intravenous line should be in place when the child arrives in the radiology department. This reduces patient agitation that otherwise would be associated with a venipuncture performed immediately prior to administration of contrast material.

Non-ionic contrast agents are recommended for CT scanning in children. Non-ionic agents have the advantages of decreasing discomfort at site of injection and patient motion during intravenous administration [6,7]. For contrast-enhanced chest CT, the volume is 1.5 to 2.0 ml/kg (not to exceed 125 ml). For abdominal CT scanning, the volume is 2.0 ml/kg, The volume is lower for chest CT than for abdominal CT scanning, since there is intrinsically higher contrast resolution in the chest than the abdomen.

Contrast may be administered by hand injection or by a mechanical injector [8]. Hand injections are used when the intravenous access is via a small antecubital catheter (e.g., 24-gauge) or a central venous catheter placed via a peripheral vein. Power injectors may be used when a 22-gauge or larger cannula can be placed in an antecubital vein. The injection rate is 1.5 to 2.0 ml/s with a 22-gauge catheter and 2.0 to 3.0 ml/s for a 20-gauge catheter. A power injection also can be used to administer contrast media via a central venous catheter if the rate of injection is slow (1 ml/s). The site of injection is closely monitored during the initial injection of contrast in order to minimize the risk of contrast extravasation. The benefit of power injection is the uniformity of contrast delivery, which allows for maximal enhancement.

Scan Delay Times

The scan delay time is the time between the start of the contrast injection administration and the start of the scan data acquisition. As a general rule, the duration of the contrast bolus should be equivalent or as close as possible to the duration of the CT scan. For routine chest CT examinations (i.e., screening for metastases, tumor staging, evaluation of a mediastinal mass or congenital lung anomaly), the scan delay after the start of contrast administration is set at 20 to 30 s. A shorter delay (20 s) is used in neonates and infants (< 2 years of age), who have higher cardiac output, with longer delay times used in older children and adolescents.

In the abdomen, the goal is to initiate scanning in or as close as possible to the portal venous phase of enhancement. In adults, a delay time of 50 to 70 s from the onset of contrast administration is employed for routine uniphase abdominal CT, using a power injector and a relatively rapid injection rate. We have found that if pediatric patients receive a volume of at least 100 ml of contrast medium at a flow rate of 2.0 ml/s or a volume of at least 80 ml at 1.5 ml/s, adult delay times are appropriate.

A standard-fixed delay approach is not possible in infants and small children because of the need to inject smaller amounts of contrast medium. Thus, most contrast-enhanced helical CT examinations in this population are based on a time delay after the completion of the contrast injection. A scan delay of 10 to 20 s after completion of contrast administration usually provides excellent hepatic enhancement [9].

One of the greatest benefits of contrast-enhanced scanning with multidetector is the ability to perform CT angiography, even in neonates and infants. An empiric delay is used for thoracic CT angiography in infants under 2 years of age, and scanning begins 12 to 15 s following the start of the intravenous contrast injection. In older children a bolus tracking method is used. This method employs a series of low-dose axial images at a predetermined level that is representative of the scan volume. Once a designated threshold has been achieved (in Hounsfield units), the low-dose scanning terminates and the diagnostic examination begins. The individual arteries are tracked and CT initiated when adequate enhancement is reached, which quantitatively is about 100 HU for thoracic CT angiography and 45 to 50 HU for abdominal angiography.

Specific CT Parameters

One of the advantages of multidetector CT is the flexibility in selecting a range of technical parameters, which enables the radiologist to customize the CT examination for each patient. Prior to initiation of the scan, the following parameters need to be selected: detector collimation (i.e., acquisition slice thickness), table fed per rotation, and slice reconstruction thickness (i.e., display thickness).

Routine chest and abdominal CT examinations on a 4-row detector (Plus 4 Volume Zoom) are performed with a 2.5-mm slice collimation and a table speed of 15 to 20 mm per rotation. The scans are reconstructed at 2.5 to 5.0 mm. For detailed assessment of small structures, such as vessels, a 1.0-mm collimation and a 2-mm reconstruction thickness should be considered. On a 16-row detector (Sensation 16), the collimation for routine studies is 1.5 mm with a table speed of 36 mm per rotation.

The field of view is chosen to cover the area of interest. A standard reconstruction algorithm usually suffices for routine studies and CT angiograms. A high-resolution algorithm is used for 3-D reconstructions of the airways.

Breathing Instructions

CT examinations are performed with breath-holding at suspended inspiration in cooperative patients, usually children over 5 to 6 years of age. Scans are obtained during quiet respiration in children who are unable to cooperate with breath-holding instructions and in patients who are sedated.

Post-Processing Techniques

Image-processing techniques include methods such as multiplanar reformation, volume rendered displays, variable-thickness viewing (sliding slabs), and shaded-surface displays [10–12].

Multiplanar reformatting, which is the simplest reformation technique, is used to assess the extent of disease processes in the craniocaudal direction. Its advantages are that it is fast; it can be easily performed at the CT scanner; and it uses all of the attentuation values in the dataset, presenting them in off-axis views. The major disadvantage of this technique is that it provides only a two-dimensional display of data; thus, it lacks depth cues.

The volume-rendering technique has largely replaced other 3-D reconstruction techniques because it uses all the original data in creating the final image, and the data can be displayed from an external or internal perspective, including the ability to fly through objects (i.e., virtual bronchoscopy). Volume-rendering techniques allow for more reliable measurements of vascular and airway stenoses. This technique is particularly useful in evaluating those branches which course perpendicular to the axial plane.

Sliding slabs are an additional technique that is used to evaluate pulmonary vessels and airways. Rather than collecting data from a series of individual sections of equivalent thickness, a series of overlapping minimum or maximum intensity projections images are combined in multiples or slabs to create a thicker image [10].

The shaded-surface representation displays data in a 3-D format based on an assigned threshold. All structures within the threshold range are displayed, while other tissues are deleted. The principle application of the shaded-surface display is the evaluation of osseous structures of the thorax.

Radiation Dose in Pediatric Multislice CT

Techniques that minimize radiation dose are mandatory for CT examinations in children. These techniques include the use of low milliamperage (mA) setting, low kilovoltage (kV) settings, appropriate slice thickness, and higher pitches [13–19]. Additionally, multiphasic studies should be performed only when necessary, rather than being used as a routine protocol.

Milliamperage (tube current) perhaps is the most recognized variable that affects radiation dose. The relationship between mA and radiation dose is linear; doubling the mA doubles the radiation dose. A 33 to 75% reduction in tube current represents a 33 to 75% decrease in radiation dose, without substantial loss of image quality [14]. The mA for pediatric CT examinations needs to be the lowest possible that maintains image quality. General guidelines for tube current based on patient weight are shown in Table 2.

Kilovoltage is another factor that affects both scan quality and radiation dose. A kV less than 120 can result in a 30% reduction in dose [20]. A kV of 80 should be considered for patients weighing less than 50 kg. In larger patients, a higher kVp should be used to compensate for the higher noise [20].

The collimation determines the nominal or effective section thickness, which can be changed after the patient has left the department provided that the raw data have been saved. For example, if the chest is scanned with a 5-mm detector configuration, the minimum slice thickness is 5 mm. If the chest is scanned with a 1.0-mm detector configuration, the raw data can be reconstructed at 1.0-, 2.5-, 3.75-, or 5.0-mm contiguous sections. Thinner slices (1.0 mm thickness or less) increase spatial resolution, but they also increase radiation exposure. The use of thinner sections requires a higher mA to maintain photon flux and image quality, which results in a higher radiation dose. Thus, most CT examinations in children

Table 2. Milliamperage and kilovoltage settings versus patient weight

Weight (kg)	Chest CT (mA)	Abdomen CT (mA)
<15	25	30
15–24	30	35
25–34	45	50
35–44	75	80
45–54	100	100–120
>54	120–140	120–140

are performed using a 2.5-mm collimation on a 4-row detector scanner and a 1.5-mm collimation on a 16-row detector scanner.

The table increment per gantry rotation (speed) has an impact on resolution and radiation dose. Faster speeds increase temporal resolution and decrease radiation dose.

Pediatric Chest CT: Clinical Applications

Specific areas in which multidetector CT of the pediatric chest have proven particularly useful are:
1. evaluation of lung metastases;
2. evaluation of the character and extent of a mediastinal or pulmonary mass:
3. assessment of cardiovascular anomalies (CT angiography);
4. assessment of airway narrowing or mass; and
5. evaluation of complex chest wall abnormalities.

Evaluation of Pulmonary Metastases (Protocol 1)

The temporal and spatial resolution afforded by helical CT improves the detection and characterization of pulmonary nodules. Of particular importance, the use of thin collimation allows retrospective reconstructions to be obtained through suspected nodules without the need to rescan. This decreases radiation dose as well as optimizing characterization of focal lesions.

Protocol 1

Indication	Standard lung/mediastinum (oncologic staging, detection of metastases, characterization of mediastinal or pulmonary mass, evaluation of trauma), and chest wall
Extent	Lung apices to caudal bases
Scanner settings:	kVp: 80 for patients weighing <50 kg; higher kVp for larger patient mA: lowest possible based on patient weight
Detector collimation	2.5 mm for 4-row scanner 1.5 mm for 16-row scanner
Table speed	15 to 20 mm/rotation for 4-row scanner 36 mm/rotation for 16-row scanner
Slice thickness	3–5 mm for 4-row scanner 2–5 mm for 16-row scanner
IV Contrast	Nonionic 280–320 mg iodine/ml
Contrast volume	2 ml/kg (maximum of 4 ml/kg or125 ml, whichever is lower)

Contrast injection rate	Hand injection: rapid push bolus Power injector: 22-gauge: 1.5–2.0 ml/s 20-gauge: 2.0–3.0 ml/s
Scan delay	20 to 30 s
Miscellaneous	Contrast medium used at discretion of radiologist in the evaluation of metastases. Routinely given for evaluation of mediastinal and pulmonary masses and trauma Use a standard reconstruction algorithm

Evaluation of a Mediastinal or Pulmonary Mass (Protocol 1)

Multidetector CT has several advantages in the evaluation of a suspected or known mediastinal or pulmonary mass. The faster acquisition times improve spatial and temporal resolution and allow consistently high levels of vascular enhancement, which can facilitate characterization of mediastinal and parenchymal lesions and definition of their extent. In general, axial images alone can provide sufficient information about the nature and extent of these masses (Fig. 1). The

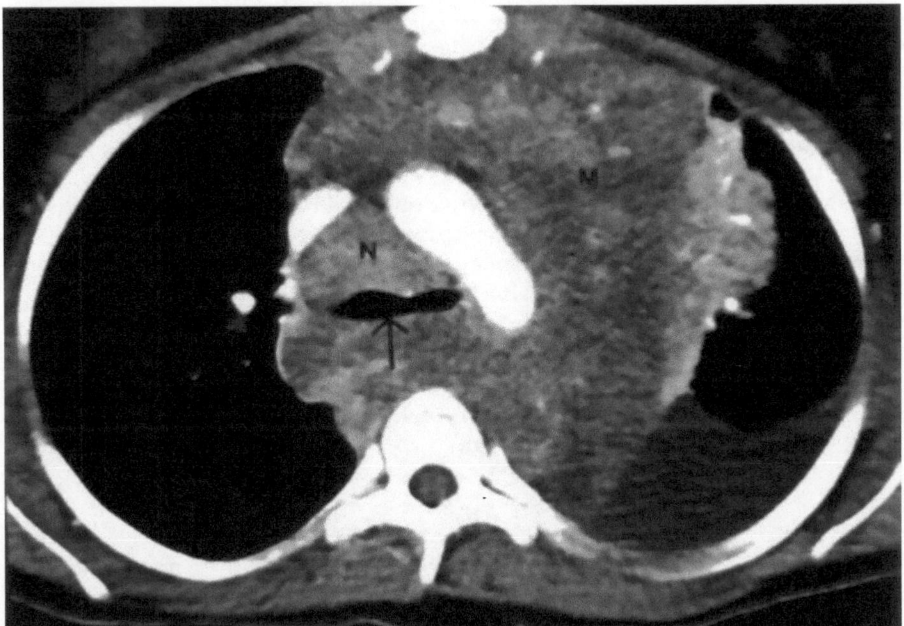

Fig. 1. Thymic Hodgkin's disease, adolescent girl. A large, soft-tissue attenuation, anterior mediastinal mass (*M*) is seen in the expected position of the thymus. The mass compresses the trachea (*arrow*). Also noted are enlarged pretracheal lymph nodes (*N*) and a left pleural effusion. The high-level of vascular enhancement allows determination of the character of this mass and its extent

ability to obtain multiplanar (coronal, sagittal, and oblique reformations) and also 3-D images can help in planning surgical or radiation therapy.

Cardiovascular Assessment (Protocol 2)

CT angiography has become a valuable technique for vascular imaging and is challenging conventional angiography and MRI for assessing anomalies of the thoracic vessels and congenital heart disease [3, 21–27]. Faster scan times afforded by multidetector CT coupled with the use of cardiac gating not only reduce artifacts, but they allow high-resolution imaging of intra- and extra-cardiac regions that previously were difficult to evaluate because of cardiac motion.

Axial images usually suffice for diagnosis, but multiplanar or 3-D reconstructions, particularly when viewed in a cine mode, provide better anatomic detail

Protocol 2

Indication	CT angiography (cardiovascular anomalies, post-operative shunts)
Extent	Lung apices to caudal bases
Scanner settings:	kVp: 80 for patients weighing <50 kg; higher kVp for larger patient mA: lowest possible based on patient weight
Detector collimation	2.5 mm for 4-row scanner 1.5 mm for 16-row scanner
Table speed	15 to 20 mm/rotation for 4-row scanner 36 mm/rotation for 16-row scanner
Slice thickness	3–5 mm for 4-row scanner 2–5 mm for 16-row scanner
IV Contrast	Nonionic 280–320 mg iodine/mL
Contrast volume	2 ml/kg (maximum of 4 ml/kg or 150 ml, whichever is lower)
Contrast injection rate	Hand injection: rapid push bolus Power injector: 22-gauge: 1.5–2.0 ml/s 20-gauge: 2.0–3.0 ml/s
Scan delay	Patient weight < 15 kg: 12 to 15 s Patient weight > 15 kg: 20 to 25 s
Miscellaneous	If sequestration is suspected, scanning should extend through the upper abdominal aorta Precontrast images are not needed for most examinations, but they are used in the evaluation of endovascular stents Use standard reconstruction algorithm

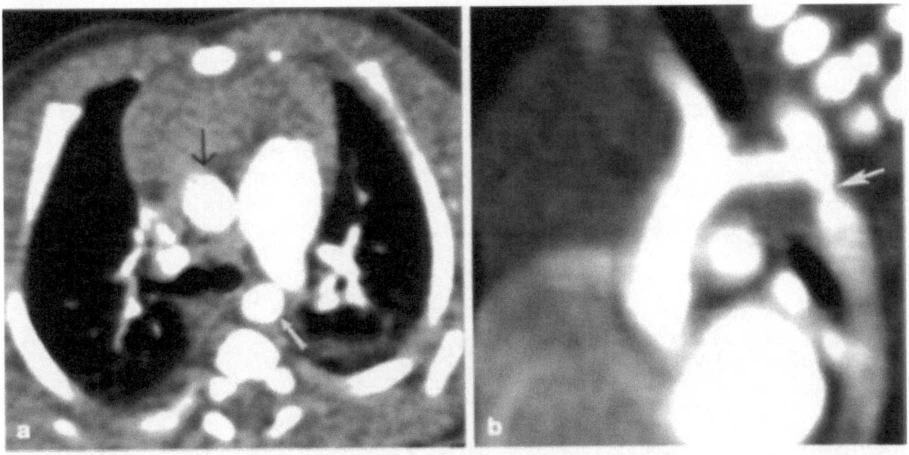

Fig. 2a,b. Aortic coarctation in an infant. **a** Axial image shows normal caliber ascending aorta (*black arrow*) and descending aorta (*white arrow*). **b** 3-D volume rendering demonstrates focal narrowing (*arrow*) of the descending aorta just beyond the left subclavian artery. This was unsuspected on the axial images

about anatomic relationships between the great vessels and tracheobronchial tree, aid in the diagnosis of mild stenoses, improve the accuracy of determining the length of vascular narrowing, and help in planning surgery or stent placement.

The common indications for CT angiography of the mediastinal vessels include:

1. characterization of congenital aortic anomalies, such as coarctation (Fig. 2), arch anomalies (double aortic arch and right arch with aberrant subclavian artery) (Fig. 3);
2. diagnosis of congenital pulmonary vascular anomalies, such as patent ductus arteriosus, pulmonary artery hypoplasia, partial anomalous pulmonary venous return and pulmonary arteriovenous malformation; and
3. evaluation of combined parenchymal and vascular anomalies, including pulmonary sequestration and hypogenetic lung syndrome (e.g., pulmonary hypoplasia and anomalous venous return; Fig. 4).

The major indications for CT evaluation of congenital cardiac anomalies include:

1. evaluation of the size and patency of the pulmonary arteries in patients with complex heart diseases, such as pulmonary atresia, tetrology of Fallot, and hemitruncus (Fig. 5);
2. detection of anomalous origin of the coronary artery;
3. evaluation of palliative extracardiac systemic-to-pulmonary artery shunts (Fig. 6);
4. assessment of residual intracardiac shunt lesions following repair of complex heart diseases;
5. evaluation of the integrity of intracardiac baffles; and
6. demonstration of collateral vessel formation.

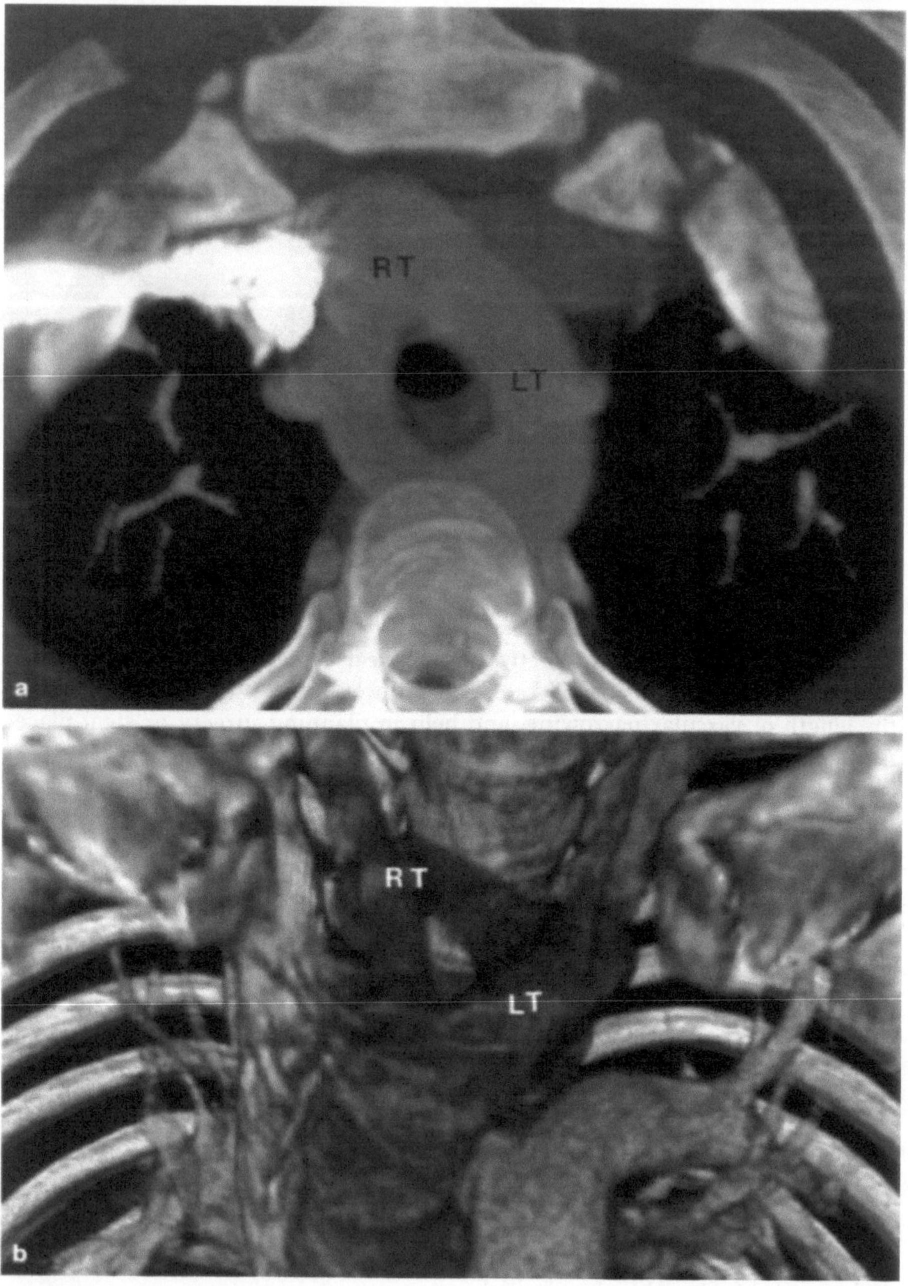

Fig. 3a,b. Double aortic arch. **a** Axial contrast-enhanced slab image shows double aortic arch surrounding the trachea without airway compression. The two arches meet posteriorly. **b** Coronal volume rendered image shows the relationship of the great vessels to both right and left arches. 3-D images often show anatomic relationships better than axial images. **Rt** right arch; **Lt** left arch (Reprinted from [3])

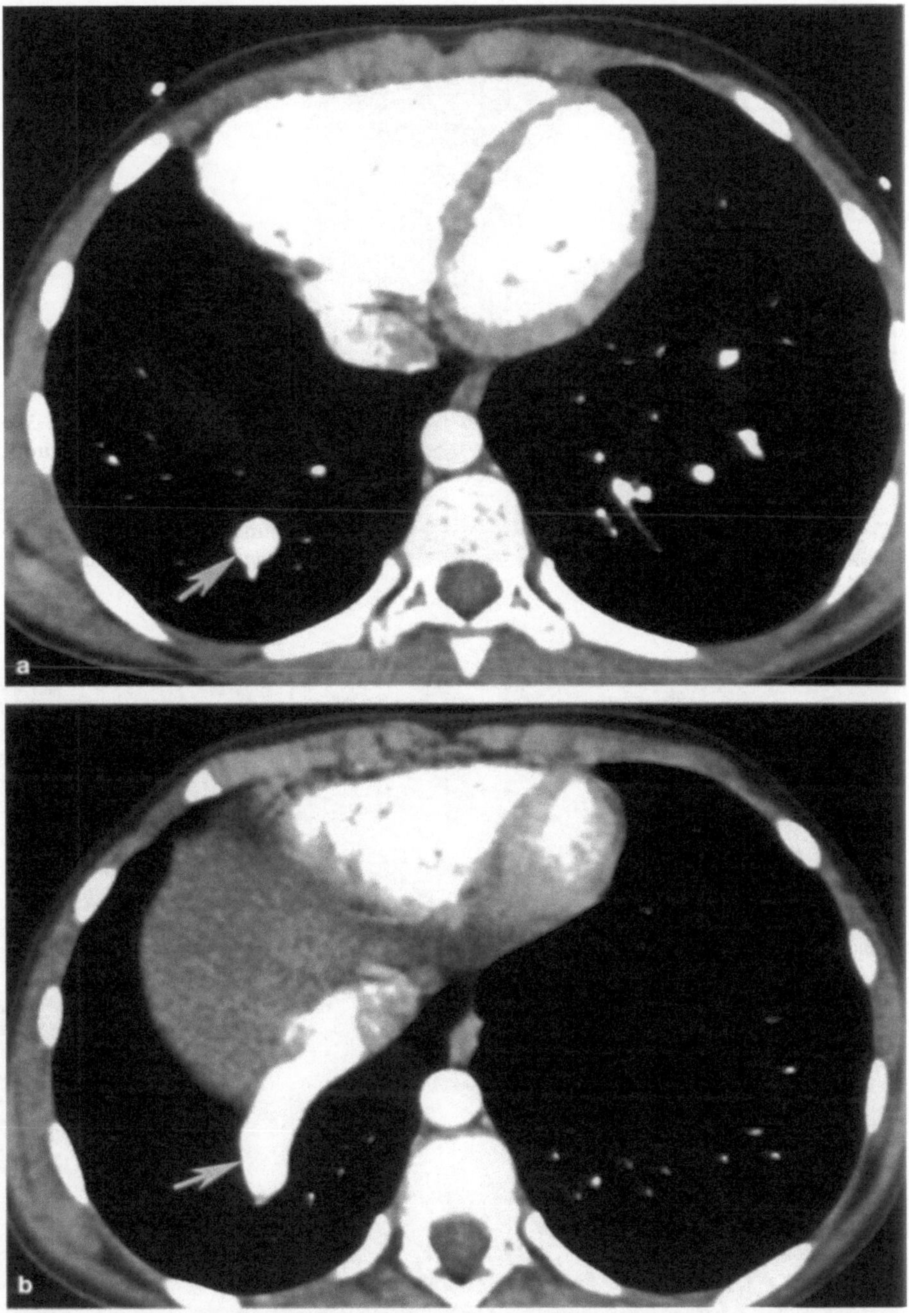

Fig. 4a–c. Pulmonary hypoplasia with partial anomalous venous return. **a** Axial CT scan at the level of the ventricles shows part of the anomalous pulmonary vein. **b** Several centimeters lower, the anomalous vessel enters the intrahepatic inferior vena cava. Note also the slightly smaller right hemithorax and the ipsilateral mediastinal shift.

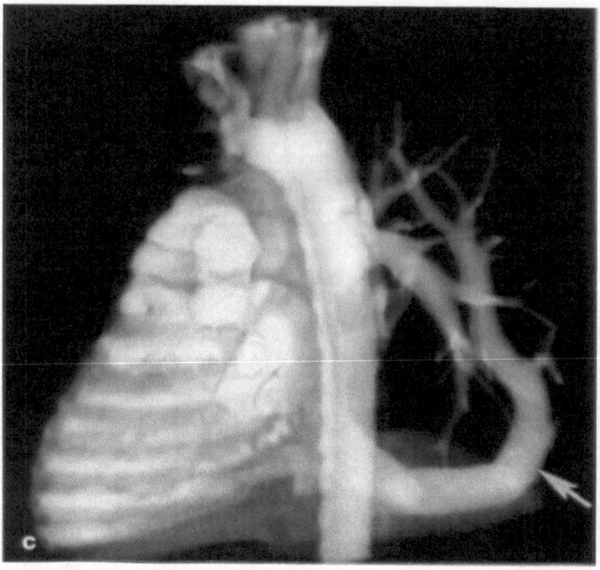

Fig. 4c. Volume-rendered 3-D display viewed posteriorly. With this technique, it is possible to depict the entire course of the vessel on one image; **arrow** anomalous pulmonary vein

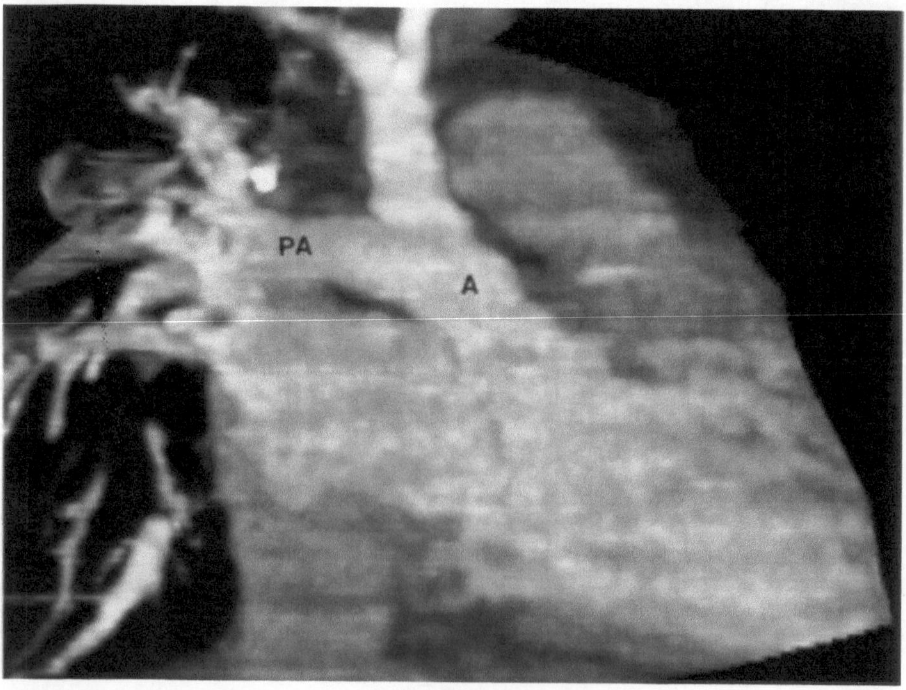

Fig. 5. Hemitruncus in a neonate. Coronal volume rendering shows the origin of the right pulmonary artery (*PA*) from the aorta (*A*). The left pulmonary artery arose as a separate branch (Reprinted from [3])

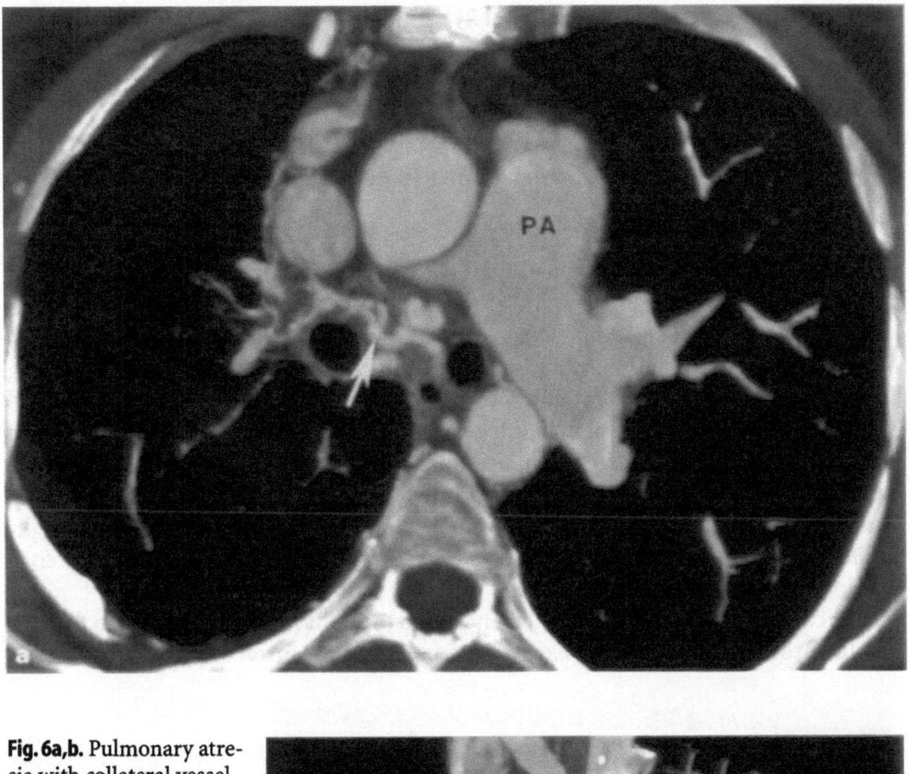

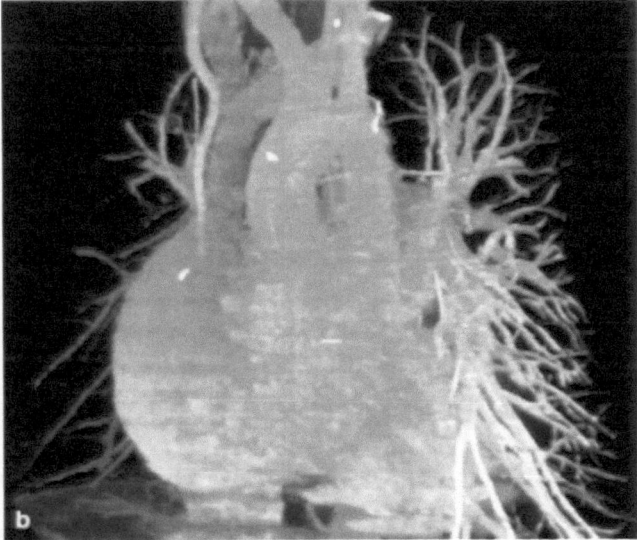

Fig. 6a,b. Pulmonary atresia with collateral vessel formation, adolescent female. Patient had a Waterston shunt (anastomosis of ascending aorta to right pulmonary artery) as an infant, and now returned with cyanosis. **a** Axial image shows a dilated main pulmonary artery (*PA*) and hypertrophied bronchial collateral vessels (*arrow*). **b** Coronal image shows normal branching of the left pulmonary vessels. The right pulmonary vessels are diminutive. The Waterston shunt was thrombosed

CT of the Central Airways (Protocol 3)

The chest radiograph is usually the initial imaging study in patients with suspected airway abnormalities. However, evaluation of the airway often is difficult because of overlapping mediastinal structures. Multidetector CT with reformatted images can allow more precise depiction of tracheobronchial abnormalities [28–31].

Axial images are indispensable for assessing the presence and extent of extraluminal disease, but multiplanar and 3-D volume-rendering aid in diagnosing subtle areas of narrowing and in assessing the craniocaudal length of an abnormality (Fig. 7). Focally short segments of narrowing may not be seen on axial images, but they will be identified on multiplanar and 3-D imaging. Long segment disease usually can be identified on axial as well as on multiplanar and 3-D reconstructions. Multiplanar images are also helpful to assess the position of endobronchial stents placed for management of stenosis.

Virtual bronchoscopy has a rather limited application in the evaluation of the pediatric airway, but it can help to evaluate the airways beyond the site of high-grade stenosis or neoplasm, which otherwise can be difficult to visualize by conventional bronchoscopy.

Indications for CT of the trachea and large bronchi include: evaluation of congenital bronchial anomalies, e.g., accessory bronchi, bronchial hypoplasia and

Protocol 3

Indication	Tracheobronchial tree (congenital anomalies, stricture, tumor, tracheomalacia)
Extent	Vocal cords to mainstem bronchi, just below carina
Scanner settings	kVp: 80 for patients weighing <50 kg; higher kVp for larger patient mA: lowest possible based on patient weight
Detector collimation	2.5 mm for 4-row scanner 1.5 mm for 16-row scanner
Table speed	15 to 20 mm/rotation for 4-row scanner 36 mm/rotation for 16-row scanner
Slice thickness	3–5 mm for 4-row scanner 2–5 mm for 16-row scanner
Patient instructions	Suspended inspiration
Contrast type	None
Comments	Select table speed so that the area of interest can be scanned in a single breath hold in cooperative patients Use high spatial resolution reconstruction (bone) algorithm Multiplanar and 3-D reconstructions are useful to provide an overview of anatomy for surgical planning If tracheomalacia is suspected, obtain scans in inspiration and expiration

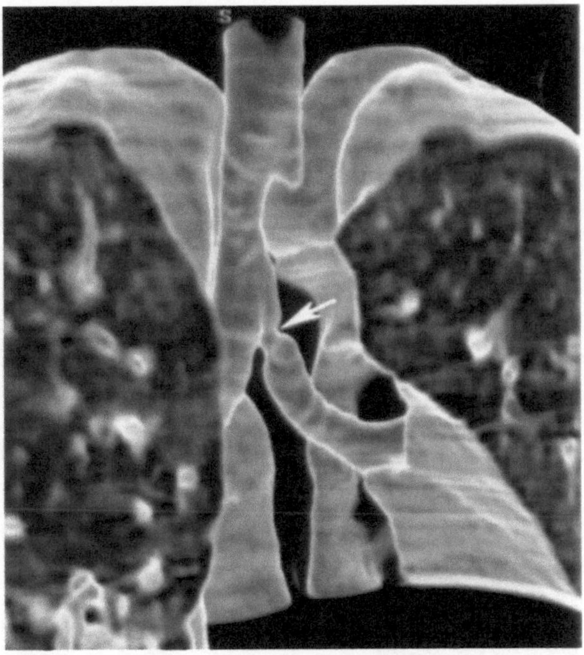

Fig. 7. Congenital tracheal strictures in a neonate. Coronal volume rendering shows an area of long segment tracheal narrowing above the carina and a focal area of narrowing (*arrow*) at the origin of the left mainstem bronchus

atresia, airway stenosis (Fig. 7), narrowing caused by extrinsic compression, and tracheomalacia.

Multiplanar and 3-D Evaluation of the Chest Wall (Protocol 1)

Multiplanar and 3-D surface rendering techniques are ideal for displaying the complex osseous structures of the thorax. The ability to display chest wall masses or thoracic wall deformities in multiple projections can improve the understanding of anatomy and assist in planning complicated reconstructive surgery. In particular, CT can help in evaluating congenital and postsurgical changes, assessing the relationship of peripheral masses to the chest wall, and planning surgical repair of pectus excavatum deformities

Abdominal CT

Four major clinical questions usually prompt CT examination of the abdomen:

1. determination of the site of origin, extent and character of an abdominal mass;
2. determination of the extent of lymphoma;
3. evaluation of the extent of injury from blunt abdominal trauma; and
4. determination of the presence or absence of appendicitis.

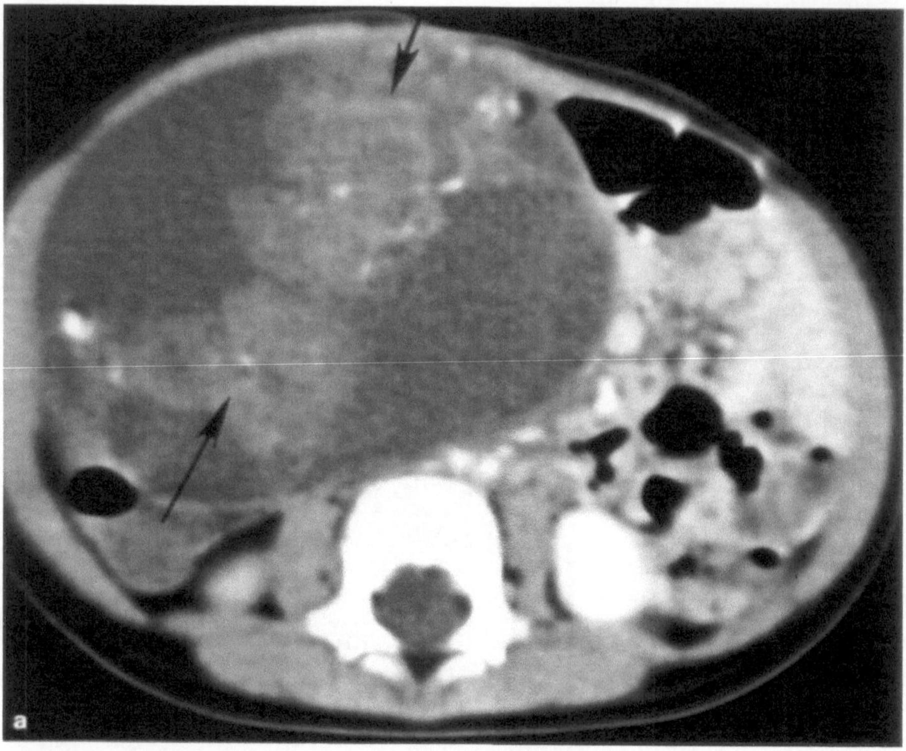

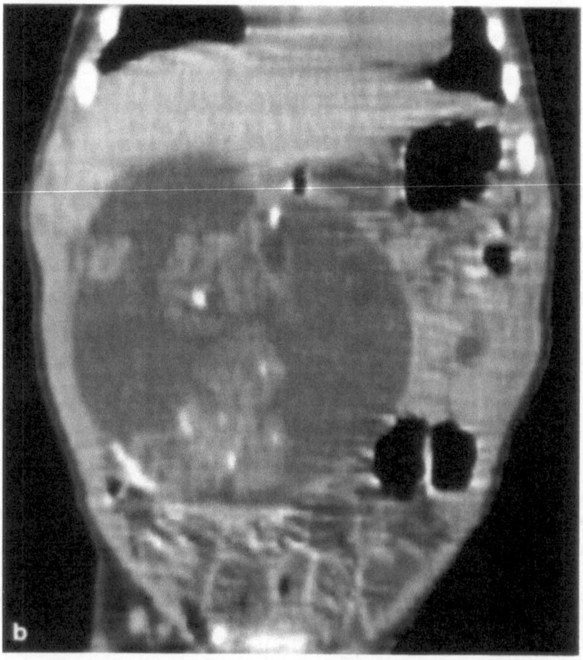

Fig. 8a,b. Cystic ovarian teratoma, 5-year-old girl. **a** Axial mass shows a large near-water attenuation mass with soft-tissue nodules (*arrows*). **b** Coronal multiplanar reconstruction. The extent of the mass and its relationships to adjacent structures are easily seen on this reconstruction

Abdomen/Pelvis Survey (Protocol 4)

The ability to scan large portions of the body in a shorter time period improves delineation of the extent of abdominal masses (Fig. 8) and lymphoma, identification of focal inflammation or abscess, and determination of the extent of trauma. Thin collimation allows multiplanar reformations and 3-D reconstructions of the dataset, which are useful in precisely localizing and defining the extent of tumor for surgical planning.

Acute Appendicitis (Protocol 4)

The ability to acquire contiguous high-resolution CT images has improved the use of CT to diagnose appendicitis and other causes of right lower quadrant pain

Protocol 4

Indication	Abdomen/pelvis survey (tumor, trauma, appendicitis)
Extent	Diaphragm to pubic symphysis
Scanner settings	kVp: 80 for patients weighing <50 kg; higher kVp for larger patient mA: lowest possible based on patient weight
Detector collimation	2.5 mm for 4-row scanner 1.5 mm for 16-row scanner
Table speed	15 to 20 mm/rotation for 4-row scanner 36 mm/rotation for 16-row scanner
Slice thickness	3–5 mm for 4-row scanner 2–5 mm for 16-row scanner
Oral contrast	Water soluble contrast material given 45 to 60 minutes prior to scan. Additional volume given 15 minutes prior to scan Oral contrast medium should be used with caution if patient has a depressed level of consciousness
Intravenous contrast volume	2 ml/kg (maximum of 4 ml/kg or125 ml)
Contrast injection rate	Hand injection: rapid bolus administration Power injector: 22-gauge: 1.5 to 2.0 ml/s 20-gauge: 2.0 to 3.0 ml/s
Scan delay	50 to 70 seconds after onset of contrast injection if patients receive at least 80 ml @ 1.5 ml/s or 100 mL @ 2.0 ml/s Otherwise, 10 to 20 s after the completion of the contrast injection The goal is to initiate the scan in or as close as possible to the portal venous phase of enhancement

Miscellaneous	Multiplanar or 3-D reconstructions can help define the full longitudinal extent of a tumor In setting of trauma, delayed images may be helpful if an abnormality of the bladder or renal collecting system is suspected Non-focused technique for appendicitis is performed with oral and intravenous contrast medium using parameters in this table Other techniques for performing appendiceal CT include 1. imaging limited to the lower abdomen and pelvis without IV, oral, or rectal contrast material, 2. imaging limited to the lower abdomen and pelvis with the use of only IV contrast material, and 3. imaging of the lower abdomen and pelvis with the use of only rectal contrast material

(Fig. 9) Although most investigators agree that appendiceal CT should incorporate thin-section scanning of the right lower quadrant, disagreement exists regarding the extent of anatomic coverage and the need for intravenous, oral, or rectal contrast material. Our standard approach is to perform CT of the entire

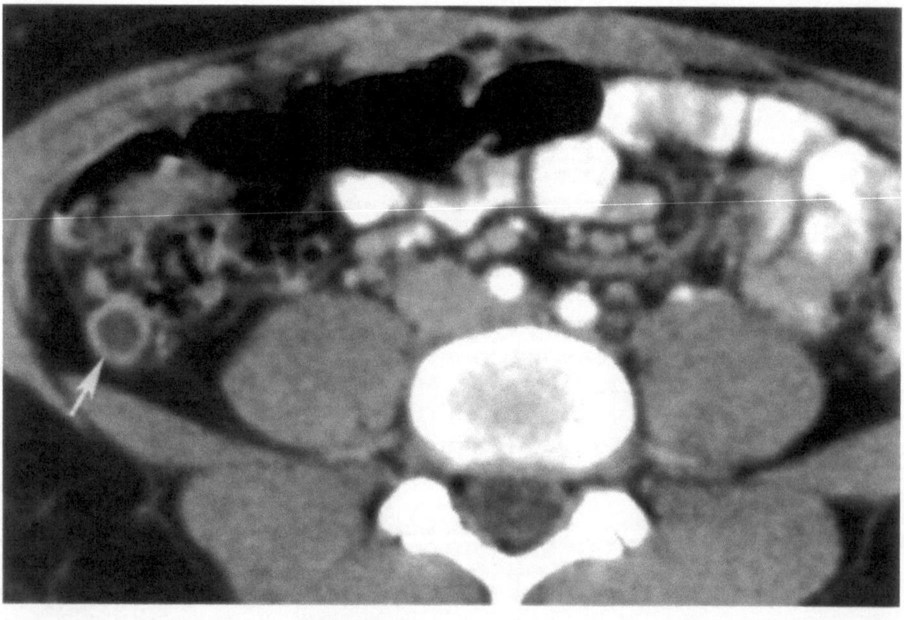

Fig. 9. Acute appendicitis, 15-year-old boy. CT image obtained after administration of both intravenous and oral contrast media show a dilated, fluid-filled appendix with thick walls (*arrow*).

abdomen and pelvis with both intravenous and oral contrast material. This non-focused technique is easy to interpret and allows the diagnosis of other inflammatory disorders that may present with abdominal pain and mimic appendicitis [32, 33]. Alternative protocols include a focused appendiceal CT technique with rectally administered contrast medium and unenhanced scanning of the lower abdomen and pelvis without intravenous, oral, or rectal contrast material [34, 35].

References

1. Bhalla S, Siegel MJ (2002) Multislice computed tomography in pediatrics. In: Silverman PM (ed) Multislice computed tomography: a practical approach to clinical protocols. Lippincott Williams & Wilkins, Philadelphia, PA pp 231–282
2. Donnelly LF, Frush DP, Nelson RC (2000) Multislice helical CT to facilitate combined CT of the neck, chest, abdomen and pelvis in children. AJR 174:1620–1622
3. Siegel MJ (2003) Multidetector CT angiography in children and adolescents. How I do it. Radiology (in press)
4. Kaste SC, Young CW, Holmes TP, Baker DK (1997) Effect of helical CT on the frequency of sedation in pediatric patients. AJR 168:1001–1003
5. Pappas JN, Donnelly LF, Frush DP (2000) Reduced frequency of sedation of young children using new multi-slice helical CT. Radiology 215:897–899
6. Cohan RH, Ellis JH, Garner WL (1996) Extravasation of radiographic contrast material: recognition, prevention and treatment. Radiology 200:593–604
7. Stockberger SM, Hickling JA, Liang Y, Ambrosius WT (1998) Spiral CT with ionic and nonionic contrast material: evaluation of patient motion and scan quality. Radiology 206:631–636
8. Kaste SC, Young CW (1995) Safe use of power injectors with central and peripheral venous access devices for pediatric CT. Pediatr Radiol 26:499–501
9. Frush DP, Donnelly LF, Bisset GS (2001) Effect of scan delay on hepatic enhancement for pediatric abdominal multislice helical CT. AJR 176:1559–1561
10. Cody DD (2002) Image processing in CT. RadioGraphics 2:1255–1268
11. Lawler LP, Fishman EK (2001) Multi-detector row CT of thoracic disease with emphasis on 3-D volume rendering and CT angiography. RadioGraphics 21: 1257–1273
12. Ravenel JG, McAdams HP, Remy-Jardin M, Remy J (2001) Multidimensional imaging of the thorax. Practical applications. J Thor Imaging 16:279–281
13. Donnelly LF, Emery KH, Brody AS, et al. (2001) Minimizing radiation dose for pediatric body applications for single-detector helical CT: strategies at a large children's hospital. AJR 176:303–306
14. Frush DP, Slack CC, Hollingsworth CL, et al. (2002) Computer-simulated radiation dose reduction for abdominal multidetector CT of pediatric patients. AJR 179: 1107–1113
15. Haaga JR (2001) Commentary. Radiation dose management weighing risk versus benefit. AJR 177:289–291
16. Lucaya J, Piqeunas J, Garcia-Pena P, et al. (2000) Low-dose high resolution CT of the chest in children and young adults: dose, cooperation artifact, incidence and image quality. AJR 2 175:985–992
17. Patterson A, Frush DP, Donnelly L (2001) Helical CT of the body: are settings adjusted for pediatric patients. AJR 176:297–301
18. Rogalla P, Stover B, Scheer I, Juran R, Gaedicke G, Hamm B (1999) Low-dose spiral CT: applicability to paediatric chest imaging. Pediatr Radiol 29: 565–569
19. Slovis TL (2002) The ALARA concept in pediatric CT: myth or reality. Radiology 223:5–6
20. Siegel MJ, Suess C, Schmit B, et al. (pending) Radiation doses and image quality for pediatric patients in multi-slice CT: comparison using different tube voltages and varying phantom sizes and shapes. Submitted AJR

21. Gupta H, Mayo-Smith WW, Mainiero MB, Dupuy DE, Abbott GF (2002) Helical CT of pulmonary vascular abnormalities. AJR 178:487–492
22. Hoffman LV, Kuszyk BS, Mitchell SE, et al. (2000) Angioarchitecture of pulmonary AVM malformation characterization using volume-rendered 3-D CT angiography. Cardiovasc Intervent Radiol 23:165
23. Hopkins KL, Patrick LE, Simoneaux SF, et al. (1996) Pediatric great vessel anomalies: initial clinical experience with spiral CT angiography. Radiology 200:811–815
24. Katz M, Konen E, Rozenman J, et al. (1995) Spiral CT and 3-D image reconstruction of vascular rings and associated tracheobronchial anomalies J Comput Assist Tomogr 19:564–568
25. Ko SF, Ng SH, Lee TY, et al. (2000) Noninvasive imaging of bronchopulmonary sequestration. AJR 175:1005–1012
26. Lawler LP, Fishman EK (2000) Arteriovenous malformations and systemic lung supply: evaluation by multidetector CT and three-dimensional volume rendering. AJR 178:493–4
27. Zwetsch B, Wicky S, Meuli R, et al. (1995) Three-dimensional image reconstruction of partial anomalous pulmonary venous return to the superior vena cava. Chest 108:1743–1745
28. Hoppe H, Walder B, Sonnenschein M, Vock P, Dinkel H-P (2002) Multidetector CT virtual bronchoscopy to grade tracheobronchial stenosis. AJR 178:1195–2000
29. Remy-Jardin M, Remy J, Artaud D, Fribourg M, Naili A (1998) Tracheobronchial tree: assessment with volume rendering – technical aspects. Radiology 208: 393–398
30. Remy-Jardin M, Remy J, Artaud D, Fribourg M, Duhamel A (1998) Volume rendering of the tracheobronchial tree: clinical evaluation of bronchographic images. Radiology 208: 761–770
31. Sorantin E, Geiger B, Lindbichler F, Eber E, Schimph G (2002) CT based virtual tracheobronchoscopy in children – comparison with axial CT and multiplanar reconstructions: preliminary results. Pediatr Radiol 32:8–15
32. Kamel IR, Goldberg SN, Keogen MR, Rosen MP, Raptopoulos V (2000) Right lower quadrant pain and suspected appendicitis: nonfocused appendiceal CT – review of 100 cases. Radiology 217:159–163
33. Raman SS, Lu DSK, Kadell BM, Vodopich DJ, Sayre J, Cryer H (2002) Accuracy of nonfocused helical CT for the diagnosis of acute appendicitis: a 5-year review. AJR 178:1319–1325
34. Rao PM, Rhea JT. Novelline RA, et al. (1997) Helical CT technique for the diagnosis of appendicitis: prospective evaluation of a focused appendix CT examination. Radiology 202:139–144
35. Lane MJ, Katz DS, Ross BA, Clautice-Engle TL, Mindelzun RE, Jeffrey RB, Jr. (1997) Unenhanced helical CT for suspected appendicitis. AJR 168:465–469

II Neuro, Head and Neck

4 Multislice Spiral CT Angiography in Vascular Neuroradiology

B. Schuknecht

Introduction

Multisclice spiral CT offers the potential to non-invasively delineate major extra- and intracranial vessels. Using an intravenous bolus injection of contrast media, CT angiography serves as an increasingly applied alternative or complimentary examination to digital subtraction angiography. In the head and neck, the anatomic regions investigated by CT angiography consist of the circle of Willis and, less frequently the vertebro-basilar territory intracranially and the carotid bifurcation extracranially.

Thin collimated acquisition of a 3-D dataset requires appropriate timing of the contrast bolus to coincide with the location and extent of the scan range. The short scan duration and limited scan range offer the potential to significantly reduce the amount of contrast material. However, this goal has been only insufficiently accomplished. A literature review of studies applying CT angiography disclosed contrast volumes in the range of 100 to 140 ml with injection rates between 2 and 3.5 ml/s.

Based on the conviction that perfect coupling of contrast bolus injection and data acquisition serve to optimize image quality and reduce contrast volume, the feasibility of fast low-contrast volume CTA was assessed.

Patients and Methods

Fast low-contrast volume CTA was performed with a four-detector row CT (Siemens Volume zoom) and applied extracranially to evaluate the carotid bifurcation in 10 patients with color duplex-proven high degree (70–90%) steno-occlusive disease. In an additional 12 patients CTA was performed to characterize saccular aneurysms.

With the aid of a CT power injector (Ulrich, Missouri) 30 ml of non-ionic contrast media (Guerbet Xenetix, 300 mg iodine/ml) were administered at an injection rate of 5 ml/s for the extracranial, 4 ml/s for the intracranial examination. Contrast application was followed by flushing with 20 ml of saline. The care bolus technique was used with the region of interest set into the aortic arch.

For the extracranial examination the scan range encompassed 50 mm focused on the carotid bifurcation. Following a delay of 6 s after initiation of contrast injection and after reaching a blood-contrast threshold of 80 HU, the scan was performed with a table feed of 6 mm/s. For the intracranial examination the scan range was reduced to 30 mm starting at the level of the sella floor covering the entire circle of Willis including the basilar tip. The threshold was set to 65 HU, the table feed was 3.5 mm per rotation in order to optimize image quality by reducing artefacts within the z direction. The rotation time for both extra- and intracranial examination was 0.5 s. Reconstruction consisted of maximum-intensity projection (MIP) and 3-D surface-shaded display (3-D SSD) images, the latter with a threshold of 100 HU. Intraarterial contrast density was visually and qualitatively assessed and objectively analyzed. Contrast-density calculations were performed in five patients extracranially and in eight patients with intracranial CT angiography. For the extracranial examination, density calculations encompassed the ipsilateral and contralateral common and internal carotid carotid artery at the lower and upper end of the scan range. Correspondingly, the density was measured in the internal jugular vein at the lower and upper (craniad) end of the scan range.

Contrast-density calculations in the intracranial examination comprised the supraclinoid internal carotid artery, the parent artery harbouring the aneurysm, the aneurysm itself and a major branch adjacent to the aneurysm. The resultant contrast density curves were graphically displayed.

Results

High-quality CT angiography was achieved in every patient with respect to DSA as standard of reference. Calculation of contrast density for the extracranial examination was between 155 and 320 HU on the arterial side in the common and internal carotid artery and 55–120 HU within the internal jugular vein (Fig. 1). Intracranial density calculations obtained from the supraclinoid internal carotid artery, the parent artery, the aneurysmal sac and a major branch were in the range of 185 and 350 HU (Fig. 2). Differences in contrast density exceeding 50 HU were noted only interindividually and not intraindividually. Interindividual differences in contrast density were attributed to different body weight and circulation times. Contrast densities in the range of 150 to 250 HU are considered optimal for the measurement of the degree of extracranial vessel stenosis [1].

For the extracranial examination the following images were assessed: axial multiplanar Reconstruction images (MPR), maximum intensity projections (MIP)and 3-D surface-shaded display images (3-D SSD).

Two mm axial MPR sections photographed at constant window and center settings (550/180) allowed assessment of:

- the location of the residual vessel lumen,
- the presence of calcifications,
- non-calcified hypodense plaque components,
- eccentricity of plaques with respect to the transverse vessel diameter.

Axial MPR images correlated well with DSA but, despite the limited number of patients, not better than MIP images. This opposes the findings of others [2]. Eccentricity of the plaque with respect to the vessel wall circumference and the

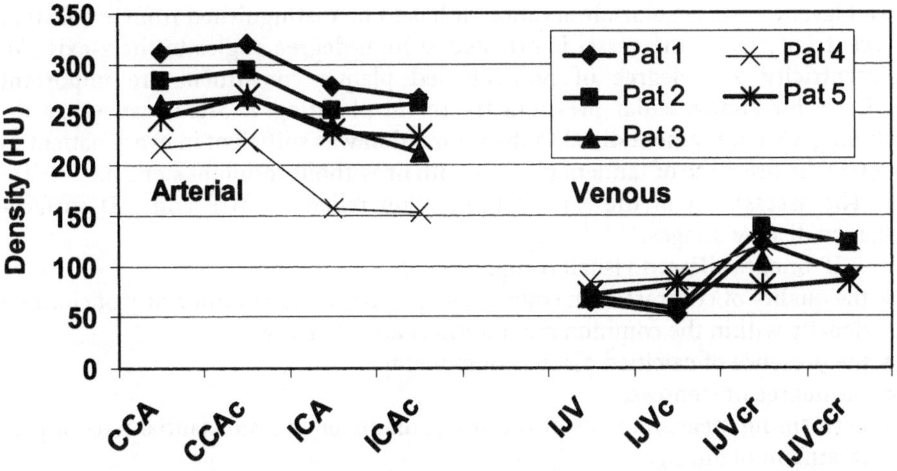

Fig. 1. Based on the 30 ml contrast volume, 5 ml flow/s, table increment 6 mm and scan range 50 mm, protocol density calculations were performed within the common carotid artery (CCA) and the internal carotid artery (ICA) ipsilateral and contralateral (c) to a high-degree stenosis. The densities were between 155 and 320 HU on the arterial side. Additionally, density calculations were obtained from the internal jugular vein (IJV) at the lower and craniad end (cr) of the scan range. Densities were in the range of 55 to 120 HU within the internal jugular vein. Density increase in IJVcr marks the beginning of venous return in caudo-craniad scan direction

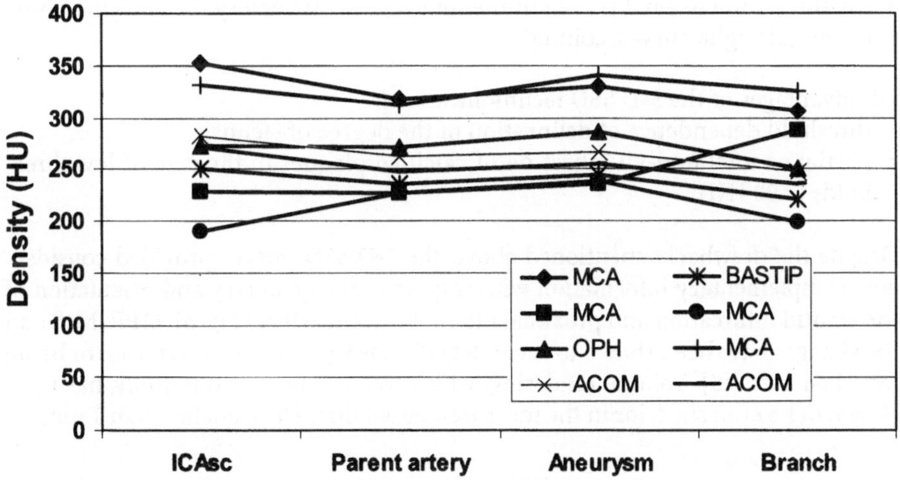

Fig. 2. Based on the 30 ml contrast volume, 4 ml flow/s, table increment 3.5 mm and scan range 30 mm, protocol intracranial density calculations were obtained from the supraclinoid internal carotid artery (ICAsc), the parent artery, the aneurysm itself and a major branch adjacent to the aneurysm. The location of the aneurysm is indicated on the right. The densities calculated were in the range from 185 to 350 HU in our protocol. Density differences were primarily noted interindividually and attributed to differences in body weight and circulation time

wall layers was a regular observation. It has to be distinguished from artefactual eccentricity when the vessel is oriented at high-degree angles to the z-axis [3]. Eccentricity and degree of non-calcified plaque constituent are important criteria for endovascular pre-stent treatment planning. A 5-cm scan range including a 3-cm segment distal to the bifurcation was sufficient in every patient to detect the presence of tandem plaques with or without resultant stenosis.

The assessment of the carotid bifurcation relied on MIP and 3-D surface-shaded display images.

MIP images allowed visuall recognition of:

- the quality of contrast/scan coupling displayed as (non)-uniformity of contrast density within the common and internal carotid artery
- the presence of calcified plaque components
- the degree of stenosis,
- performing measurements of the vessel diameter as a substantial part of pre-treatment planning.

MIP images displayed high-degree stenosis and subtotal occlusion to better advantage than threshold-dependent 3-D SSD images (Fig. 3). Careful adjustment of centre and window setting when photographing the MIP images window is important to avoid under- or overestimation of the degree of stenosis [4].

MIP allowed determination of the »profile« of the maximum degree of stenosis by rotation of the images along the vessel axis. This is a particular advantage compared to DSA (with the only exception being rotational DSA).

3-D surface-shaded display images demonstrate:

- the geometry of the carotid bifurcation, in particular, the angulation between the common and internal carotid carotid artery,
- the three-dimensional course of the internal carotid artery distal to the bifurcation (straight, curves, coiling).

Disadvantages of the 3-D SSD technique are:

- threshold dependence of delineation of the degree of stenosis,
- partial or total non-visualization of calcified plaques in the case of low thresholds (<90 HU).

Despite the drawbacks mentioned above, the 3-D SSD images provided considerable complementary information with respect to the geometry and orientation of the carotid bifurcation and proximal internal carotid artery (Fig. 3). MPR, MIP and SSD images have been shown to accurately display vessel diameters, the error being less than 2.5% [5]. Volume rendering, which was not part of this study, has been shown to be even superior in the measurement of diameters smaller than 1 mm.

Examination of Intracranial Aneurysms

CT angiography was performed either following DSA in ruptured aneurysms or prior to DSA in the case of suspicion of an aneurysm incidentally detected during cranial contrast-enhanced CT. Application of CT angiography in these

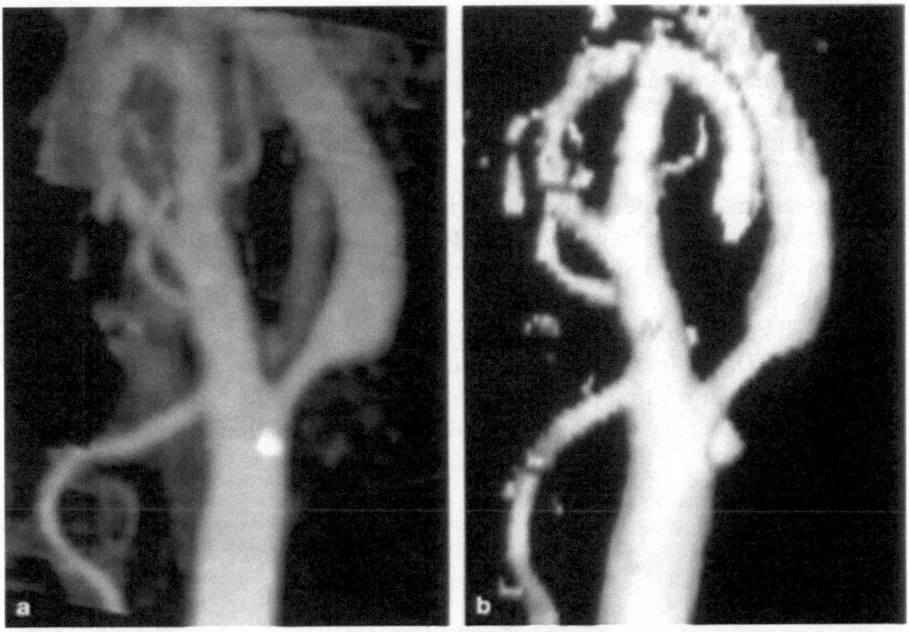

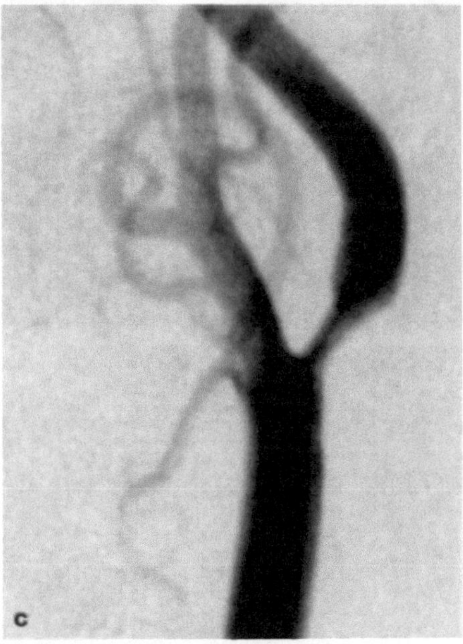

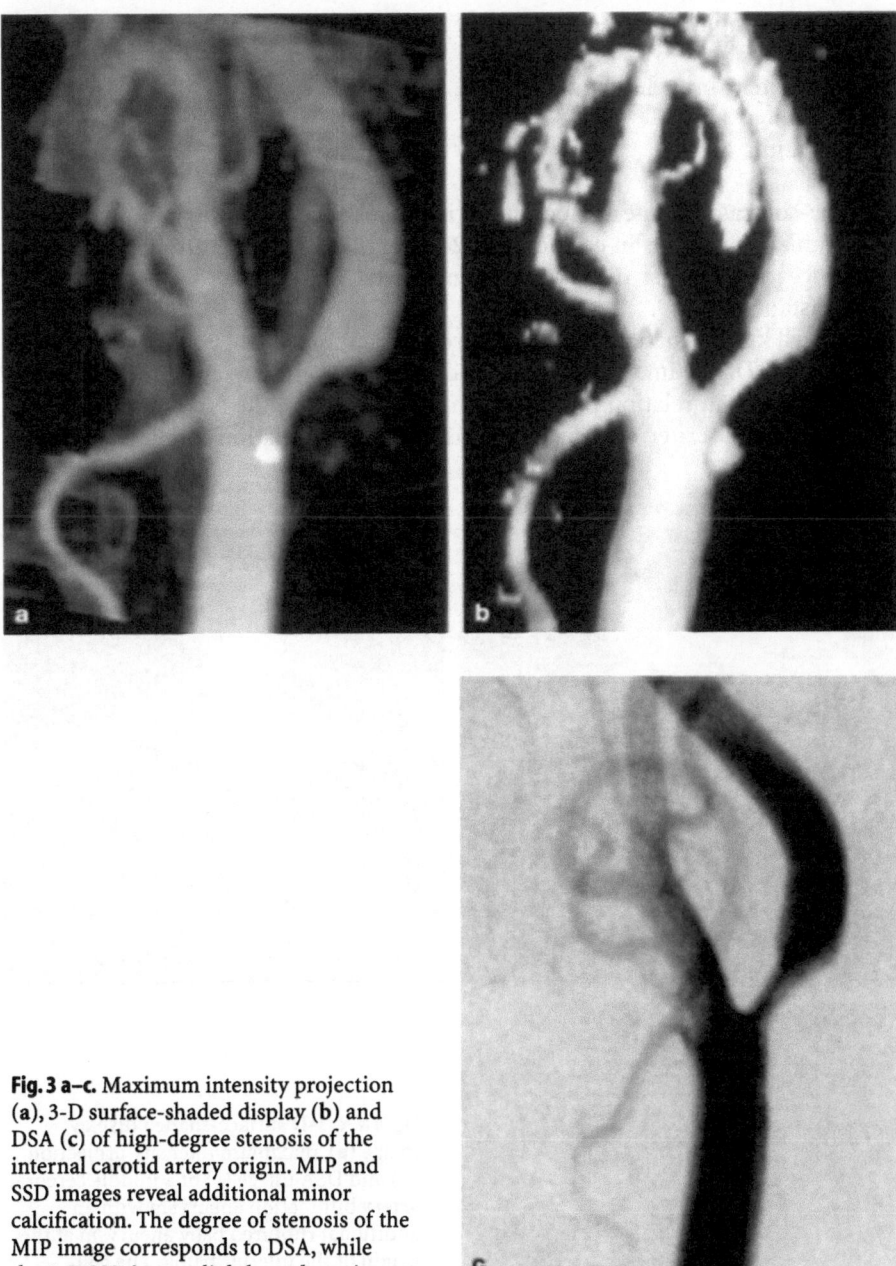

Fig. 3 a–c. Maximum intensity projection (**a**), 3-D surface-shaded display (**b**) and DSA (**c**) of high-degree stenosis of the internal carotid artery origin. MIP and SSD images reveal additional minor calcification. The degree of stenosis of the MIP image corresponds to DSA, while the 3-D SSD image slightly underestimates the degree of narrowing

two conditions is based on the concept that DSA is the most sensitive technique to detect intracranial aneurysms and is therefore required in every patient with subarachnoid haemorrhage. Only in incidental aneurysms was CT angiography performed prior to DSA [1].

CT angiography in intracranial aneurysms serves to define the

- location,
- parent artery/branch relationship,
- morphology and
- orientation.

Fast low-contrast volume angiography with 30 ml of contrast was able to delineate intracranial aneurysms in each of the 12 patients investigated. Despite individual differences in contrast density, high-quality CT-angiograms were obtained in every instance (Fig. 4).

It is well known that characterization of intracranial aneurysms is best accomplished by 3-D SSD images [6,7]. For the decision if endovascular is feasible, the size of the base in relation to the maximum diameter of the sac of the aneurysm is the important criterion. This relationship and the relation to major branches

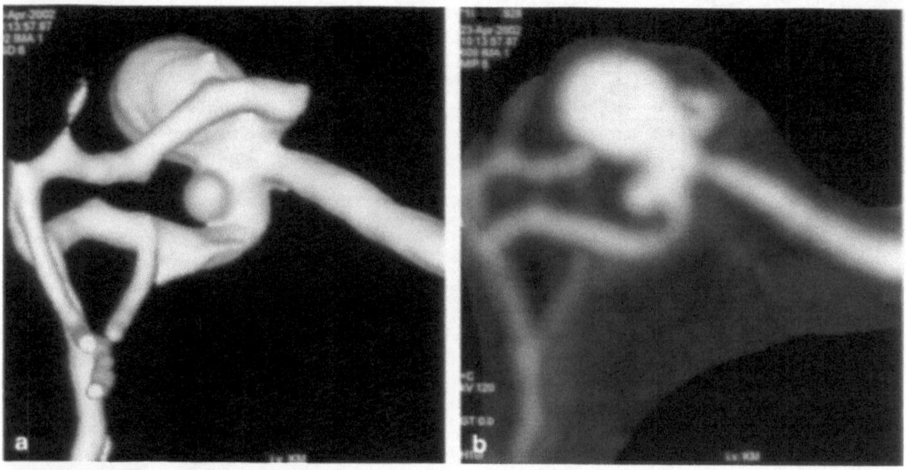

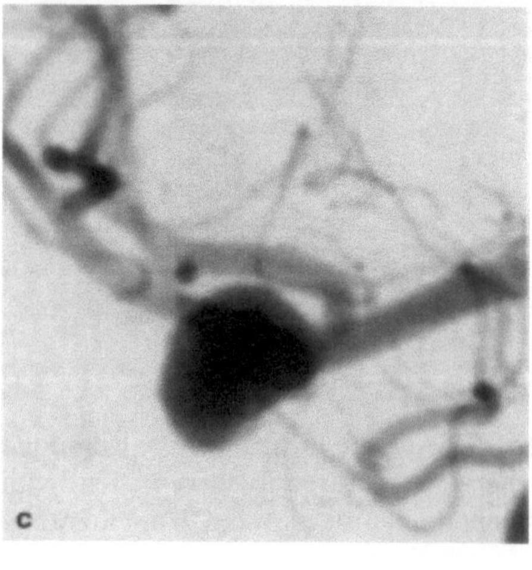

Fig. 4 a–c. 3-D surface-shaded display image (**a**), maximum intensity projection (**b**) and DSA image (**c**) of a middle cerebral artery bifurcation aneurysm with an additional ruptured baby aneurysm at the origin of the inferior trunk. The configuration, orientation and relationship of the main aneurysm to the inferior and superior trunk are best delineated by 3-D SSD. MIP precisely depicts the incorporation of the origin of the inferior trunk into the base of the baby aneurysm. Limitation of rotation precluded recognition of the baby aneurysm on DSA arising close to the aneurysm are occasionally better displayed by 3-D SSD and MIP images than by DSA (Fig. 4). Aneurysms with a large base or »neck« are usually not amenable to endovascular treatment.

For surgical treatment planning, 3-D SSD images offer the additional advantage of demonstrating the anatomic relationship of aneurysms to the anterior clinoid process, the dorsum sellae and the relationship of the middle cerebral artery bifurcation to the silvian fissure. Furthermore information about the calibre and connections of vessels contributing to the circle of Willis is available. Careful interactive adjustment of the threshold is required to delineate smaller vessels and not to miss small aneurysms [8]. Operator dependence therefore holds true for both SSD images with respect to threshold and even more for MIP images [8].

MIP images delineate the constituents of the circle of Willis and allow measurements to be obtained from the maximum dimension of the aneurysm sac (longitudinal and transverse) and along the presumed »neck« of the aneurysm.

Therefore, MIP and 3-D SSD images serve the same purpose for both the examination of the carotid bifurcation and the delineation of intracranial aneurysms. While MIP images play the major role in assessing steno-occlusive disease of the internal carotid artery, 3-D SSD images are of primary importance for the characterization of intracranial aneurysms.

Fast low-contrast volume angiography provides insight into the morphology of intracranial aneurysms and extracranial high degree stenoses at significantly reduced contrast volumes. High-quality CT angiograms thus facilitate comprehension and treatment planning of these common vascular lesions.

References

1. Claves JL, Wise SW, Hopper KD, et al. (1997). Evaluation of contrast densities in the diagnosis of carotid stenosis by CT angiography. AJR Am J Roentgenol 169:569–573
2. Anderson GB, Ashford R, Steinke D, et al. (2000) CT Angiography for the detection and characterization of carotid artery bifurcation disease. Stroke 31:2168–74
3. Wise SW, Hopper KD, Ten have T, Schwartz T (1998) Measuring carotid artery stenosis using CT angiography: the dilemma of artifactual lumen eccentricity. AJR Am J Roentgenol. 170:919–23
4. Liu Y, Hopper KD, Maugher DT, Addis KA (2000). CT angiographic measurement of the carotid artery: optimized visualization by manipulating window and level settings and contrast material attenuation. Radiology 217:494–500
5. Addis KA, Hopper KD, Lyriboz TA, et al. (2001) CT angiography: in vitro comparison of five reconstruction methods. AJR Am J Roentgenol 177: 1171–1176
6. Schuknecht B, Wichmann W, Valavanis A (1994) Hochauflösende Angio-Computertomographie intrakranieller vaskulärer Läsionen. Klinische Neuroradiol 4:62–72
7. Aoki S, Sasaki T, Machida T et al. (1992) Cerebral aneurysms:detection and delineation using 3-D CT angiography. AJNR-Am J Neuroradiol 13:115–1120
8. Casey S-Oalberico RA, Azsvath R-R (1997) Operator dependence of cerebal CT angiography in the detection of aneurysms. AJNR Am J Neuroradiol 18: 790–792

5 Multislice CT of the Head and Neck

M. Lell, H. Greess, U. Baum, W. Römer, W. Bautz

Introduction

Assessing the head and neck region makes great demands on the imaging modality:

- delineation of tiny structures (auditory ossicles, inner ear),
- delineation of complex anatomy (compartments of the neck),
- short examination time (decreased ability in cooperation of patients with advanced cancer).

MSCT facilitates multiplanar imaging in CT due to increased z-resolution with isotropy of the volume data. In contrast to MR imaging, image planes in anatomically adapted orientation are acquired not by additional examination sequences but with reformating a single 3-D volume dataset. The rapid development in scanner technology brought 4, 6, 8, 10, and 16 slice systems on the market. With the latest scanners large regions (350 mm) can be examined with submillimeter slice collimation (0.75 mm) in 10–15 s. Motion artifacts can be eliminated in virtually all patients, because even patients with advanced head and neck tumors can avoid swallowing or coughing within this short examination time. In head and neck imaging there are three major fields for CT imaging:

1. Temporal bone
CT is the method of choice in imaging osseous changes in temporal bone disease due to the high spatial resolution. Fractures, inflammatory disease, and depiction of congenital abnormalities are major clinical indications.

2. Midface and paranasal sinuses
Sinusitis is a major indication for CT, especially in the preoperative setting or in the detection of complications. It is the basis for new technologies like computer-assisted surgery. CT of the midface and cervical spine has become part of the imaging protocol in the initial evaluation of multitrauma patients.

3. Head and neck
Tumor staging is the major indication for CT or MRI. Multidimensional image planes can be acquired with both techniques. The advantage of MRI is the superior soft tissue resolution, while the advantage of CT is the high spatial resolution and short examination time

Temporal Bone

Assessment of the skull base and the temporal bone requires two or more image planes. With single-slice scanners it was customary to perform both axial and coronal scans. Studies with multislice spiral CT [1, 2] demonstrated that direct coronal scans can be replaced with coronal multiplanar reformations (MPR) from axial submillimeter spiral CT. This reduces both examination time and radiation exposure for the patient. Apart from this, images in additional planes can be achieved to improve the diagnostic confidence. Sagittal images are used to delineate the vestibular aqueduct and the vertical portion of the bony canal of the facial nerve. The nerve itself is best visualized with MRI.

For the CT examination, the patient should be positioned in a comfortable supine position. If the head is tilted slightly backwards, the eye lenses are not

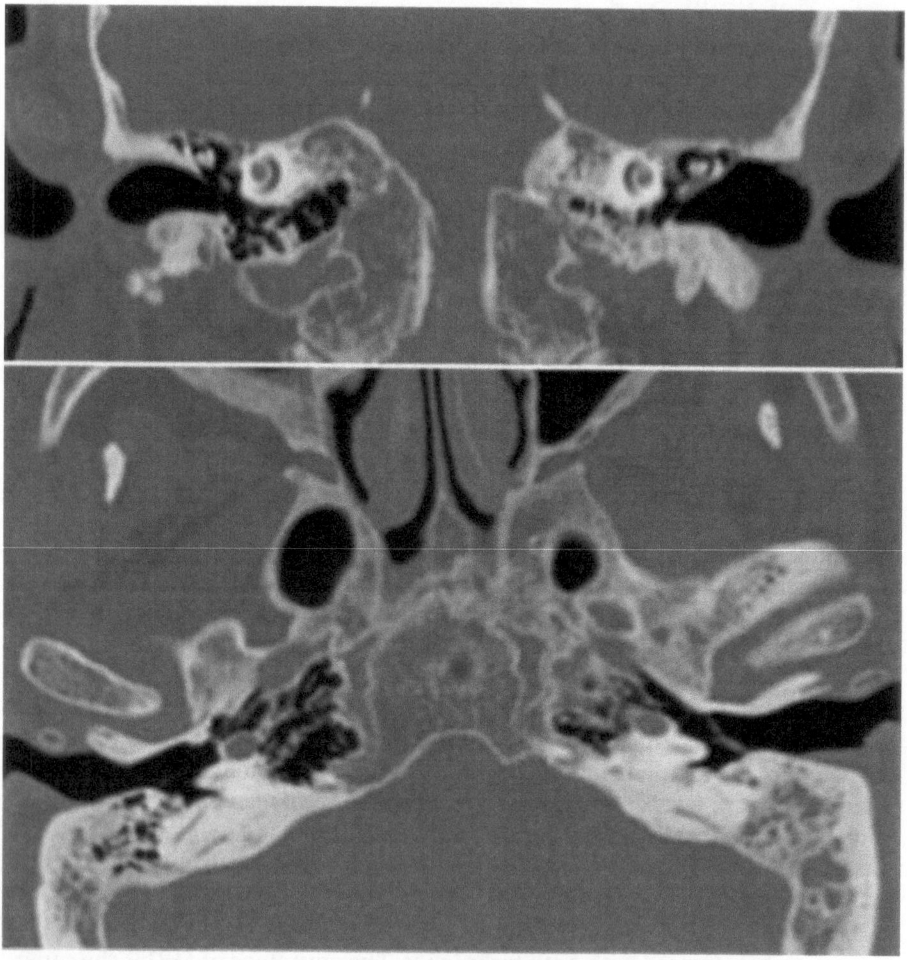

Fig. 1a,b. Sclerosis of the left tympanic membrane. **a** Coronal MPR. **b** Axial slice

Table 1. Scan protocol for the temporal bonea

Scan parameter	Sensation 4	Sensation 10	Sensation 16
Scan length (mm)		50	
Scan direction		Caudocranial	
Slice collimation (mm)	2 x 0.5	10 x 0.75	16 x 0.75
Table feed (mm/rot)	1	7.5	9
Rotation time (s)		0.75	
mAs_{eff}[b]		120	
Tube voltage (kV)		120	
Contrast material:	120 ml, flow rate: 2.5 ml/s; start delay: 80 s		
Image reconstruction			
Slice width (mm)	0.5	0.75	0.75
Reconstruction increment (mm)		0.3	
Slice width of MPR (mm)		0.5–0.8	
Kernel		U70u – U90u and U40u	

[a]UHR: ultra high resolution
[b]mAs_{eff}: the effective current-time-product, the so-called effective mAs value, is a measure of the number of quanta contributing to a given z-position. It is normalized according to the degree of scan overlap (pitch value): mAs_{eff} = (mA x rotation time)/pitch

within the scan range. A high resolution mode is used to increase the spatial resolution (~22 lp/cm; 2% MTF). We perform overlapping image reconstruction with a large field of view (FOV = 200 mm) to cover both temporal bones and a small FOV (70–90 mm) for the affected temporal bone. In routine examination the administration of contrast material is not necessary (Fig. 1). Contrast material should be injected in the evaluation of vascular lesions, tumor, or intracranial complications such as brain abscess [3, 4]. Therefore image reconstruction is done with a soft tissue kernel and slice thickness of the reformated images is increased to 3 mm to reduce image noise. The scan protocol is shown in Table 1.

Midface and Paranasal Sinuses

Chronic sinusitis may be associated with asthma, allergies, analgetic intolerance, eosinophila, cystic fibrosis, and Karthagener's syndrome. Anatomical variants of the sinonasal or ostiomeatal complex predispose the ostia to occlusion. Polyps are associated with the Churg–Straus syndrome, allergic fungal sinusitis, and cilia dyskinetics. High-resolution CT of the paranasal sinuses is an alternative to plain film radiographs, providing superior delineation of all anatomical structures. Because the majority of the patients are young, otherwise healthy, individuals, radiation exposure is an important issue. Increasing the number of detector rows utilized for imaging improves the dose efficiency by reducing the »penumbra« due to postpatient collimation. To demonstrate both the anatomy and inflammatory disease low-dose CT scanning provides sufficient information. Figure 2 shows coronal MPR of an anthropomorphic head phantom examined with different tube currents at 120 kV. The images obtained with an effective current-time product of 25 mAs_{eff} are noisy, but noise can be reduced if the thick-

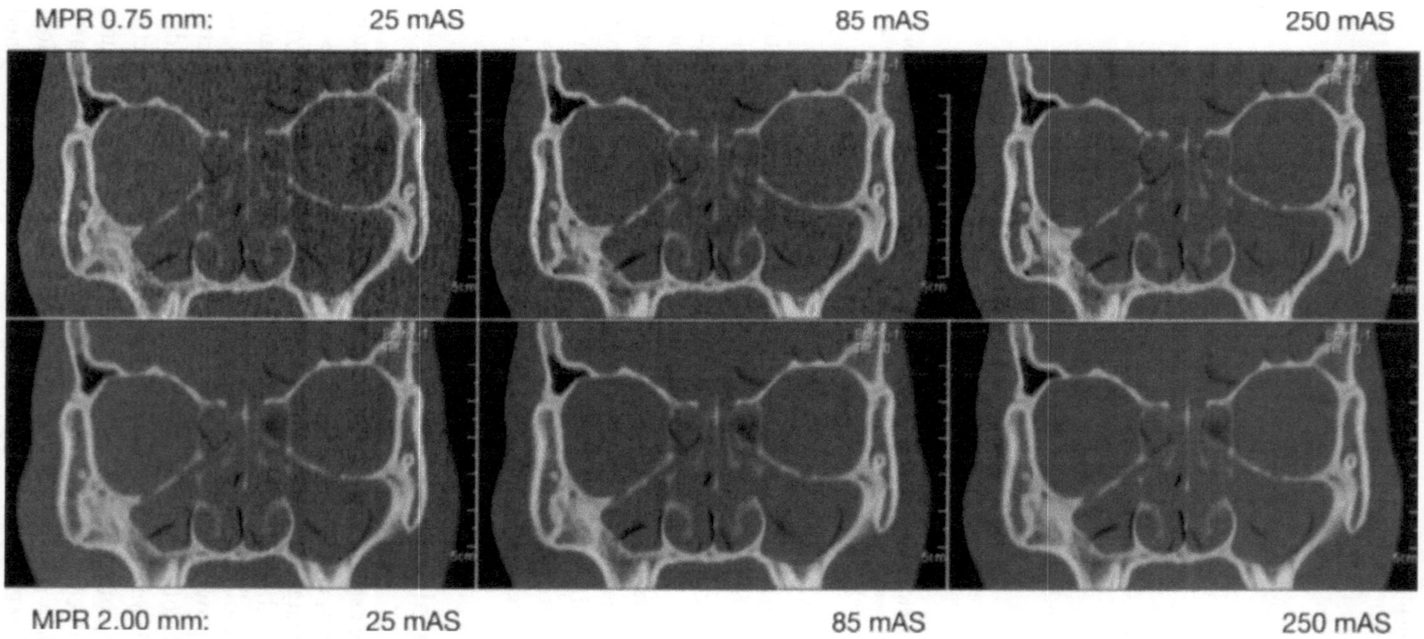

Fig. 2a–c. Phantom study: *upper row* thin MPR, *lower row* 2.0-mm-thick MPR: 25 mAs_{eff} (**a**); 85 mAs_{eff} (**b**); 250 mAs_{eff} (**c**)

Table 2. Scan protocol for the paranasal sinuses (low dose)[a]

Scan parameter	Sensation 4	Sensation 10	Sensation 16
Scan length (mm)		250	
Scan direction		Craniocaudal	
Slice collimation (mm)	4 x 1	10 x 0.75	16 x 0.75
Table feed (mm/rot)	6	11	18
Rotation time (s)[a]		0.75	
mAs_{eff}		150	
Tube voltage (kV)		120	
Contrast material	120 ml, flow rate: 2.5 ml/s; start delay: 80 s		
Image reconstruction			
Slice width (mm)	1.25	1.0	1.0
Reconstruction increment (mm)		0.5	
Slice width of MPR (mm)		1.0	
Kernel		B31s – B40s and B70s	

[a]*UHR* ultra-high resolution

ness of the MPR is increased, thus leading to a sufficient image quality for most questions regarding sinusitis. The scan protocol we use routinely in adult patients is shown in Table 2. CT is superior in demonstrating complicated sinusitis like orbital periostitis or abscess. To evaluate intracranial abscess or sinus thrombosis, contrast-enhanced CT or MRI should be performed. Information of anatomical variants like a low cribriform plate or an abnormal course of the carotid artery are crucial for the ENT surgeon. High-resolution CT is the basis for advanced surgical procedures like computer-assisted surgery (CAS). If tumors of the paranasal sinuses need to be evaluated, the application of contrast material and reconstruction with soft tissue kernels is mandatory. To achieve reasonable image quality (low noise level), higher tube currents are necessary (Table 3). This protocol is also suitable in the evaluation of patients from high-speed accidents

Table 3. Scan protocol for head and neck cancer

Scan parameter	Sensation 4	Sensation 10	Sensation 16
Scan length (mm)		120	
Scan direction		Caudocranial	
Slice collimation (mm)	2 x 0.5	10 x 0.75	16 x 0.75
Table feed (mm/rot)	1	7.5	9
Rotation time (s)		0.75	
mAs_{eff}		35	
Tube voltage (kV)		120	
Image reconstruction			
Slice width (mm)	0.5	0.75	0.75
Reconstruction increment (mm)		0.3	
Slice width of MPR (mm)		0.5–0.8	
Kernel		U70u – U90u	

[a]0.5 s rotation time can be used alternatively to reduce the scan time

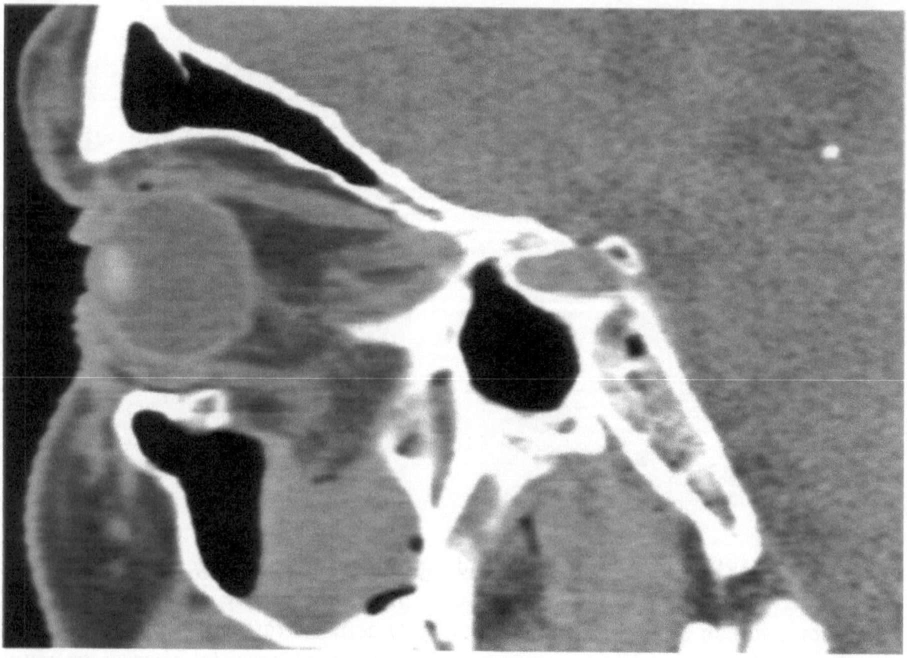

Fig. 3. »Blow out« fracture: sagittal MPR aligned to the orbital muscles show herniation of the inferior rectus muscle into the maxillary sinus

to search for midface or cervical spine fractures. In the setting of adequate trauma conventional radiography in the emergency room is limited to chest X-ray and CT scans of the cerebrum, the midface, and cervical spine, as well as thorax and abdomen, are performed immediately at our institution. The scan is performed in a supine position and coronal MPR are reformated from the 3-D dataset, avoiding both motion artifacts from the patient and beam-hardening artifacts from dental fillings. In patients with fractures of the orbital floor, parasagittal images aligned to the course of the optical nerve can be reconstructed to detect retrobulbar haematoma (Fig. 3).

Tumor Staging – Compartments of the Neck

The major role of CT and MRI in the evaluation of head and neck tumors is to delineate the tumor extent and infiltration depth rather than to search for the tumor. Squamous cell carcinoma arising from the mucosal surface can be visualized with mirror examination and endoscopy, and tissue can be collected for histologic verification. The deep compartments of the neck – mucosal space, parapharyngeal space, masticator space, carotid space, parotid space, retropharyngeal space, prevertebral space – can only be assessed with cross-section-imaging modalities. These compartments are oriented in an cranio-caudal direction, thus best evaluated on coronal and sagittal images.

To assess the lymphatic pathways, the scan range should cover the region from the skull base to the aortic arch. Criteria for malignant nodes are a size over 10–15 mm in diameter, grouping of nodes under 10 mm, quotient of longitudinal and transversal diameter (L/T quotient) less than 2, rim enhancement and central inhomogeneity or necrosis, as well as extracapsular spread [3]. The lymphatic drainage varies with the anatomic subsite of the neck, but within a certain subsite, the drainage occurs in a predictable manner. In nasopharyngeal carcinoma, spread to the retropharyngeal nodes and to nodal group II and V is most common. These retropharyngeal nodes are embedded deeply in the neck and are usually not accessible to palpation and ultrasound. Tumors of the oropharynx and oral cavity spread to the ipsilateral group I, II, and III. Group II nodes are fre-

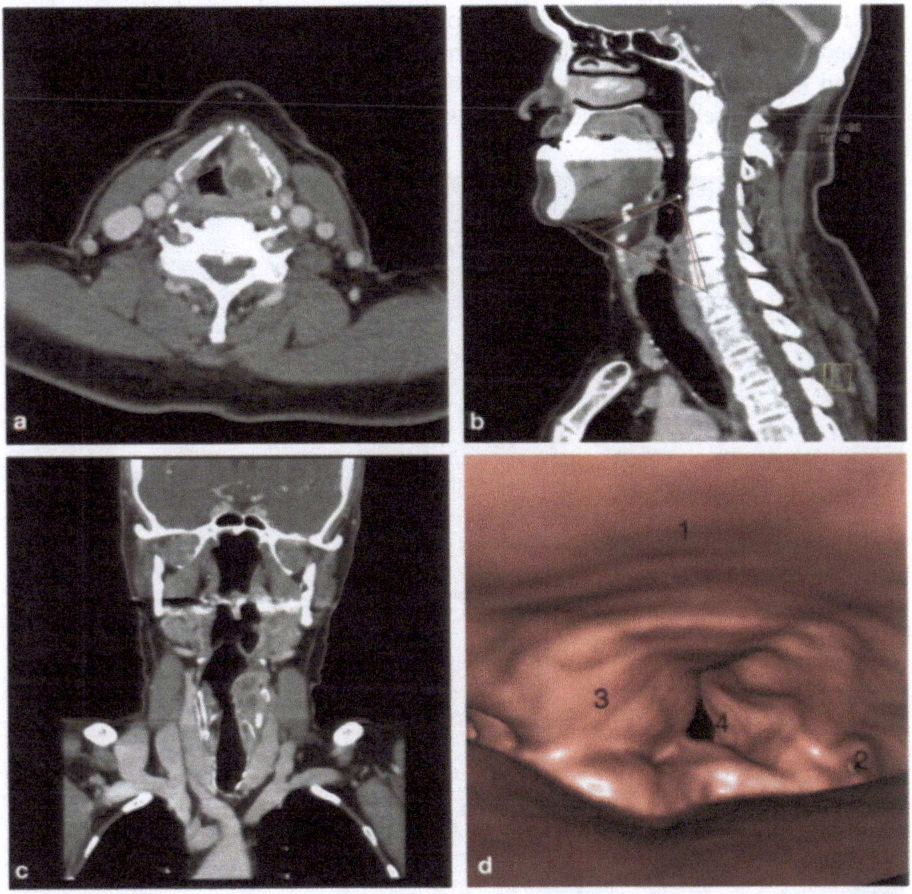

Fig. 4a–d. Laryngeal carcinoma invading the paralaryngeal space and thyroid cartilage: axial slice (**a**); sagittal MPR (with position of the »virtual endoscope«) excludes tumor spread to the tongue base (**b**); coronal MPR delienates craniocaudal extent of the tumor and invasion of the paralaryngeal space and the cartilage (**c**); virtual endoscopy: **d** *1* epiglottis, *2* piriform sinus; *3* tumor; *4* glottis

quently involved ipsi- and contralateral in tongue base and tonsillar carcinoma. Group II and III nodes are commonly involved in laryngeal carcinoma, group II, III, and IV in hypopharyngeal carcinoma [6, 7]. Comprehensive information of most lymph nodes can be obtained from coronal images; sagittal images are best suited to display retropharyngeal nodes.

Nasopharyngeal carcinoma and tumors of the paranasal sinuses cause unspecific symptoms and therefore patients often present with advanced tumor stages with osseous destruction (skull base, orbital floor, palate) being present. These structures cannot be assessed sufficiently on axial images, therefore additional coronal images are necessary. Pharyngeal cancer, infiltrating the masticator space, can spread to the medial cranial fossa via the 3rd branch the trigeminal nerve through the oval foramen. The course of the nerve is best evaluated on coronal images. Laryngeal carcinomas may infiltrate the paralaryngeal fat space and reach the tongue base via the preepiglottic space, compartments which are connected with each other (Fig. 4). Thus tumor invasion of the tongue base beyond an intact mucosal surface is possible. The rapid data acquisition with MSCT allows excellent functional studies of the larynx [8].

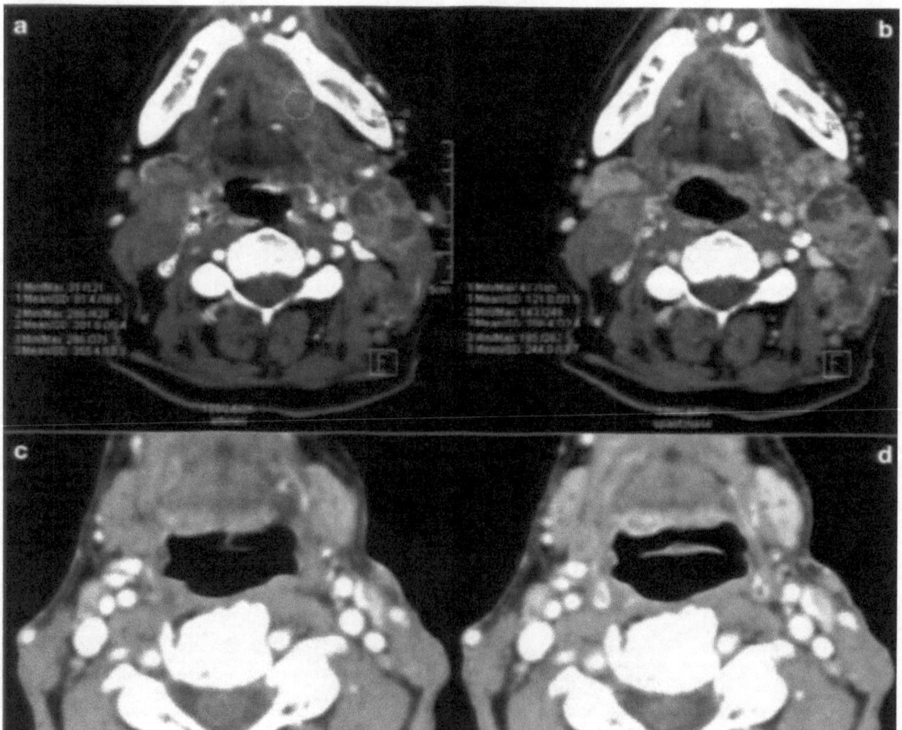

Fig. 5a–c. Comparison of arterial phase (**a,c**) and late venous phase (**b,d**) images. Attenuation measurement for the tumor (ROI 1), the internal carotid artery (ROI 2) and the internal jugular vein (ROI 3). Better delineation of the tumor and lymph node metastasis (*arrow*) with the necrotic areas due to higher contrast enhancement in the late phase

The application of intravenous contrast material is mandatory to demarcate tumor from surrounding soft tissue and to display internal morphologic changes in both the tumor and lymph nodes. The delay between the injection of contrast material and the scan is discussed controversially. We prefer a long delay of 80–90 s. The direct comparison of images acquired in an arterial phase (35 s) and a late venous phase (80 s) from biphasic examinations of the neck did not reveal any advantages for the arterial phase. Drawback of the arterial phase images were severe beam-hardening artifacts at the level of the lung apex because of the inflow of highly concentrated contrast material in the subclavian vein and lower enhancement values of the tumors compared with the late venous phase images (Fig. 5).

To detect osseous or cartilage destruction, images are reconstructed also with a high-resolution kernel (Table 3).

Conclusion

Multislice spiral CT offers the potential for 3-D imaging of the head and neck region in 10 to 15 s with excellent spatial resolution. Therefore MSCT is the imaging modality of choice in the assessment of pharyngeal tumors as well as osseous pathology of the midface and skull base. For the evaluation of diseases of the inner ear, the internal auditory canal and the cerebello-pontine angle MRI is preferable. MRI should also be preferred in patients with cancer of the oral cavity and extensive dental hardware. PET-CT, an evolving new technique, will further improve the diagnostic accuracy in the evaluation of head and neck malignancies, especially in patients with lymph node metastases of unknown primary tumor (CUP syndrome).

References

1. Baum U, Lell M, Noemayr A et al. (2000): Ultrahochauflösende Diagnostik des Felsenbeines mit einem Mehrzeilen Spiral CT (MSCT). Röfo 172: pp151
2. Venema HW, Phao SSKS, Mirck PGB, Hulsmans FJH, Majoie CBLM, Verbeeten B (1999) Petrosal bone: coronal reconstructions from axial spiral CT data obtained with 0.5-mm collimation can replace direct coronal sequential CT scans. Radiology 213: 375–382
3. Valvassori GE, Mafee MF, Carter BL (1995) Imaging of the head and neck. Thieme Medical Publishers, Stuttgart
4. Greess H, Baum U, Römer W, Bautz W (2002) CT und MRT des Felsenbeins. HNO 50: 906–919
5. Sakai O, Curtin HD, Romo LV, Som PM (2000) Lymph node pathology. Benign proliferative, lymphoma, and metastatic disease. Radiol Clin North Am 38:979–98
6. Som PM, Curtin HD, Mancuso AA. (2000) Imaging-based nodal classification for evaluation of neck metastatic adenopathy. AJR 174: 837–844
7. Mukherji, SK, Armao D, Joshi VM (2001) Cervical nodal metastases in squamous cell carcinoma of the head and neck: what to expect. Head Neck 23: 995–1005
8. Lell M, Baum U, Köster M et al. (1999): Morphologische und funktionelle Diagnostik der Kopf-Halsregion mit der Mehrzeilen-Spiral-CT. Radiologe 39: 932–938

III Abdomen and Chest

6 State of the Art MSCT in the Abdomen: Emphasis in Liver and Pancreas

H. Ji, P. R. Ros

»You can't be too rich or too thin...« (Hollywood proverb)
»You can't be too fast or too thin...« (Tuebingen proverb)

Introduction

With the development of multislice or multidetector row computed tomography (MSCT) at the end of the 20th century, CT has regained its place as the most exciting technique in abdominal imaging, a position it lost to magnetic resonance imaging in the mid-1980s. Now it appears that there is nothing MRI can do that multislice CT cannot. With increased spatial resolution in the **z** plane, MSCT makes feasible isotropic imaging, interactive multiplanar imaging, and improved three-dimensional imaging for surgical planning. It is driving a transition from two-dimensional to three-dimensional imaging in abdominal radiology.

MSCT in the Abdomen

MSCT has several advantages over conventional helical CT. The most significant is shorter acquisition times. The core of multislice technology is to replace the single row of detectors used in conventional helical CT with multiple detector rows, thereby allowing the depiction of multiple slices with a single pass of the X-ray tube.By combining the multirow detector with increased gantry rotation speed, the new generation of MSCT scanners can acquire 32 slices/s, and this number increases continually [1,2]. Typically, to scan the abdomen with conventional CT, one must sacrifice resolution to cover the desired volume in one pass, as the area of interest stretches from the base of the lungs to the pubis and may be 40–60 cm in length. MSCT, however, can cover this entire volume at thinner slice thickness than single-row detector CT. A second advantage of MSCT technology is the ability to acquire the dataset at a high resolution especially in the z-plane (S–I axis). Slice reconstruction uses helical reconstruction weighting algorithms that interpolate between adjacent detector rows. With high **z**-axis resolution, multiplanar and 3-D volume-rendering images are routinely acquired (Fig. 1). Finally, MSCT helps prevent tube overheating. The X-ray beam used in CT heats the tube through which it is transmitted to the patient. Since the beam is wider in MSCT than conventional helical CT and a wider area is being covered in a shorter time, the tube is less likely to overheat during scanning and the cooling time between patients is shorter [3]. Unfortunately, MSCT has several potential disadvantages as well. One disadvantage of MSCT is the increased radiation dose to patients. To acquire at the thin slice thicknesses possible with MSCT at

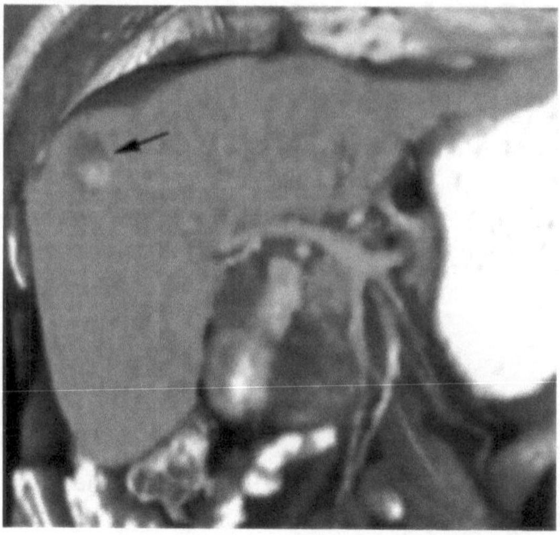

Fig. 1. 3-D volume rendered image of abdomen using multislice CT. 3-D volume rendered image demonstrates a hemangioma in right lobe of liver (*arrow*) and the upper abdominal vasculatures

high resolution, higher tube current and resulting radiation dose are required, particularly when the arterial and venous phases of contrast are captured (multiphasic scanning). To minimize this disadvantage, image thicknesses and multiphasic scanning are chosen carefully based on the clinical objectives of the study [4]. In some cases, thin slice thickness is necessary, such as to detect small focal lesions or for CT angiography. In other cases, thicker slices may be used. Another drawback of MSCT is the large datasets that are generated by reconstructing at a thin slice thickness, typically between 500 and 1000 images for an abdominal study. This high number of images makes it necessary to use workstations rather than film to analyze abdominal MSCT data. Still, implementation of MSCT can have a significant impact on PACS resources by increasing the average number of images per study [5].

Some other drawbacks are related to the basic physical principles of MSCT. Since the X-rays are tilted in the outer rows of the detector array, a cone angle is created. The X-rays wobble like a top in the circumferential rotation, and as a result, cone artifacts form. In the outer rows, the cone-beam artifact may be as high as 1 mm. In clinical practice, however, cone beam artifacts have not limited the applications of MSCT in the abdomen.

Clinical Applications

MSCT in the Liver

Scan Techniques

The liver has complex hemodynamics. Approximately 80% of the hepatic blood supply is derived from the portal venous system and 20% from the hepatic artery. The injected bolus of contrast material initially enhances the liver via inflow

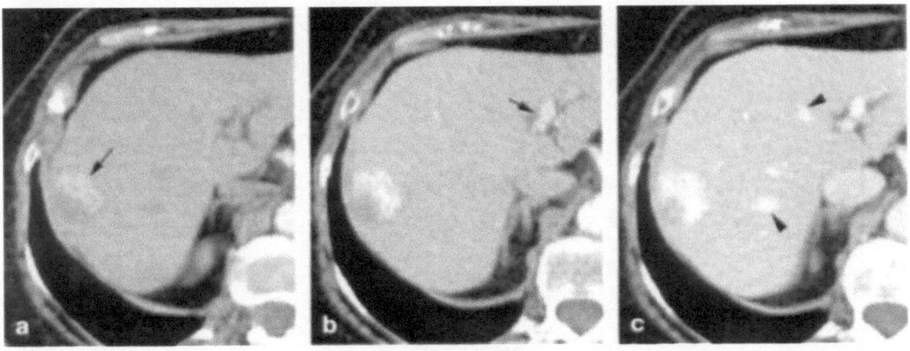

Fig. 2a–c. Triphasic contrast enhancement of hepatic hemangioma with multislice CT (MSCT). **a** Axial MSCT image during the early arterial phase of enhancement demonstrates eccentric enhancement of the hemangioma (*arrow*). **b** Image during late arterial phase of enhancement demonstrates further enhancement of the lesion. **c** Image during hepatic phase demonstrates further contrast fill-in of the lesion. Hepatic veins enhance during this phase (*small arrows*). This phase of enhancement has been described as portal venous phase

through the hepatic arteries. The patient would receive a bolus injection of 100 ml of 60% iodinated contrast material administered at the 3 ml/s rate. Acquisition parameters – specifically, table speed per rotation and scan rotation speed – are set to allow full coverage of the liver in less than 8 s [6]. (Table 1)

With multislice systems, the initial admixed arterial dominant phase used with a single-detector CT system can be subdivided into an early arterial phase and a late arterial phase. Each of these phases has a temporal window of approximately 8–10 s [7]. The phase of maximum hepatic parenchymal enhancement and hepatic venous opacification occurs about 45 s after the beginning of the early arterial phase. An imaging pass performed during this circulatory phase has been entitled the hepatic phase, and corresponds to the portal venous phase of the conventional biphasic protocol used with a single-detector row helical CT (Fig. 2).

Accurate acquisition timing for multipass imaging depends on the assessment of circulation time in individual patients. The arrival time of an intravenously injected contrast material bolus in the aorta can vary between 12 and 25 s. Because the temporal window for the initial early arterial phase is only 8 s, both accurate circulation timing and rapid image acquisition are mandatory if a defined early arterial phase image is to be acquired in individual patients.

Water, as the enteric contrast agent in the upper gastrointestinal tract, allows a three-dimensional volume dataset to be used for multiplanar CT angiography. The patient should receive 8 oz of water 15 min before the study and an additional 8 oz immediately before the bolus injection.

Malignant Hepatic Neoplasm

Murakami et al. [7] demonstrated a distinct benefit of early arterial phase imaging for tumor detection and reduction of false positive diagnosis. Several clinical imaging trials, however, have demonstrated that hypervascular hepatic neoplasms, either primary or metastatic, are best demonstrated during the late

Table 1. A multislice CT (Sensation 16) protocol for liver and pancreas

Protocol	Indications	p.o.	IV rate/vol.	Delay (s)	Area	Collimation (mm)	Reconstruction (thk/inc)[d]	MPR[e]	Remarks
Liver									
Basic liver	Trauma, suspect liver metastasis	C+[a]	3/100	70	A/P[c]	1.5	5/5		For trauma, clamp Foley
Hypervascular liver lesion	Hypervascular mass search (HCC, FNH, hemangioma, etc.)	H_2O[b]	3/100	25 45 70	Liver Liver A/P	1.5 0.75 1.5	5/5 5/5 5/5	3/1.5	
Pancreas									
Basic pancreas	Pancreatitis, suspect pancreatic necrosis	C+	3/100	40	A/P	0.75	5/5	3/1.5	
Pancreatic mass	Suspect pancreatic cancer: jaundice	H_2O	3/100	25 40 70	Pancreas Pancreas A/P	0.75 0.75 1.5	3/1.5 3/1.5 5/5	3/1.5	

[a] *C+* 2.1% dilution of barium sulfate.
[b] *H_2O* water.
[c] *A/P* abdomen to pelvis.
[d] *thk* thickness, inc increment.
[e] *MPR* multiplanar reconstruction

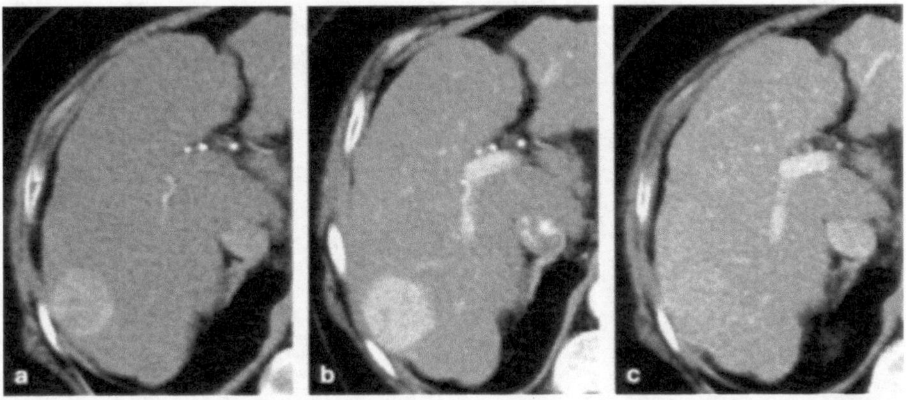

Fig. 3a–c. Triphasic CT images of a hepatocellular carcinoma. **a** Axial CT during early arterial phase demonstrates a hypervascular mass in right lobe of the liver. **b** During late arterial phase, the lesion shows more dense enhancement and increase of the enhancing area comparing with early arterial phase. **c** The image obtained during the hepatic phase, however, demonstrates no visible mass because the temporal window for this lesion has passed

arterial/portal venous inflow phase rather than during the early arterial phase [8, 9]. Early arterial phase imaging is reserved for CT angiography, which would be of benefit for the preoperative detection of vascular anomalies in patients who are candidates for hepatic resection, ablation (radiofrequency and cryoablation), and arterial chemoembolization. CT angiography is useful for therapy planning by defining arterial stenosis and anomalies, particularly aberrant or replaced right and left hepatic arteries arising from the superior mesenteric and left gastric arteries, respectively.

A combined CT angiogram/CT portogram can be obtained adding the late arterial/portal venous inflow phase. This study is valuable for mapping the extrahepatic portal venous system in patients with suspected pancreatic or bile duct malignancy and in patients who are potential transplant recipients. Venous compression, venous stenosis or thrombosis, and portal systemic venous collateral vessels can be displayed. Hypervascular neoplasms are more clearly visible in this phase (Fig. 3).

The third imaging pass, the hepatic phase, corresponds in timing to what is conventionally labeled as the portal venous phase. In this imaging pass, the hepatic parenchyma achieves the maximum level of enhancement. Patients with hypovascular primary or metastatic neoplasms are best identified on this phase as a hypoattenuating tumor [10]. Hypervascular neoplasms, however, often become iso-attenuated and therefore hard to detect (Fig. 4).

Focal Benign Hepatic Tumors and Tumor-Like Lesions

The characteristic imaging features of benign hepatic lesions observed with multislice CT, such as cyst, hemangioma, focal nodular hyperplasia, or hepatic adenoma, are the same as those seen with single-detector CT. CT angiography with volume rendering shows the anomalous feeding artery and draining veins

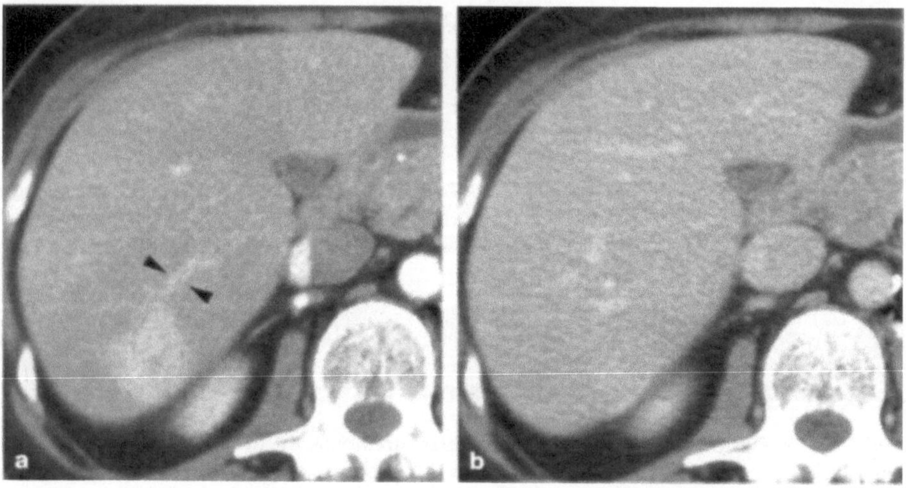

Fig. 4a,b. Focal nodular hyperplasia of the liver. **a** Axial CT scan taken on late arterial phase demonstrates an enhancing mass on right lobe of the liver. Note the early enhancement of draining hepatic vein from the lesion (*arrows*). **b** During hepatic phase, the lesion is not detectable. All the hepatic vessels are now enhanced

characteristic of focal nodular hyperplasia. These features may be helpful in distinguishing focal nodular hyperplasia from other lesions [11].

Hepatic perfusion anomalies occur in patients with focal interruptions to the liver blood supply and venous drainage and in patients with vascular hepatic neoplasms, both before and after ablative therapy. Perfusion anomalies are most pronounced during arterial phase imaging. Hypervascular tumors often demonstrate similar findings (Fig. 5). In patients with vascular hepatic neoplasms, the

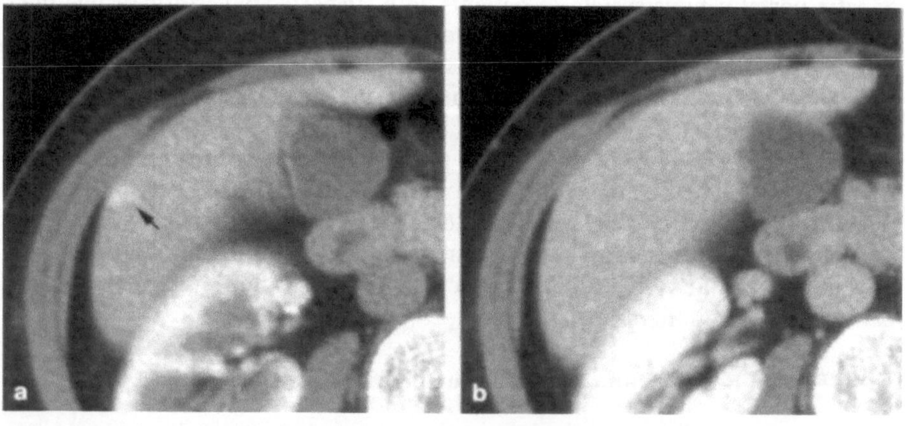

Fig. 5a,b. Focal nodular hyperplasia mimicking hepatic perfusion abnormality. **a** Axial CT scan during early arterial phase demonstrates a focal nodular hyperplasia in right lobe of the liver (*arrow*). **b** Image during hepatic phase, however, shows no visible mass. Differential diagnosis should include hypervascular mass and hepatic perfusion abnormality for this lesion surrounding normal hepatic parenchyma may also be relatively hyper-enhanced due to a »sump« effect, in that the liver tumor produces increased hepatic arterial inflow in a segmental or lobar distribution [12]. Arterial perfusion anomalies should be distinguished from hepatocellular carcinoma.

Diffuse Liver Disease

The most common diffuse liver diseases identified in clinical practice include fatty change, cirrhosis, hemosiderosis, sarcoidosis, and Budd-Chiari syndrome (Fig. 6). The utility of MSCT is most apparent in the evaluation of patients with underlying hepatic cirrhosis who are at risk for hepatocellular carcinoma. The appropriate CT technique is a combination of late arterial/portal venous inflow phase and hepatic phase imaging. This approach maximizes the detection of hepatocellular carcinoma, a lesion that occurs with 20% prevalence in patients with chronic cirrhosis [7, 12]. Lesions that simulate hepatocellular carcinoma include coincidental hemangiomas, focal nodular hyperplasia, adenomas, and localized vascularized fibrous scars.

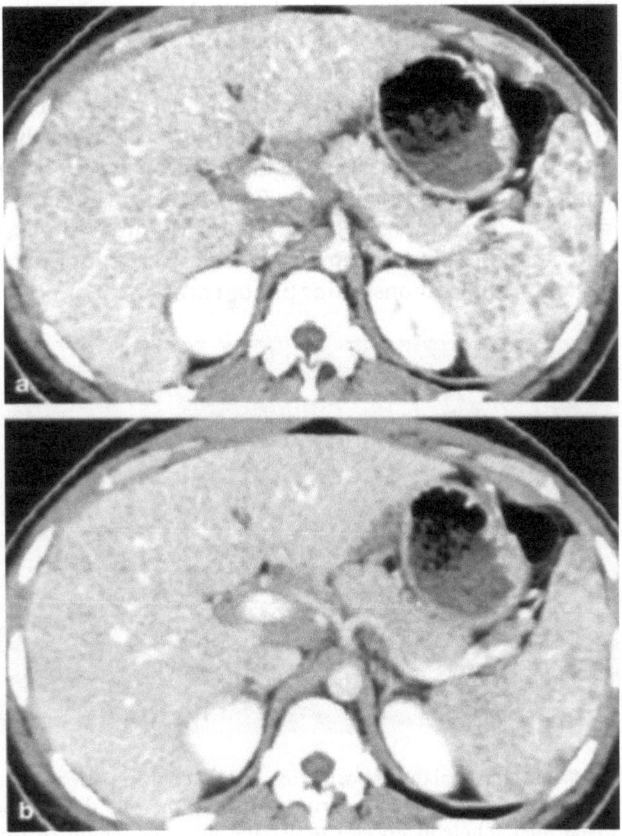

Fig. 6a,b. Multislice CT of a patient with sarcoidosis using **a** 3-mm and **b** 5-mm slice thickness. Multislice CT demonstrates numerous tiny low attenuation nodules in liver and spleen. Note the improved image resolution with thin slice thickenss

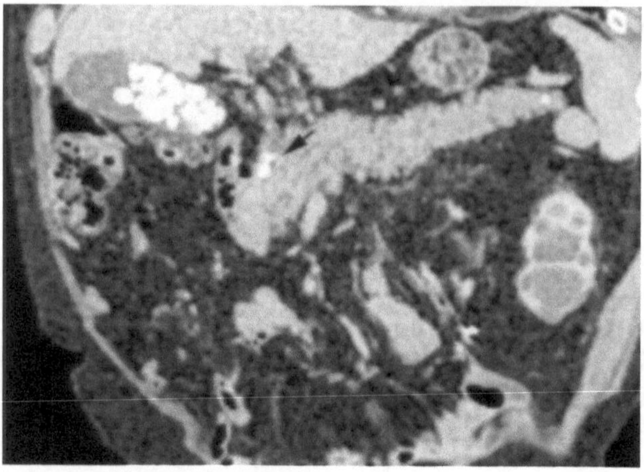

Fig. 7. Coronal curved planar reconstruction along the bile duct. Coronal curved planar reconstruction of MSCT shows multiple stones in gallbladder and distal common bile duct (*arrow*)

Biliary Disease

Use of thin-section hepatic CT techniques with MSCT results in better demonstration of the intrahepatic and extrahepatic biliary tree than can be achieved with the thicker slices used in single-slice CT. Thin-section imaging performed before the administration of contrast material (precontrast) may be useful in detecting partly calcified ductal stones and assessing the cause of bile duct obstruction [13, 14] (Fig. 7). Postcontrast imaging is useful in defining the extent of biliary tract obstruction and, in cases of malignant duct obstruction, the location of lymphadenopathy and hepatic metastases. Enhanced thin-section late arterial/portal venous phase or hepatic phase CT may provide three-dimensional CT cholangiography and curved planar reformation, which is useful for defining the site of biliary obstruction and demonstrating tumor encasement of periductal vessels [15] (Fig. 8).

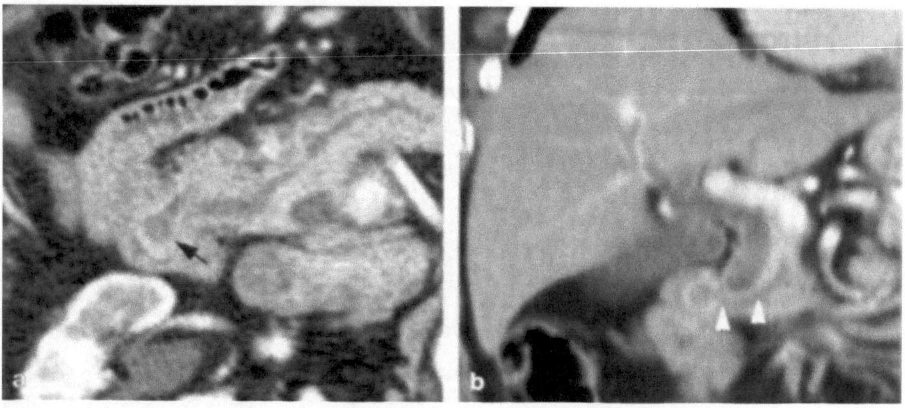

Fig. 8a,b. Curved planar reformation of bile duct in patient with choledochocele. **a** Axial and **b** coronal curved planar reformation along the bile duct demonstrates cystic dilatation of distal duct (choledochocele) projecting into duodenum (*arrow*). Note the pancreatic duct joining into the choledochocele (*arrowheads*)

MSCT in the Pancreas

Pancreatic cancer remains the fourth leading cause of cancer-related death. Surgery is the only option for cure. Accurate detection and staging of pancreatic adenocarcinoma are major challenges in pancreatic imaging [16]. MSCT and advanced postprocessing techniques can provide solutions for difficult problems in diagnosing and staging disease, and can aid radiologists in communicating findings to surgeons and oncologists. Multiplanar reformats provide additional information on the involvement of the pancreatic duct, common bile duct, and peripancreatic vessels. Maximum intensity projection (MIP) images and volume rendered images can aid in identification of important vascular variants. MIP images can show the relationship of tumor to the pancreatic duct or biliary tree. Curved reformatted images can show the relationship of tumor to the pancreatic duct or vascular structures [17, 18] (Fig. 9).

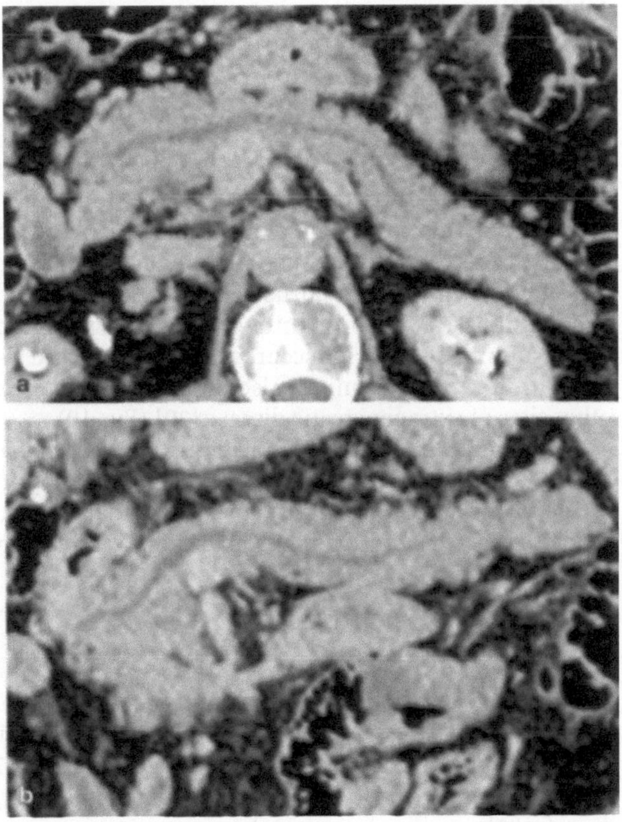

Fig. 9a,b. Curved multiplanar reformation images along the pancreatic duct. **a** Axial and **b** coronal curved planar image of the pancreatic duct

Scan Techniques

A triple phasic imaging technique using MSCT includes an early arterial phase, pancreatic phase [19] (corresponding in timing to the late arterial/portal venous inflow phase of the liver), and subsequent hepatic phase. Thin-section technique (1.5 mm in the early arterial phase and pancreatic phase) and rapid coverage are used in conjunction with rapid intravenous bolus injection of the standard 42-g iodine load delivered at 3–5 ml/s. The early arterial phase is used in patients with suspected pancreatic carcinoma who are potential candidates for surgery, and it can be used to produce a CT angiogram for a vascular road map. Focal tumor, focal pancreatitis, and pseudocyst are best delineated in the pancreatic phase. In addition, this phase provides data for a reformatted CT angioportogram. As with triple phasic hepatic CT, water is used as the enteric contrast material for triple phasic pancreatic CT in patients with suspected pancreatic carcinoma in order to provide a suitable imaging template for CT arteriography and venography (see Table 1).

Pancreatic Adenocarcinoma

Pancreatic adenocarcinoma presents a hypoattenuating mass associated with pancreatic ductal dilatation proximal to the tumor mass. An important characteristic for determining potential resectability is perivascular tumor invasion, particularly in relation to the celiac and mesenteric arteries, the splenic and superior mesenteric veins, and the portal vein confluence. With the use of thin collimation and multiphase acquisition through the whole pancreas, MSCT provides a detailed vascular mapping with accuracy that may exceed that of classic angiography. Use of thin-section technique also improves the detection of metastasis as well as other sites of extrapancreatic disease [20] (Fig. 10).

Multiplanar reformations, including curved planar reformations, optimize display of pancreatic tumors and local metastases by providing a high-resolution image of the whole organ in planes other than the axial plane, which help demonstrate peripancreatic tumor extension, vascular invasion, and lymphadenopathy [18, 21].

Other Tumors

In patients with localized cystic neoplasms, the relationship of the neoplasm to the surrounding vessels and adjacent organs is well displayed [22]. The major advantage of thin-section multislice CT technique (1.25 or 2.5 mm) is that the thinner slices permit better visualization of the duct, aiding detection of the extent of the tumor. Intraductal mucinous tumors may also be found as small cystic pancreatic lesions with ductal dilatation. Most small side-branch ductectatic tumors are benign, but the appearance on CT does not allow differentiation of benign from malignant disease [23]. Focal chronic pancreatitis with associated pseudocysts should be considered as the most common and important differential diagnosis.

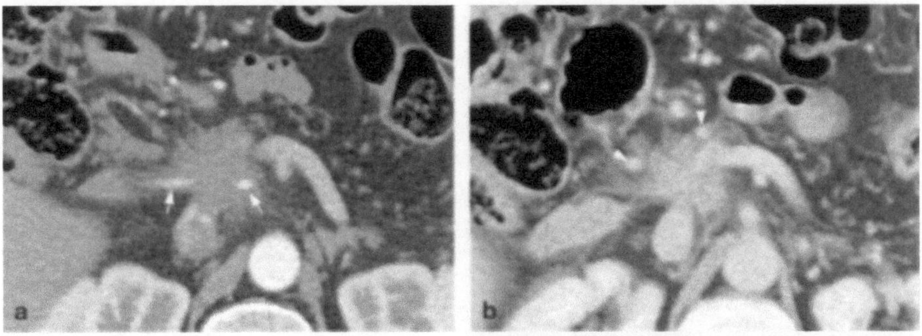

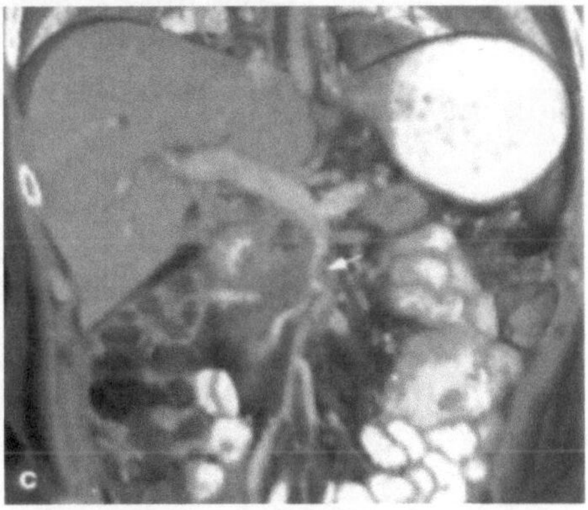

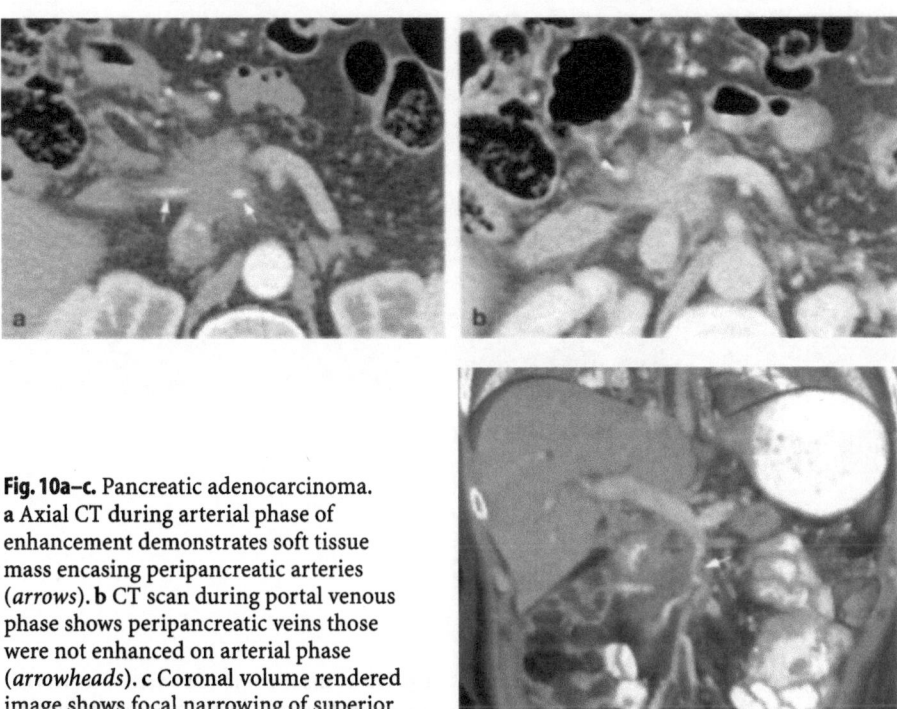

Fig. 10a–c. Pancreatic adenocarcinoma. **a** Axial CT during arterial phase of enhancement demonstrates soft tissue mass encasing peripancreatic arteries (*arrows*). **b** CT scan during portal venous phase shows peripancreatic veins those were not enhanced on arterial phase (*arrowheads*). **c** Coronal volume rendered image shows focal narrowing of superior mesenteric vein by tumor encasement (*arrow*)

Islet cell tumors are often found as focal hypervascular pancreatic lesions, either functional or nonfunctional. Patients with suspected islet cell tumors are evaluated by using a triple pass pancreatic/hepatic technique [24] (Fig. 11). A major advantage of multiphasic abdominal imaging in patients with islet cell tumor is detection and localization of vascular hepatic metastases. As with other vascular hepatic lesions, the optimal phase for detecting these hepatic metastases is the late arterial/portal venous inflow phase. When resection is being considered, triple phasic MSCT is important in the preoperative planning.

Pancreatitis

Management of patients with acute pancreatitis is based on the early assessment of severity of disease. Initial staging is established on clinical and laboratory grounds and on the findings of contrast-enhanced CT imaging. Individual clinical parameters and laboratory indices, although sometimes helpful, are not sufficiently accurate to reliably assess the severity of an acute attack. Numerical grading systems (Ranson's, Apache II) are available with sensitivities of about 70%, and are commonly used today as indicators of systemic failure and predictors of disease severity.

CT staging of pancreatitis is assessed according to the degree of pancreatic enlargement, pancreatic necrosis, the number and size of pancreatic pseu-

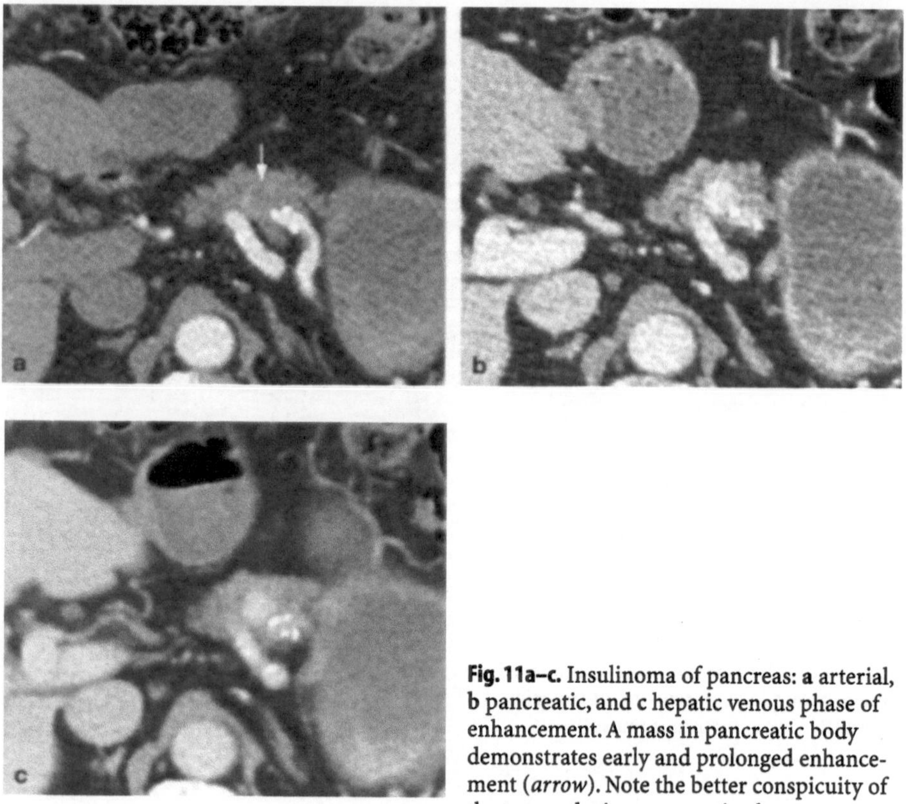

Fig. 11a–c. Insulinoma of pancreas: **a** arterial, **b** pancreatic, and **c** hepatic venous phase of enhancement. A mass in pancreatic body demonstrates early and prolonged enhancement (*arrow*). Note the better conspicuity of the tumor during pancreatic phase

docysts, peripancreatic effusion [25]. The CT severity index has proved to be a reliable indicator of disease severity, having shown an excellent correlation with the risk of death and the development of local complications. Associated complications include peripancreatic vascular thrombosis and gastrointestinal fistulization [26]. In patients with acute pancreatitis, a double pass helical imaging technique that includes pancreatic and hepatic phase acquisitions is potentially beneficial for outlining focal areas of pancreatic necrosis. In patients with recurrent pancreatitis or chronic pancreatitis, MSCT can demonstrate the underlying causes, which include ductal anomalies, ampullary tumors, and intraductal/biliary calculi (Figs. 8, 12).

Conclusions

MSCT offers exciting new tools in abdominal imaging. MSCT has had a tremendous impact on imaging of the abdomen, and has ensured that CT will remain the main imaging tool in abdominal radiology. Radiologists should be well versed in imaging technology, vascular physiology, and contrast material

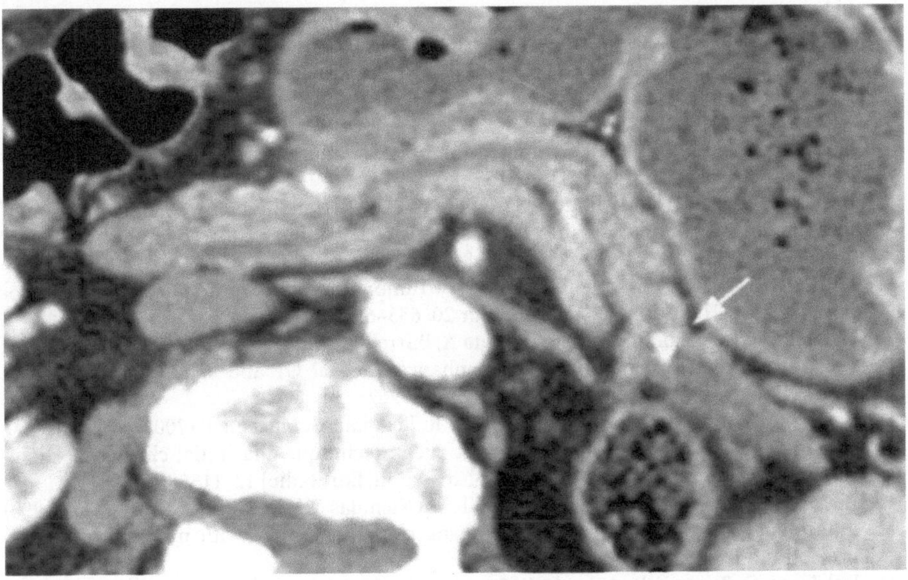

Fig. 12. Focal chronic pancreatitis. Axial curved planar reformation along the pancreatic duct shows an intraductal calcification (*arrow*) and distal low-density pancreatic parenchyma suggesting chronic pancreatitis

pharmacokinetics. To be successful, they must also understand evolving clinical needs like tumor detection and staging in abdominal visceral imaging. Radiologists with this background will be able to apply, MSCT technology effectively in the evaluation of suspected hepatic and pancreatic pathologic conditions. State-of-the-art MSCT will continue to have new applications in liver and pancreas imaging.

References

1. Ros PR, Ji H (2002) Special focus session: multisection (multidetector) CT: applications in the abdomen. Radiographics 22: 697–700
2. Rydberg J, Buckwalter KA, Caldemeyer KS et al (2000) MSCT: scanning techniques and clinical applications. Radiographics 20: 1787–1806
3. Foley WD (2002) Special focus session: multidetector CT: abdominal visceral imaging. Radiographics 22: 701–719
4. Baker SR (2003) Musings at the beginning of the hyper-CT era. Abdom Imaging 28: 110–114
5. Tamm EP, Thompson S, Venable SL, McEnery K (2002) Impact of multislice CT on PACS resources. J Digit Imaging 15 Suppl 1: 96–101
6. Ji H, McTavish JD, Mortele KJ, Wiesner W, Ros PR (2001) Hepatic imaging with multidetector CT. Radiographics 21 Spec no: S71–80
7. Murakami T, Kim T, Takamura M et al. (2001) Hypervascular hepatocellular carcinoma: detection with double arterial phase multi-detector row helical CT. Radiology 218: 763–767

8. Foley WD, Mallisee TA, Hohenwalter MD, Wilson CR, Quiroz FA, Taylor AJ (2000) Multiphase hepatic CT with a multirow detector CT scanner. AJR Am J Roentgenol 175: 679–685
9. Laghi A, Iannaccone R, Rossi P et al. (2003) Hepatocellular carcinoma: detection with triple-phase multi-detector row helical CT in patients with chronic hepatitis. Radiology 226: 543–549
10. Sica GT, Ji H, Ros PR (2002) Computed tomography and magnetic resonance imaging of hepatic metastases. Clin Liver Dis 6: 165–179
11. Brancatelli G, Federle MP, Katyal S, Kapoor V (2002) Hemodynamic characterization of focal nodular hyperplasia using three-dimensional volume-rendered multidetector CT angiography. AJR Am J Roentgenol 179: 81–85
12. Lin JP, Lu DS (1996) Early enhancement of tumor thrombus in the portal vein on two-phase helical CT. J Comput Assist Tomogr 20: 653–655
13. Neitlich JD, Topazian M, Smith RC, Gupta A, Burrell MI, Rosenfield AT (1997) Detection of choledocholithiasis: comparison of unenhanced helical CT and endoscopic retrograde cholangiopancreatography. Radiology 203: 753–757
14. Zandrino F, Benzi L, Ferretti ML, Ferrando R, Reggiani G, Musante F (2002) Multislice CT cholangiography without biliary contrast agent: technique and initial clinical results in the assessment of patients with biliary obstruction. Eur Radiol 12: 1155–1161
15. Raptopoulos V, Prassopoulos P, Chuttani R, McNicholas MM, McKee JD, Kressel HY (1998) Multiplanar CT pancreatography and distal cholangiography with minimum intensity projections. Radiology 207: 317–324
16. Del Frate C, Zanardi R, Mortele K, Ros PR (2002) Advances in imaging for pancreatic disease. Curr Gastroenterol Rep 4: 140–148
17. Tamm E, Charnsangavej C, Szklaruk J (2001) Advanced 3-D imaging for the evaluation of pancreatic cancer with multidetector CT. Int J Gastrointest Cancer 30: 65–71
18. Nino-Murcia M, Jeffrey RB Jr, Beaulieu CF, Li KC, Rubin GD (2001) Multidetector CT of the pancreas and bile duct system: value of curved planar reformations. AJR Am J Roentgenol 176: 689–693
19. Lu DSK, Vedantham S, Krasny RM, Kadell B, Berger WL, Reber HA (1996) Two-phase helical CT for pancreatic tumors: pancreatic versus hepatic phase enhancement of tumor, pancreas, and vascular structures. Radiology 199: 697–701
20. Fishman EK, Horton KM (2001) Imaging pancreatic cancer: the role of multidetector CT with three-dimensional CT angiography. Pancreatology 1: 610–624
Shioyama Y, Kimura M, Horihata K et al. (2001) Peripancreatic arteries in thin-section multislice helical CT. Abdom Imaging 26: 234–242
21. Procacci C, Megibow AJ, Carbognin G et al. (1999) Intraductal papillary mucinous tumor of the pancreas: a pictorial essay. RadioGraphics 19: 1447–1463
Sugiyama N, Atomi Y (1998) Intraductal papillary mucinous tumors of the pancreas: imaging studies and treatment strategies. Ann Surg 228: 685–691
22. VanHoe L, Gryspeerdt S, Marchal G, Baert AL, Mertens L (1995) Helical CT for the preoperative localization of islet cell tumors of the pancreas: value of arterial and parenchymal phase images. AJR Am J Roentgenol 165: 1437–1439
23. Paulson EK, Vitellas KM, Keogan MT, Low VH, Nelson RC (1999) Acute pancreatitis complicated by gland necrosis: spectrum of findings on contrast-enhanced CT. AJR Am J Roentgenol 172: 609–613
24. Balthazar EJ (2002) Staging of acute pancreatitis. Radiol Clin North Am 40: 1199–1209

7 3-D Imaging of the Pancreas with the Siemens Volume Zoom CT Scanner

A. J. Megibow

Introduction

Fundamental observations concerning the appearance and gross pathologic alterations of the pancreas were described with the 27–30 s per slice scanners prevalent in the late 1970s and early 1980s. With the advent of 2–10 s per slice scanners, batch acquisitions (dynamic scanning) utilizing slice collimation between 4–5 mm improved image quality allowing the development of optimized protocols [1]. With the introduction of spiral/helical CT in the late 1980s, much emphasis was placed on the increasing ability to optimize the timing of the imaging sequence in order to evaluate organ pathology during the most clinically relevant phase of contrast enhancement. Further, continuous acquisitions allowed the initial exploration of 3-D applications for image analysis and display [2]. Widespread acceptance of 3-D was limited by slice-broadening effects which were more pronounced with thinner slices at higher pitch [3, 4]. For example, the effective slice width of a 3 mm slice collimation at a table feed of 6 mm/s (pitch 2), yielded z-axis resolution equivalent to a 3.9-mm slice (almost 30% increase in the anticipated slice width).

Multidetector row CT acquires near isotropic voxels which are favorable for 3-D imaging [5–7]. This allows for detailed evaluation of the pancreas, peripancreatic tissues, peripancreatic vessels, duct and surrounding bowel, by both conventional and interactive 3-D reading [8, 9].

Protocol Considerations

The goal of pancreatic imaging is to detect intraparenchymal lesions, assess their relation to the pancreatic ducts and surrounding vessels, and provide a global survey of the surrounding structures. In order to achieve these goals, protocol elements regarding the timing of the acquisition, the slice width, the slice output, and proper contrast administration, must all be carefully considered. Because the pancreatic parenchymal enhancement is based on its arterial supply, and peak hepatic enhancement is based on portal venous supply, the two organs cannot be simultaneously interrogated; therefore, dual-phase acquisitions are recommended [10, 11]. The significant increase in acquisition speed must be factored into protocol decisions because the most common source of error is beginning the scan too early. McNulty and associates have shown that an acquisition beginning

Table 1. Multidetector row CT of pancreas

Indications	Pancreatic mass, jaundice, epigastric pain, weight loss, acute or chronic pancreatitis
Acquisition	Dual phase protocol (pancreatic and portal)
Phase 1	4 x 1 mm or 16 x 0.75 mm from dome of liver to top l–4
Phase 2	4 x 2.5 mm or 16 x 1.5 mm from liver dome to pubic symphysis
Reconstructions	
Phase 1	3-D evaluation: All images recon at 1.25 mm and sent to Leonardo for InSpace rendering Film/PACS Evaluation: All images reconstructed at 3 mm thickness with 2 mm overlap B40 kernel Abdominal windows
Phase 2	Film PACS evaluation only: All images acquired in phase 2 (portal phase) reconstructed at 5 mm and sent to PACS
Oral contrast	Three part water:1part methylcellulose, total 900 ml. (Final cup given *on table immediately before scan*)
IV contrast	4 ml/s (minimal) total 150 cc LOCM
Scan delay	4-slice: 40 s pancreatic/70 s portal 16-slice: 50 s pancreatic/80–90 s portal
KvP	120
MAs	180
Gantry rotation	0.5

approximately 40 s following the initiation of a contrast bolus will provide maximal parenchymal enhancement and more than adequate enhancement of peripancreatic vessels. This can be followed by a second acquisition at 70–80 s designed to survey the liver during peak hepatic parenchymal enhancement as well as the remainder of the abdomen [12]. With 16-detector row scanners, the initiation time may need to be even later (see Table 1).

In single-slice scanning, the collimator width directly determines the slice width. However, with multidetector row CT, the term slice width now has two meanings; the acquisition collimator (or collimator width – similar to single-slice CT) and display slice width (created independently from the collimation chosen). With single-slice pancreatic a 3 mm collimator width is most frequently utilized, yielding reconstructed slices that have a **z**-axis resolution of or close to 3 mm, depending on the pitch. With multidetector row CT, the collimator width chosen for the protocol (acquisition thickness) may or may not be identical to the width of the reconstructed slices displayed as diagnostic images on film or PACS. We choose either a 4 x 1 mm or 16 x 1.5 mm collimator (detector configuration). These acquired slices may be reconstructed with overlap to further reduce slice broadening at higher pitch. The reconstruction slice thickness is the term reserved for the displayed slices. We »sandwich« our 1-mm slices together to make 3-mm slices which are filmed and archived similar to standard CT examinations. Therefore we do not film or directly evaluate our 1–1.25 mm slices. These are utilized in an entirely different fashion.

We appreciate that the increasing numbers of slices by current 4, 8,10, and 16 detector row scanners are a challenge to workflow and image management across networks and/or film. As volume rendering (or newer) 3-D reconstruction and reading techniques become available, we anticipate that traditional slice-by-slice viewing will become less and less prevalent. Using 3-D protocols, one can perform a single reconstruction, send the dataset to the workstation, and view the image data not only in the axial plane, but in virtually any plane imaginable. Selected images can be archived and preserved, and the entire dataset can be archived as a single data block. This image set can be reproduced for future comparison to assess treatment response. In the future, it can be anticipated that successful radiologists will perform all reading in a PACS environment into which is embedded functionality which can facilitate 3-D analysis. Image quality from 3-D, even today, is remarkably good and should continue to improve. Presently, we perform 3-D analysis only in the pancreatic phase of the protocol. For detection of liver lesions and a survey of the upper abdomen where **z**-axis coverage requirement is greater, we choose a wider collimation. Therefore in the second phase, we choose an acquisition collimation of 2.5 and create 5-mm-thick images. We do not send this phase of the study for 3-D processing, and we rely on standard reconstruction algorithms to produce classical CT images.

Two advantages of multidetector row CT become evident during this second phase. First, the acquisition speed through the upper abdomen assures images obtained during peak hepatic enhancement. Second, the speed can be realized with significant improvement in individual slice profiles minimizing volume averaging effects. The same coverage time with single-slice technology is only possible by using variable pitch acquisitions with resultant slice broadening.

We utilize water as an oral contrast agent to identify the stomach and duodenum [13]. Because water is rapidly absorbed, the patient must be asked to drink at least one cup (7 oz) immediately prior to the initiation of scanning. We emphasize that the water is to be given, after the IV site has been secured, after the localizing image has been obtained, and after the injector has been armed. We administer 0.1 mg of IV Glucagon between completion of the water and initiation of the injection. Buscopan, popular in Europe as an antispasmolytic, is not available in the United States; were it available, we would routinely employ it.

Pancreatic Anatomy with Multidetector row CT

The 3-D capabilities of multidetector row CT allow for more detailed, simultaneous evaluation of both the pancreas and surrounding vessels [14].

Using multidetector row CT, the improved **z**-axis resolution can be exploited by applying a variety of 3-D reconstructions such as maximum intensity projection (MIP), volume rendering (VRT), and minimum intensity projections (MinMIP) to the datasets. The advantages and disadvantages of each technique

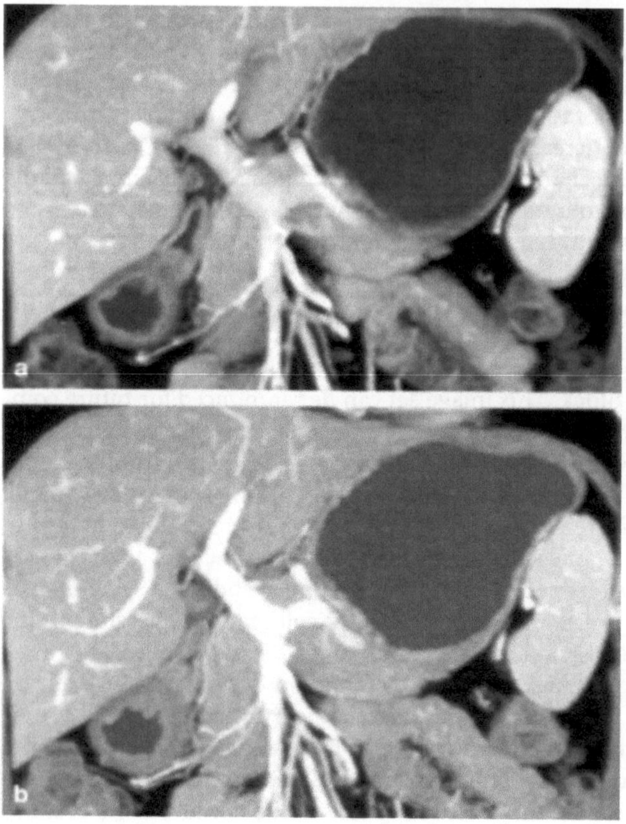

Fig. 1a,b. Narrowing the clip planes in the same patient as Fig. 1 allows visualization of abdominal anatomy in any plane and with any rendering technique. **a** 6-mm slab presented in VRT technique on Leonardo using InSpace rendering. The relationship of the portal vein, pancreas and liver are demonstrated. **b** The rendering was changed to maximum intensity projection (MIP), which allows greater visualization of hepatic vessels. The MIP rendering is useful in CT angiography surrounding the pancreas and elsewhere in the abdomen. Branches of the SMV are clearly visualized.

are familiar. In terms of routine arterial visualization, multislice CT displays the anterior and posterior pancreaticoduodenal arcades and the dorsal pancreatic artery [15, 16]. The CT anatomy of the main superior mesenteric vein (SMV), first described using single-slice technology [17], is more reliably depicted. The gastrocolic trunk, right gastroepiploic vein, and first jejunal vein branch are all reliably visualized (Fig. 1) [18, 19].

The ability to acquire thin sections and inherent improvements in z-axis resolution also results in optimized depictions of the pancreatic and bile ducts. Investigators have termed this CT cholangiopancreatography or CTCP. Visualization of duct structures is enhanced by utilizing a MinMIP projection. MinMIP projects the darkest pixel along the line of site (the exact opposite of MIP used in CT angiography). Most investigators have utilized a curved multiplanar reformating technique to display the pancreatic dust throughout its entire length [9, 20]. Our approach has been to investigate the use of 3-D volume rendering in MinMIP, which allows differentiation of masses arising from the duct or adjacent to the duct.

Pancreatic Neoplasms

Adenocarcinoma

Improved CT angiographic anatomy has implications in the evaluation of resectability of pancreatic and periampullary adenocarcinoma. The ability to perform dual-phase acquisitions timed more precisely within the period of maximal pancreatic and hepatic parenchymal enhancement will hopefully increase the level of confidence in the recognition of smaller lesions [21]. Several investigators have shown improved survival in lesions which measure less than 2 cm. Furthermore, newer surgical techniques, such as the pylorus-sparing Whipple resection, have resulted in a more aggressive approach to marginally nonresectable masses. It is possible, although not rigorously proven, that aggressive resection of periampullary and pancreatic lesions may be stimulated by the more precise road map of peripancreatic arterial and venous anatomy which is a byproduct of multidetector row CT acquisitions [16].

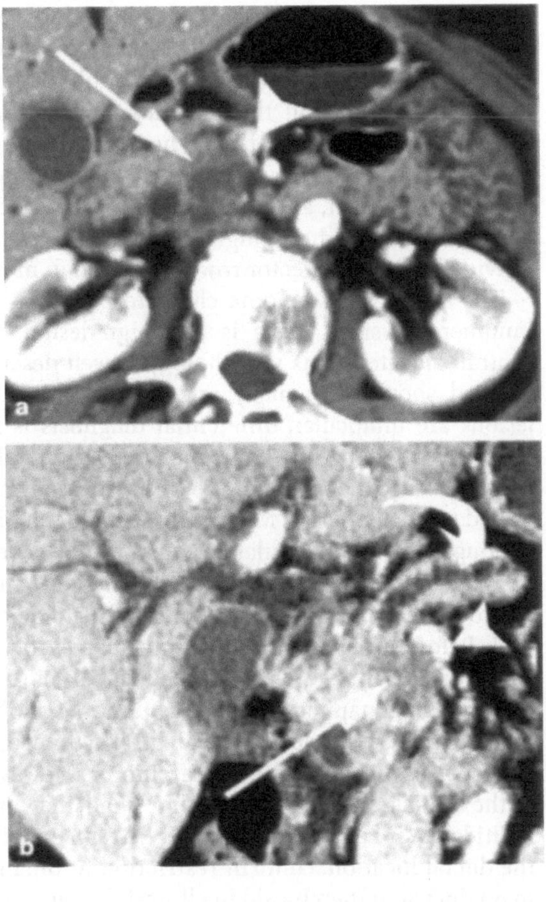

Fig. 2a,b. Two views from a different patient than in Figs. 1 and 3. The patient has an adenocarcinoma in the pancreatic head (*arrow*). Although small, it deforms the superior mesenteric vein (*arrowhead*) rendering it unresectable. **a** Created from a 4 x 1 mm acquisition using InSpace on a Leonardo workstation. **b** Created using a minimum intensity projection (MinMIP) option available within InSpace, which optimizes visualization of duct structures. Note the dilated main pancreatic duct (*curved arrow*) which ends abruptly at the tumor (*straight arrow*). Dilated intrahepatic ducts can be recognized in the liver. All of these representations of the data are created from a single patient acquisition using the protocol described in the text

Multiple studies using single-slice technology have shown that continuous-motion CT datasets can accurately detect major peripancreatic arterial encasement by extrapancreatic neoplasm. Most investigators have concluded that the degree of circumferential involvement of the vessel correlates with surgical verification of nonresectability, a threshold value of 50% circumferential contact being most sensitive and specific for encasement (Fig. 2) [22–24]. For larger masses, multidetector row CT offers little advantage over well performed single slice helical/spiral CT scanning.

The accuracy of helical computed tomography (CT) and CT angiography with three-dimensional reconstruction in predicting resectability has been extensively studied [10, 24–26]. The benefit to patient survival afforded by multidetector row CT will result from the (hopefully) increasing reliable detection rates of tumors in the range of 1 cm.

Cystic Pancreatic Neoplasms

These tumors are becoming increasingly recognized as more people undergo imaging for a greater variety of clinical indications. Detection of these lesions raises a significant management issue because it is unclear in an individual case if the lesion is benign or malignant. Multidetector row CT can add information by reliably displaying the morphologic features which aid in discriminating benign or malignant forms. These morphological changes include size and number of cysts, appearance of the wall of the cyst, origin from either the parenchyma or the duct, and location within the duct system. Each of these features has been described on single-slice CT; however, the improved **z**-axis resolution provided by multidetector row CT can aid in more precise characterization.

The serous cystadenoma characterized by a dense fibrous stroma delimiting innumerable small cysts is a benign lesion. When calcification occurs it is centrally located. This morphology is well described in single-slice helical spiral CT and should be equally appreciated on multidetector row scanning. When lesions are unilocular, differential diagnosis is impossible. Features which help predict malignant histology include peripheral calcification and nodular soft tissue density thickening of the cyst wall. Many cystic lesions will present as thin-walled unilocular cysts. Most of these unilocular cystic masses will contain mucin, although serous unilocular lesions have also been described. Regardless of the fluid content, these lesions are problematic when detected because imaging alone cannot reliably predict the presence of histologic changes of epithelial carcinoma [27]. Before any patient with unilocular cystic pancreatic neoplasm undergoes resection, it is imperative that the diagnosis of pancreatic pseudocyst be excluded.

Intraductal papillary mucinous tumors (IPMT) are also troubling in that they may contain a full spectrum of histologic change within the epithelium from hyperplasia through invasive carcinoma. However, these lesions, when confined to the branch ducts and remaining small, may have a benign clinical course [28]. Multidetector row CT scanning is extremely useful in these patients to establish the ductal location, confirm restriction to the branch duct or extension into the main duct, and thereby aid in clinical decision-making.

Pancreatitis

Acute Pancreatitis

The role of CT scanning in pancreatitis is well established [29, 30]. The Balthazar–Ranson CT severity index is used to describe both increasing severity of peripancreatic change but also, with the use of IV iodinated contrast, accurate prediction of the presence and degrees of necrosis in patients with acute pancreatitis [31, 32]. Multidetector row CT expands diagnostic utility by facilitating 3-D image display. The ability to display complex fluid collections in multiple planes, and particularly to aid a surgeon or interventional radiologist in planning debridement or drainage, is the major value added by the technology.

Chronic Pancreatitis

CT is considered the best initial noninvasive imaging test in patients suspected of chronic pancreatitis [33]. Certainly, evaluation of complications such as pseudocyst is well established. Because the diagnosis and classification of

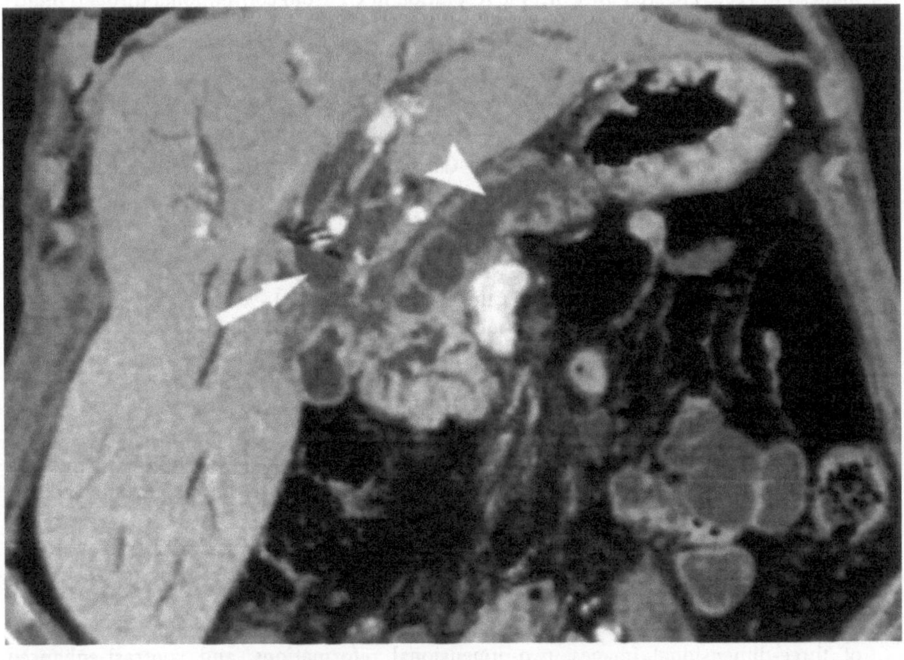

Fig. 3. CT cholangiopancreatographic (CTCP) image created on InSpace using a MinMIP rendering of a 4 x 1 mm acquisition through the pancreas. Both the CBD (*arrow*) and the pancreatic ducts (*arrowhead*) are dilated. At surgery, there was marked chronic pancreatitis. A 1 cm focus of adenocarcinoma was found within the substance of the gland. The infiltrating mass at the porta hepatis was benign fibrosis.

patients with chronic pancreatitis is so dependent on duct morphology and pattern of main versus branch duct dilatation, MR has become increasingly utilized. Using thin-slice multidetector row CT we have been able to visualize the pancreatic duct in more cases (Fig. 3). In isolated cases, we have been able to display the anatomic changes of entities such as pancreas divisum which may be causative in attacks of recurrent acute pancreatitis. Because MR is insensitive to calcification, as CTCP grows, CT will reestablish its role in evaluation of chronic pancreatitis.

References

1. Megibow AJ, Zhou XH, Rotterdam H et al. (1995) Pancreatic adenocarcinoma: CT versus MR imaging in the evaluation of resectability-report of the Radiology Diagnostic Oncology Group. Radiology 195(2):327–32
2. Fishman EK, Wyatt SH, Ney DR, Kuhlman JE, Siegelman SS (1992) Spiral CT of the pancreas with multiplanar display. AJR Am J Roentgenol 159(6):1209–15
3. Kalender WA (1994) Technical foundations of spiral CT. Semin Ultrasound CT MR 15(2):81–9
4. Polacin A, Kalender WA, Brink J, Vannier MA (1994) Measurement of slice sensitivity profiles in spiral CT. Med Phys 21(1):133–40
5. Mahesh M (2002) Search for isotropic resolution in CT from conventional through multiple-row detector. Radiographics 22(4):949–62
6. Fuchs T, Krause J, Schaller S, Flohr T, Kalender WA (2000) Spiral interpolation algorithms for multislice spiral CT, part II. Measurement and evaluation of slice sensitivity profiles and noise at a clinical multislice system. IEEE Trans Med Imaging 19(9):835–47
7. Schaller S, Flohr T, Klingenbeck K, Krause J, Fuchs T, Kalender WA (2000) Spiral interpolation algorithm for multislice spiral CT, part I. Theory. IEEE Trans Med Imaging 19(9):822–34
8. Tazawa S, Gotoh Y, Takahashi S, Zuguchi M, Maruoka S (2001) Cine viewing of abdominal CT. Comput Methods Programs Biomed 66(1):105–10
9. Nino-Murcia M, Jeffrey RB Jr. (2002) Multidetector-row CT and volumetric imaging of pancreatic neoplasms. Gastroenterol Clin North Am 31(3):881–96
10. Diehl SJ, Lehmann KJ, Sadick M, Lachmann R, Georgi M (1998) Pancreatic cancer: value of dual-phase helical CT in assessing resectability. Radiology 206(2):373–8
11. Nino-Murcia M, Olcott EW, Jeffrey RB Jr. (1998) Dual-phase helical CT of locally invasive pancreatic adenocarcinoma. J Comput Assist Tomogr 22(2):282–7
12. McNulty NJ, Francis IR, Platt JF, Cohan RH, Korobkin M, Gebremariam A (2001) Multidetector row helical CT of the pancreas: effect of contrast-enhanced multiphasic imaging on enhancement of the pancreas, peripancreatic vasculature, and pancreatic adenocarcinoma. Radiology 220(1):97–102
13. Winter TC, Ager JD, Nghiem HV, Hill RS, Harrison SD, Freeny PC (1996) Upper gastrointestinal tract and abdomen: water as an orally administered contrast agent for helical CT. Radiology 201(2):365–70
14. Takeshita K, Furui S, Takada K (2002) Multidetector row helical CT of the pancreas: value of three-dimensional images, two-dimensional reformations, and contrast-enhanced multiphasic imaging. J Hepatobiliary Pancreat Surg 9(5):576–82
15. Shioyama Y, Kimura M, Horihata K et al. (2001) Peripancreatic arteries in thin-section multislice helical CT. Abdom Imaging 26(3):234–42
16. Fishman EK, Horton KM, Urban BA (2000) Multidetector CT angiography in the evaluation of pancreatic carcinoma: preliminary observations. J Comput Assist Tomogr 24(6):849–53

17. Graf O, Boland GW, Kaufman JA, Warshaw AL, Fernandez del Castillo C, Mueller PR (1997) Anatomic variants of mesenteric veins: depiction with helical CT venography. AJR Am J Roentgenol 168(5):1209–13
18. Yamada Y, Mori H, Kiyosue H, Matsumoto S, Hori Y, Maeda T (2000) CT assessment of the inferior peripancreatic veins: clinical significance. AJR Am J Roentgenol 174(3):677–84
19. Lepanto L, Arzoumanian Y, Gianfelice D et al. (2002) Helical CT with CT angiography in assessing periampullary neoplasms: identification of vascular invasion. Radiology 222(2):347–52
20. Sugiyama M, Haradome H, Takahara T et al. (2003) Anomalous pancreaticobiliary junction shown on multidetector CT. AJR Am J Roentgenol 180(1):173–5
21. Ariyama J, Suyama M, Satoh K, Sai J (1998) Imaging of small pancreatic ductal adenocarcinoma. Pancreas 16(3):396–401
22. Lu DS, Reber HA, Krasny RM, Kadell BM, Sayre J (1997) Local staging of pancreatic cancer: criteria for unresectability of major vessels as revealed by pancreatic-phase, thin-section helical CT. AJR Am J Roentgenol 168(6):1439–43
23. O'Malley ME, Boland GW, Wood BJ, Fernandez-del Castillo C, Warshaw AL, Mueller PR (1999) Adenocarcinoma of the head of the pancreas: determination of surgical unresectability with thin-section pancreatic-phase helical CT. AJR Am J Roentgenol 173(6):1513–8
24. Valls C, Andia E, Sanchez A et al. (2002) Dual-phase helical CT of pancreatic adenocarcinoma: assessment of resectability before surgery. AJR Am J Roentgenol 178(4):821–6
25. Saldinger PF, Reilly M, Reynolds K et al. (2000) Is CT angiography sufficient for prediction of resectability of periampullary neoplasms? J Gastrointest Surg 4(3):233–7; discussion 238–9
26. Raptopoulos V, Steer ML, Sheiman RG, Vrachliotis TG, Gougoutas CA, Movson JS (1997) The use of helical CT and CT angiography to predict vascular involvement from pancreatic cancer: correlation with findings at surgery. AJR Am J Roentgenol 168(4):971–7
27. Sarr MG, Kendrick ML, Nagorney DM, Thompson GB, Farley DR, Farnell MB (2001) Cystic neoplasms of the pancreas: benign to malignant epithelial neoplasms. Surg Clin North Am 81(3):497–509
28. Terris B, Ponsot P, Paye F et al. (2000) Intraductal papillary mucinous tumors of the pancreas confined to secondary ducts show less aggressive pathologic features as compared with those involving the main pancreatic duct. Am J Surg Pathol 24(10):1372–7
29. Banks PA (1997) Practice guidelines in acute pancreatitis. Am J Gastroenterol 92(3):377–86
30. Balthazar EJ (2002) Staging of acute pancreatitis. Radiol Clin North Am 40(6):1199–209
31. Balthazar EJ, Robinson DL, Megibow AJ, Ranson JH (1990) Acute pancreatitis: value of CT in establishing prognosis. Radiology 174(2):331–6
32. Jacobs JE, Birnbaum BA (2001) Computed tomography evaluation of acute pancreatitis. Semin Roentgenol 36(2):92–8
33. Etemad B, Whitcomb DC (2001) Chronic pancreatitis: diagnosis, classification, and new genetic developments. Gastroenterology 120(3):682–707

8 Multislice CT of the Thorax: Opportunities, Challenges and Solutions

M. Das, P. Herzog, J. M. Martensen, J. E. Wildberger, U. J. Schoepf

Introduction

The scan speed of current generation multislice CT (MSCT) scanners with simultaneous acquisition of up to 16 slices translates into the ability to scan the entire chest in a breath-hold time of 10 s or less. Despite submillimeter resolution, this results in motion-free images even in the most critically ill patients. Use of thin slices was shown to significantly improve the detection of minute pathology, small lung nodules or visualization of peripheral pulmonary vessels. For a comprehensive diagnosis of focal and diffuse lung disease, both contiguous images and high-resolution CT can be reconstructed from the same single acquisition, without scanning the patient twice. ECG synchronization with MSCT is a valuable tool to improve image quality and diagnostic accuracy by reducing motion artefacts as potential sources of error. However, while MSCT provides innumerable opportunities, its unique characteristics also pose hitherto unknown challenges to its users. The large volume datasets generated by 4-, 10-, 16-, or more-slice MSCT are a logistical problem that threatens to overburden the radiologist with diagnostic information. Also, although MSCT can be used in ways which result in a reduction of patient radiation dose, with many applications the patient dose is likely to increase moderately. Solutions, however, are on the horizon: the practice of radiology is quickly adapting to novel concepts of data visualization embracing 2-D and 3-D visualization techniques. The performance of tools for the detection, visualization and characterization of lung lesions with MSCT is being continuously improved. Sophisticated means for reducing radiation dose are being implemented. In the following we discuss specific improvements, novel challenges and sophisticated solutions, which the advent of ever-faster MSCT acquisition techniques has brought about with a special focus on disease entities of great socioeconomic importance: imaging of focal lung disease and vascular imaging of the thoracic aorta and pulmonary circulation.

MSCT of Focal Lung Disease

Pulmonary nodules are one of the most common findings in chest CT. As an incidental finding they often cause a cascade of diagnostic procedures including biopsy or surgery which, in many cases, is neither cost-effective nor beneficial for the patient. Nodules found at follow-up CT in patients with a history of

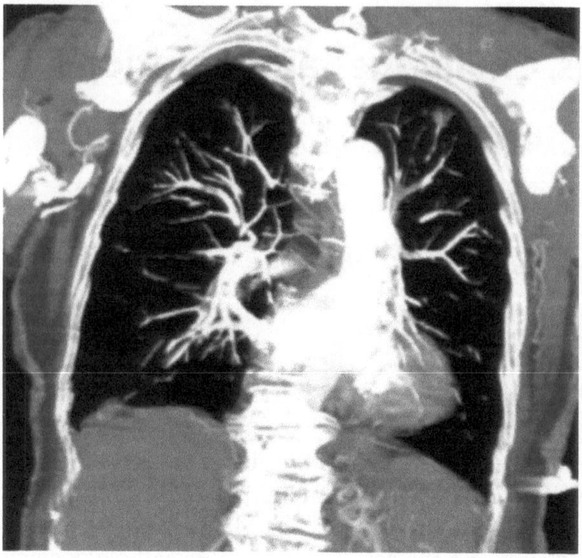

Fig. 1. Indeterminate pulmonary nodule in the left upper lobe of the lung in a patient with acute multiple pulmonary embolism as an incidental finding. Subsequent workup revealed small-cell lung cancer

malignant disease have a higher likelihood of representing metastatic spread, and require adequate therapeutic measures. However, there is an abundance of incidental nodular findings in chest CT in patients without known underlying malignancy, e.g. those undergoing CT angiography to exclude pulmonary embolism (Fig. 1). Of late, a plethora of indeterminate incidental findings in patients undergoing lung cancer screening has aggravated this general phenomenon.

Occasionally, incidental indeterminate pulmonary nodules can be compared with previous scans or radiographs and classified as unchanged over time. However, classifying a nodule as unchanged can be treacherous ground. When evaluating nodules with diameters below 5 mm, a doubling in volume within 3 or 6 months, suggesting malignant growth, cannot be diagnosed by simply measuring the diameter of the lesion in two dimensions. This is due to the fact that the volume increases with the third power of the diameter. This is also the reason why a significant increase in volume can go along with only a minor increase in diameter, which often cannot be measured on a 2-D image, particularly in a thick-slice dataset. Also, it is important to keep in mind that a nodule can grow unevenly in different dimensions. It can grow by filling out grooves on its surface, which would be challenging to detect in a 2-D image, or it can grow only in the Z direction, which would be missed when evaluating thick sections only.

If there are no previous examinations to compare or if the nodule is new, showing no signs of benignity, many clinical algorithms call for immediate invasive workup of the lesion, such as CT-guided biopsy or even surgery (see Fig. 2, 3).

Experience from previous screening programs for the early detection of lung cancer using radiography show that with algorithms where every soft-tissue nodule is evaluated by invasive means, the screening arm has no advantage regarding mortality or morbidity compared to a population in which no screening and invasive workup of suspicious findings was performed. This is mainly attributable to the overall low prevalence of cancer and the morbidity and mortality incurred by invasive procedures.

MSCT, with the ability to examine the whole thorax with thin sections in a single breath-hold, helps in the non-invasive evaluation of indeterminate pulmonary nodules (Fig. 4). Therefore a collimation of 1 mm or less should be selected for scanning. Pitch can be increased up to 1.75, depending on the capabilities of the scanner and the number of detector rows. Scan time should not exceed 25 s for a comfortable breath-hold time. If only the lung parenchyma is to be evaluated for pulmonary nodules, tube current and the resulting radiation dose can be drastically reduced compared to a staging CT of the thorax. In such cases, no

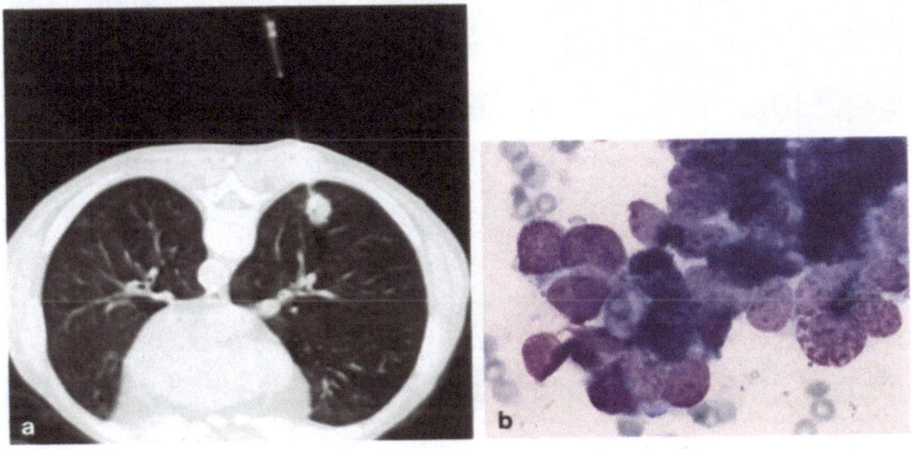

Fig. 2a,b. Highly suspicious pulmonary nodule. Workup with CT-guided biopsy. Histology reveals small cell lung cancer

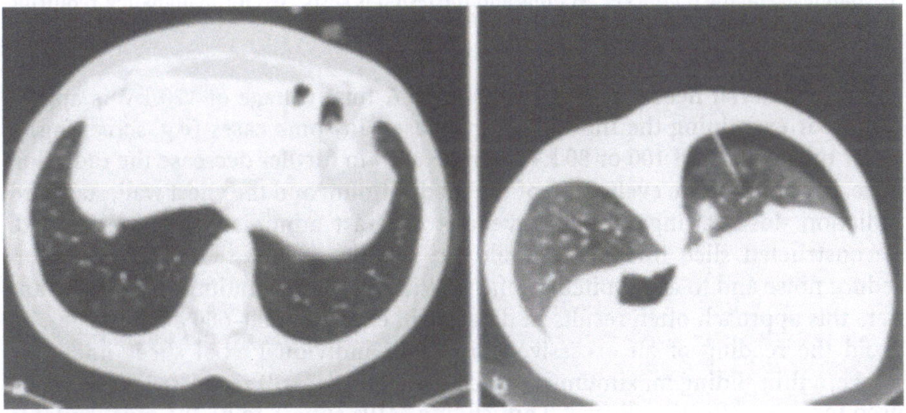

Fig. 3a,b. Indeterminate pulmonary nodule in a patient with emphysema, wait-listed for lung transplantation. Biopsy was required to rule out malignant disease as a contraindication for lung transplantation. Pneumothorax occurred as a complication of the invasive approach

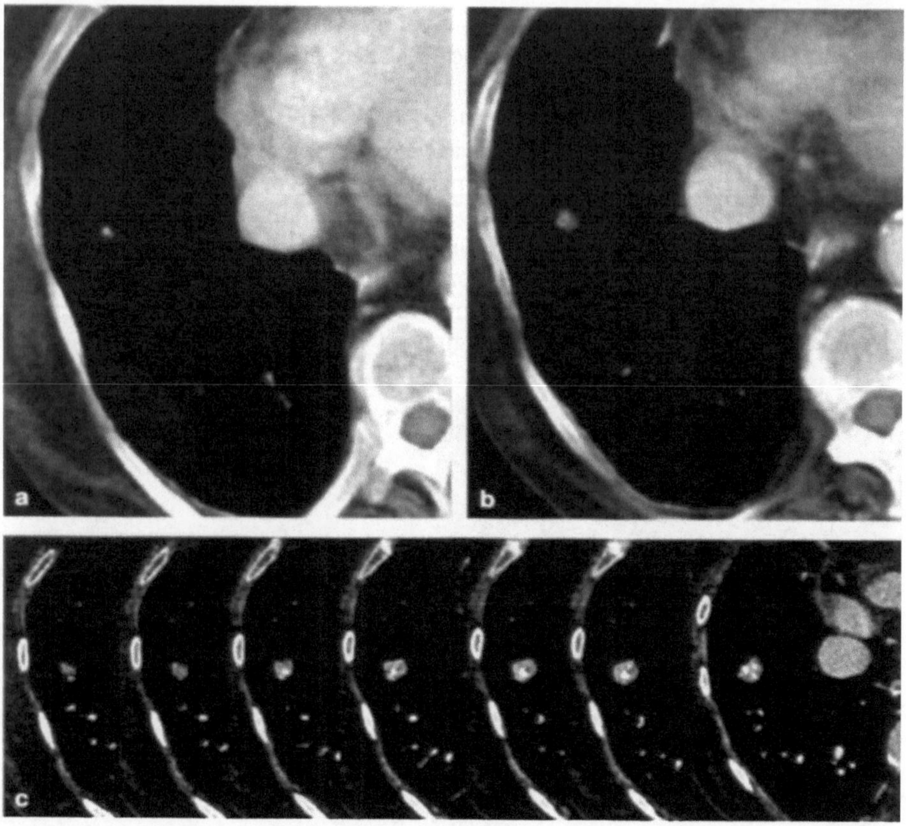

Fig. 4a–c. Indeterminate nodule reconstructed with 10 mm sections *above* and with 1 mm sections *below*. Calcification and fatty components allow diagnosis of a hamartoma and rule out malignancy when the nodule is interrogated using thin slices. Signs of benignity are obscured by volume averaging on thicker sections and the lesion is suspected for malignancy, requiring invasive workup

contrast material needs to be administered. A tube voltage of 120 kV is appropriate for examining the thorax in most cases. In some cases (e.g. screening) a lower tube voltage of 100 or 80 kVp can be used to further decrease the radiation dose. For appropriate evaluation of the mediastinum and the chest wall, standard radiation dose settings and intravenous contrast administration are needed. Reconstructed slice thickness should be slightly greater than collimation to reduce noise and to avoid pitch artefacts. With recent generations of MSCT scanners this approach often results in datasets in excess of 500–600 axial images. To avoid the reading of an excessive number of individual axial slices image by image, a thin sliding maximum-intensity projection (MIP) reconstruction can be used for more effective display. Thin sliding MIPs appear to be the most suitable visualization method of all secondary reconstruction techniques for delineating small pulmonary nodules and for differentiation of lesions from pulmonary vessels.

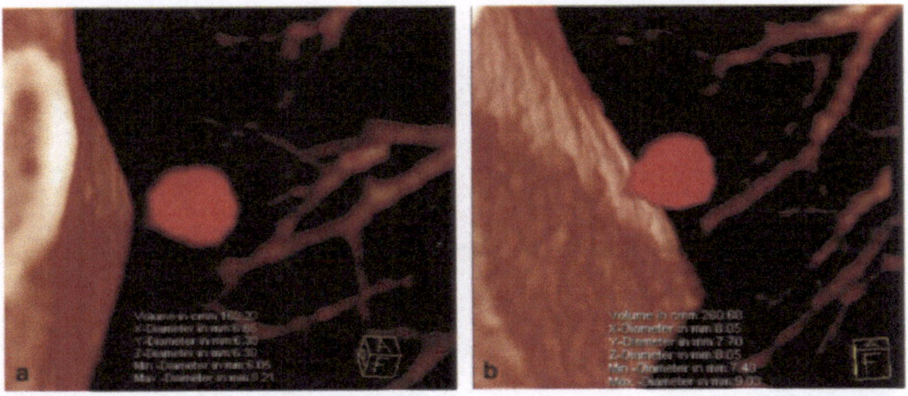

Fig. 5a,b. Squamous cell carcinoma. Initial scan on the *left* and 3-month follow-up on the *right*. The lesion exhibits a malignant growth pattern with an increase from 160 to 260 mm^3

Typical patterns of calcification or fatty areas in a previously indeterminate nodule can be used as approximate markers for benignity or malignancy.

Thin slices better enable the reader to evaluate the internal structure of a nodule while thick slices often obscure fatty or small calcified areas due to partial volume effect. However, these subtle features are often an important sign or even proof of benignity (Fig. 4).

A nodule without obvious signs of benignity must be considered as indeterminate; however, only a small portion of all incidental nodules are malignant and an invasive evaluation in every case would incur unnecessary complications and costs. Therefore other methods of non-invasive evaluation need to be devised.

Contrast media uptake has been used for sensitive differentiation between benign and malignant lesions. A threshold of enhancement of 15 HU has been found to be a sensitive but unspecific marker for differentiating benign and malignant lesions.

The most efficient way of evaluating the dignity of an indeterminate nodule is perhaps to assess lesion growth. Active malignancy ordinarily shows a distinct growth pattern depending on the tissue type, especially when untreated (Figs. 5, 6). Small-cell lung cancers have the highest growth rate with a doubling time of about 70 days (Fig. 6). Lung cancers other than small-cell lung cancer tend to have an intermediate growth rate with a doubling time of about 100 days, while adenocarcinoma exhibit slower growth with a doubling time of about 130–160 days. Nodules with faster growth rates and doubling times of less than 50 days usually represent acute inflammatory lesions, which should recede under antimicrobial therapy. Nodules with doubling times of more than 300–500 days usually represent benign or subacute inflammatory lesions when histology is obtained.

Using thin-slice MSCT data, accurate CT volumetry can be performed based on automated segmentation algorithms. Since growth is the very hallmark of malignancy, such tools may be the most suitable method for the non-invasive characterization of lung lesions in the future and help avoid unnecessary invasive procedures and the morbidity and mortality inherent to them.

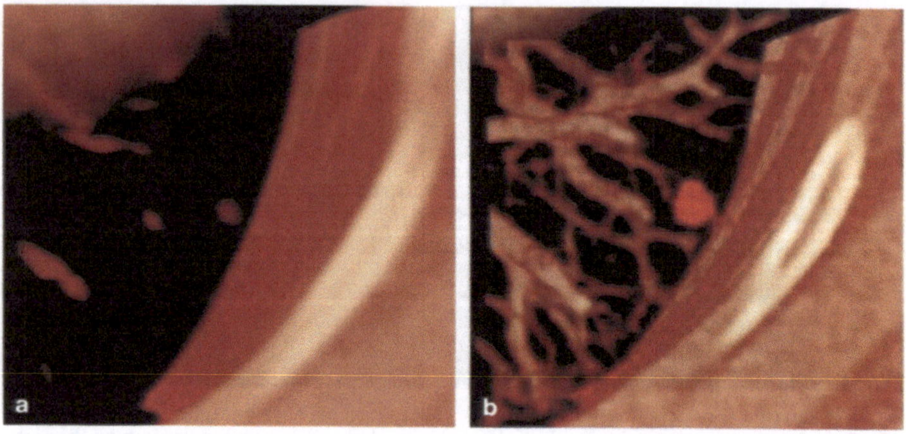

Fig. 6. Small-cell carcinoma. Initial scan (37 mm³) on the *left* with 6 months follow up (152 cmm) on the *right*

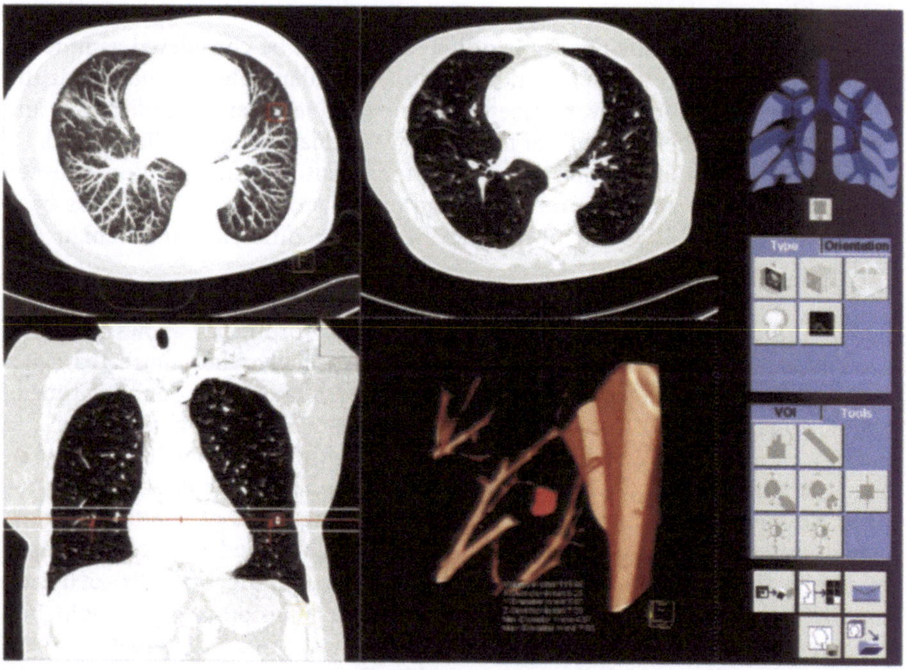

Fig. 7. Example of a dedicated software platform for visualization and analysis of focal lung disease. The LungCARE (Siemens AG, Erlangen, Germany) software platform enables intuitive visualization of focal lung disease using MIP, VRT or MPR reconstructions in various imaging planes. If focal lung disease is found, accurate lesion volumetry can be performed

While use of thin-slice MSCT data improves our capabilities for lesion detection and non-invasive characterization, this approach is inherently associated with a vast data load, routinely resulting in datasets comprising several hundred images. These large-volume datasets represent a logistical challenge that has been enhanced with the advent of 8-slice and 16-slice CT scanners. In many instances, the radiologist is overburdened with diagnostic information and it becomes increasingly time-consuming and difficult for radiologists to visualize and interpret patient data. This reduces the sensitivity for lesion detection, so that lung lesions in large-volume MSCT datasets are easily missed by radiologists. This situation is being aggravated by the lack of diagnostic radiologists that has lately been observed in several countries, including the US. The widespread application of and increasing demand for novel diagnostic tests, such as CT lung cancer screening, further increase the need for new development to cope with increasing case volumes. Computer-aided diagnosis tools, dedicated to the automated detection of lung lesions, may increase the effectiveness and accuracy for reading large-volume datasets, and may have the potential to offset some of the case burden and limited human resources that we currently witness (Figs. 7, 8, 9).

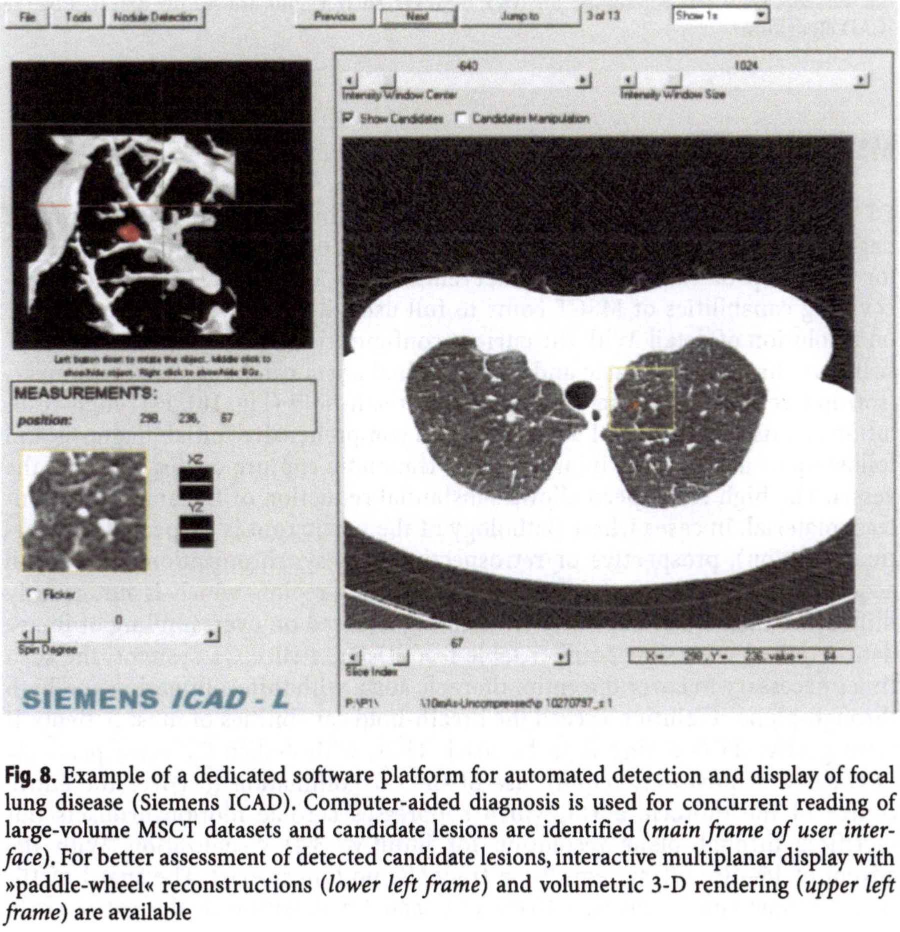

Fig. 8. Example of a dedicated software platform for automated detection and display of focal lung disease (Siemens ICAD). Computer-aided diagnosis is used for concurrent reading of large-volume MSCT datasets and candidate lesions are identified (*main frame of user interface*). For better assessment of detected candidate lesions, interactive multiplanar display with »paddle-wheel« reconstructions (*lower left frame*) and volumetric 3-D rendering (*upper left frame*) are available

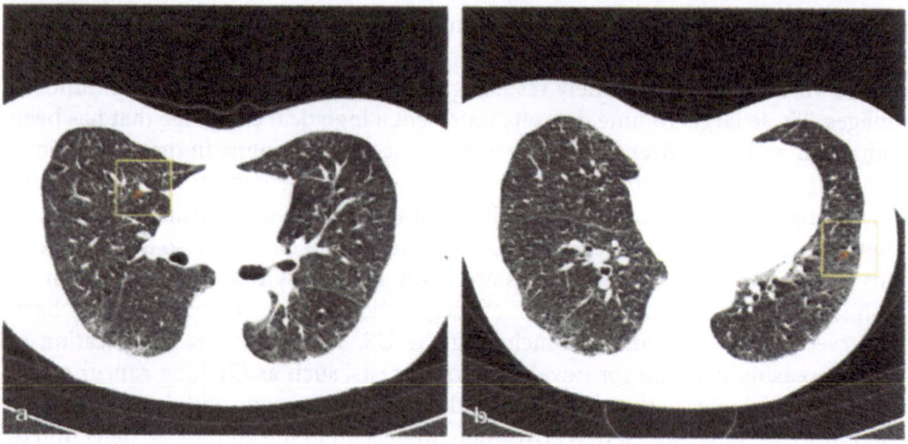

Fig. 9. Examples of ICAD-detected lesions. While peripheral lung lesions (*right*) are ordinarily more easily detected by radiologists, more centrally located lesions (*left*) frequently remain undetected even by experienced radiologists, due to their vicinity to surrounding anatomy (i.e. vessels). With 3-D volumetric analysis, however, such lesions are readily detected by the ICAD algorithm

MSCT of the Thoracic Aorta

CT angiography has been established as the first line modality for evaluation of degenerative or congenital aortic disease and for surgical planning prior to and for follow-up of cardiovascular interventions. In aortic imaging, the volume-covering capabilities of MSCT come to full use without having to compromise on resolution of detail. With the current configuration of 4-, 10- and 16-slice CT scanners the entire thoracic and/or abdominal aorta can be covered with near-isotropic resolution within a single, short breath-hold (Fig. 10). Fast high-resolution acquisition is crucial for a quick and comprehensive initial diagnosis and follow-up of acute aortic injury, such as traumatic rupture or dissection of the vessel. The high scan speed allows substantial reduction of the amount of contrast material. In cases where pathology of the aortic root is suspected (i.e. aortic dissection), prospective or retrospective ECG synchronization of the scan acquisition allows artifact-free evaluation of this region, which is notoriously difficult to image. Retrospective ECG gating is based on oversampling of image data acquired with slow scanner table feed. Using 4-slice CT systems, the scan times necessary to cover the entire thoracic aorta with thin collimation and high through-plane resolution exceed the breath-hold capabilities of most patients, if retrospective ECG gating is to be used. Thus, with 4-slice CT retrospectively ECG-gated acquisitions require use of thicker collimation to cover the entire course of the thoracic aorta, which suppresses cardiac motion artefacts but sacrifices through-plane resolution for intuitive 3-D visualization. With the advent of 16-slice CT systems, such tradeoffs no longer exist. The speed of 16-slice CT now allows retrospectively ECG gated acquisition of the entire aorta

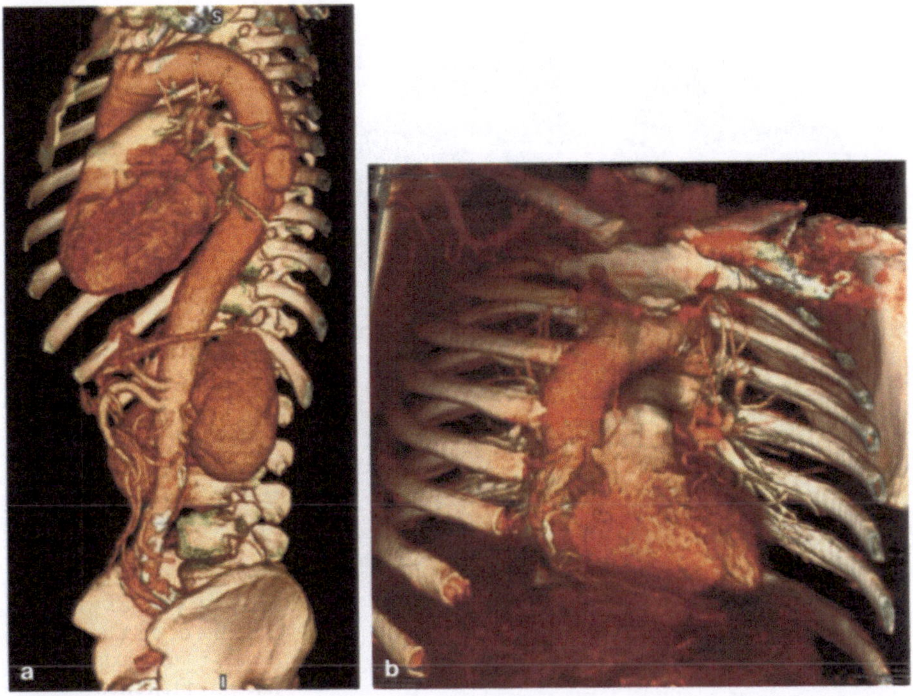

Fig. 10a,b. Patient with circumscribed penetrating aortic ulcer/type-B aortic dissection in the descending aorta. Colored volume-rendered display. A 16-slice MSCT acquisition with retrospective ECG gating covers the entire aorta and its branches from arch to bifurcation in a single breath-hold, effectively eliminating cardiac pulsation artefacts. Potential sources of diagnostic pitfalls arising from cardiac motion are thus avoided. b Systemic imaging for systemic disease – same dataset as in 10a. Focused volume rendered reconstruction of the heart seen from a right oblique inferior perspective. Note clear delineation of peripheral segments of the right coronary artery. The high resolution of a 16-slice MSCT acquisition with retrospective ECG gating enables performance of non-invasive CT coronary angiography from a full-body CT angiogram

with submillimeter resolution, which effectively eliminates cardiac motion as a source of potential diagnostic pitfalls and preserves the near-isotropic nature of MSCT datasets.

MSCT of the Pulmonary Circulation

The ability to cover substantial anatomic volumes with high in-plane and through-plane spatial resolution has brought with it a number of clear advantages (Fig. 11). Shorter breath-hold times were shown to benefit imaging of patients with suspected PE and underlying lung disease reducing the percentage of non-diagnostic CT pulmonary angiography investigations.

The near-isotropic nature of high-resolution MSCT data lends itself to 2-D and 3-D visualization. This may, in some instances, improve PE diagnosis, but is

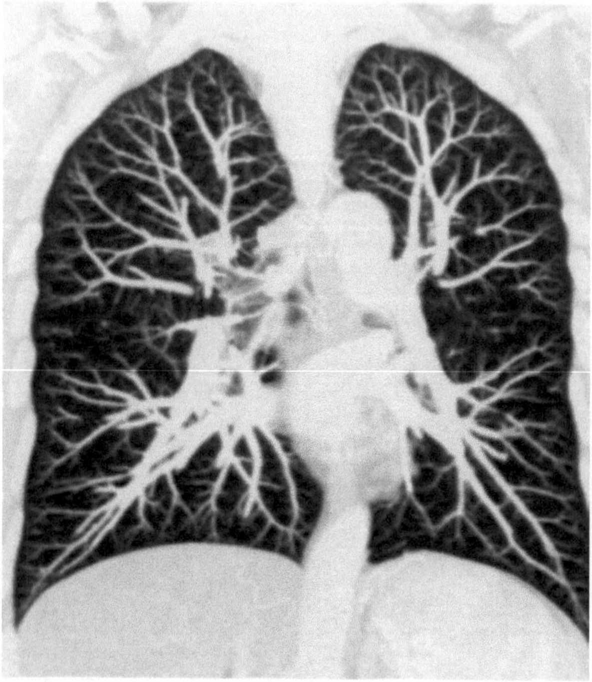

Fig. 11. Normal pulmonary vasculature. Contrast-enhanced 16-slice CT examination covers the entire chest within a scan time of 10 s allowing analysis of even the most peripheral pulmonary vessels with exquisite detail. Coronal display using maximum intensity projection

generally of greater importance for conveying information on localization and extent of embolic disease to referring clinicians in a more intuitive display format (Fig. 12).

Probably the most important advantage is improved diagnosis of small peripheral emboli. With single-slice CT it has been shown that superior visualization of segmental and subsegmental pulmonary arteries can be accomplished with thinner slice widths (e.g. 2 mm versus 3 mm). However, with single-slice CT the range of coverage with thin slice widths within one breath-hold was limited. The high spatial resolution of 1-mm or submillimeter collimation datasets now allows evaluation of pulmonary vessels down to 6th order branches and significantly increases the detection rate of segmental and subsegmental pulmonary emboli (Fig. 13). This improved detection rate is most likely due to reduced volume averaging and the accurate analysis of progressively smaller vessels by use of thinner sections.

While traditional technical limitations of CT in the diagnosis of pulmonary emboli appear successfully overcome by multidetector row CT, we are now facing new challenges that are a direct result of our high-resolution imaging capabilities. Small peripheral clots that might have gone unnoticed in the past are now frequently detected, often in patients with minor symptoms. While, based on a good quality MSCT scan, there may be no doubt in the mind of the interpreting radiologists as to the presence of a small isolated clot, such findings will be increasingly difficult to prove in a correlative manner. Animal experiments that use artificial emboli as an independent gold standard indicate that high-resolution 4-slice MSCT is at least as accurate as catheter pulmonary angiography for

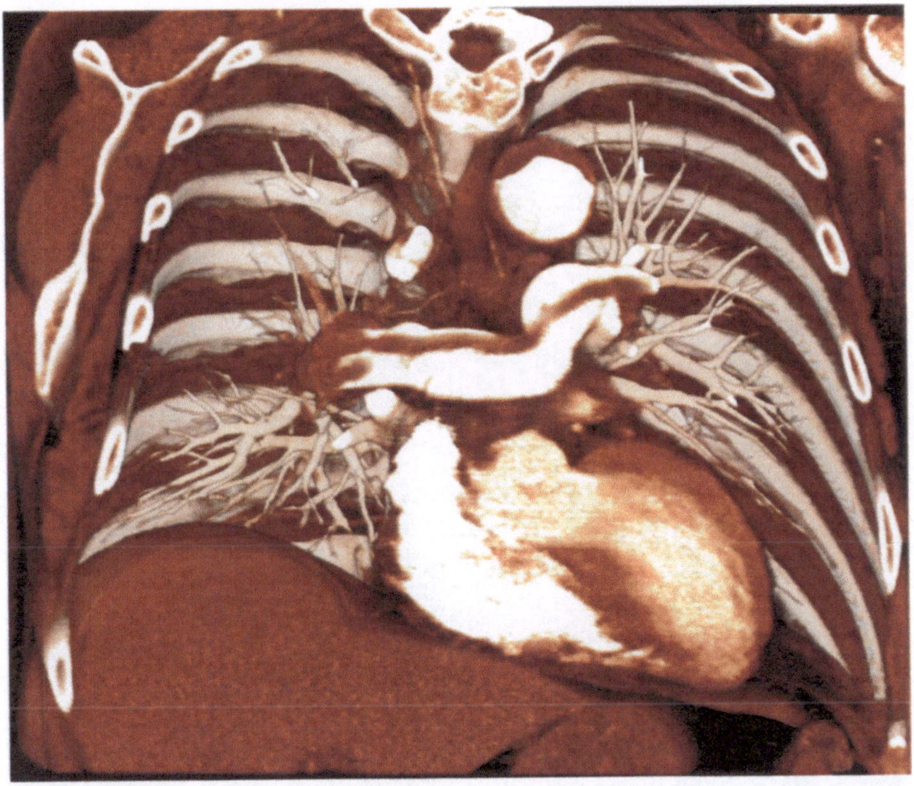

Fig. 12. Extensive, acute central pulmonary embolism with saddle embolus extending into both central pulmonary arteries. Contrast-enhanced 16-slice CT examination. Coronal colored volume-rendering technique seen from an anterior perspective allows intuitive visualization of location and extent of embolism

the detection of small peripheral emboli. However, it appears highly unlikely that pulmonary angiography will be performed on a patient merely to prove the presence of a small (2–3 mm) isolated embolus. Additionally, given the limited interobserver correlation of pulmonary angiography it appears doubtful that this test, even if performed, would provide as useful and conclusive proof as high-resolution multidetector row CT (Fig. 13).

Perhaps more importantly, there is a growing sense of insecurity within the clinical community as to how to manage patients in whom a diagnosis of isolated peripheral embolism has been established. There is little disagreement that the presence of peripheral emboli may be an indicator for current deep vein thrombosis, thus potentially heralding more severe embolic events. A burden of small peripheral emboli may also have prognostic relevance in individuals with cardiopulmonary restrictions and for the development of chronic pulmonary hypertension in patients with thromboembolic disease. Despite advances in CT technology, there are still several factors that can render CT pulmonary angiography inconclusive. The most common reasons for non-diagnostic CT studies are poor

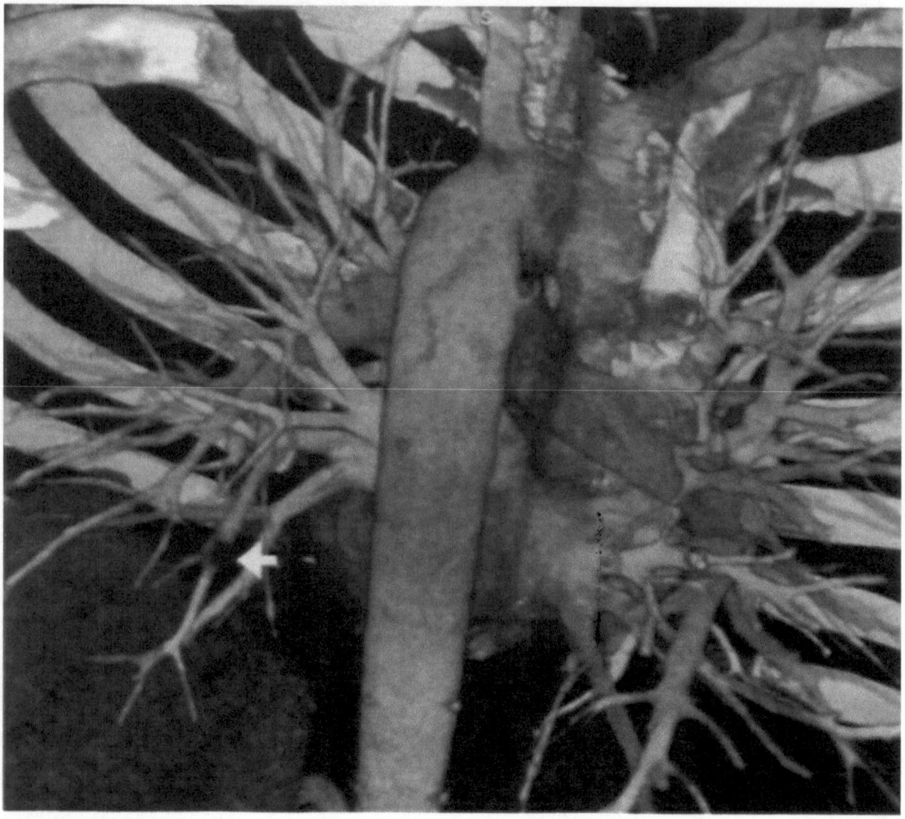

Fig. 13. Contrast-enhanced 16-slice CT examination with 0.75-mm collimation in a patient with mild pleuritic chest pain. Isolated peripheral pulmonary embolus (*arrow*) in a subsegmental pulmonary artery in segment 9 of the left lung is visualized by volume-rendered display seen from posterior within otherwise normal pulmonary vasculature

contrast opacification of pulmonary vessels, patient motion and increased image noise due to excessive patient obesity. Use of high-resolution MSCT protocols was shown to improve visualization of pulmonary arteries and the detection of small subsegmental emboli. In suspected PE, establishing an unequivocal diagnosis as to the presence or absence of emboli or other disease based on a high-quality MSCT examination may reduce the overall radiation burden of patients, since further workup with other tests that involve ionizing radiation may be less frequently required. However, if a 4-slice MSCT protocol with 4 x 1-mm collimation is chosen to replace a single-detector CT protocol based on a 1 x 5-mm collimation, the increase is radiation dose ranges between 30 and 100%. Similar increases in radiation dose, however, are not to be expected with the introduction of 16-slice multidetector-CT technology with submillimeter resolution capabilities. The addition of detector elements improves tube output utilization compared to current 4-slice CT scanners and reduces the ratio of excess radiation

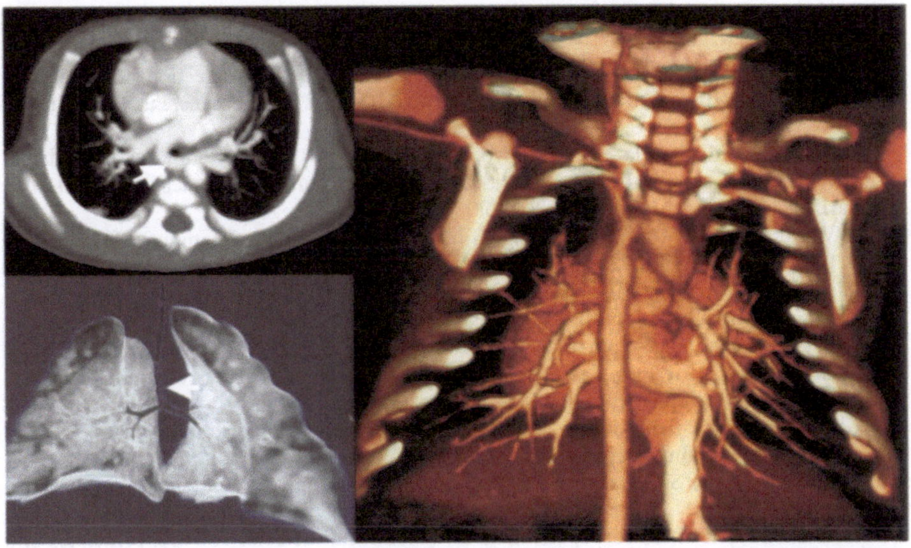

Fig. 14. Infant presenting with acute shortness of breath. Contrast-enhanced 16-slice CT demonstrates the left pulmonary artery taking an aberrant course posterior to the trachea (*arrow*, axial MIP image *left upper panel*) forming a pulmonary artery »sling« compressing the trachea. 3-D volume-rendered displays of the thoracic vessels (right panel) and of the airways (left lower panel) demonstrate anomalous vessel course and subsequent compression of the trachea (*arrow, left lower panel*). (CT scan data courtesy of Dr. R. Fischbach, University of Muenster)

dose that does not contribute to actual image generation. As sophisticated technical devices move into clinical practice, that modulate and adapt tube output relative to the geometry and X-ray attenuation of the scanned object, i.e. the patient, substantial dose savings can be realized without compromising diagnostic quality. The most important factor, however, for ensuring responsible utilization of multidetector-row CT's technical prowess is the increased awareness of protocols used by technologists and radiologists. It has been shown that diagnostic quality of chest CT is not compromised if tube output is adjusted to the body type of the individual patient (Fig. 14).

Also, with MSCT radiologists are more and more adapting to the concept of volume imaging. There is a tradeoff between increased spatial resolution and image noise, when thinner and thinner sections are acquired with fast CT techniques.

Given the great flexibility and diagnostic benefit that a high-resolution, near-isotropic MSCT dataset provides, radiologists are increasingly willing to compromise on the degree of image noise in an individual axial thin-section image which they are willing to accept in order to keep radiation dose within reasonable limits.

Further Reading

1. Das M, Schneider AC, Anderson M et al. (2003) Computer-aided detection (CAD) of lung nodules in high-resolution multidetector-row CT (MDCT) chest scans. Eur Radiol 13(S): 169
2. Das M, Schneider AC, Jacobson FL, Wood SA, Schoepf UJ (2003) Computer-aided detection (CAD) of lung nodules on multidetector-row CT (MDCT): impact on readers with variable levels of experience. Eur Radiol 13(S): 315
3. Dawn SK, Gotway MB, Webb WR (2001) Multidetector-row spiral computed tomography in the diagnosis of thoracic diseases. Respir Care 46:912–21
4. Diederich S, Lentschig MG, Overbeck TR, Wormanns D, Heindel W. (2001) Detection of pulmonary nodules at spiral CT: comparison of maximum intensity projection sliding slabs and single-image reporting. Eur Radiol 11:1345–50
5. Fuchs TO, Kachelriess M, Kalender WA (2000) System performance of multislice spiral computed tomography. IEEE Eng Med Biol Mag 2000; 19: 63–70
6. Ghaye B, Remy J, Remy-Jardin M (2002) Non-traumatic thoracic emergencies: CT diagnosis of acute pulmonary embolism: the first 10 years. Eur Radiol 12: 1886–905
7. Herold CJ (2002) Spiral computed tomography of pulmonary embolism. Eur Respir J Suppl 35: 13s–21s
8. Horton KM, Sheath S, Corl F, Fishman EK (2002) Multidetector row CT: principles and clinical applications. Crit Rev Comput Tomogr 43: 143–81
9. Kauczor HU, Heussel CP, Thelen M (1999) Update on diagnostic strategies of pulmonary embolism. Eur Radiol 9: 262–75
10. MacMahon H, Engelmann R, Behlen FM et al. (1999) Computer-aided diagnosis of pulmonary nodules: results of a large-scale observer test. Radiology 213: 723–6
11. Ravenel JG, McAdams HP, Remy-Jardin M, Remy J (2001) Multidimensional imaging of the thorax: practical applications. J Thorac Imaging 16: 269–81
12. Reeves AP, Kostis WJ (2000) Computer-aided diagnosis for lung cancer. Radiol Clin North Am 2000; 38: 497–509
13. Remy-Jardin M, Remy J (1999) Spiral CT angiography of the pulmonary circulation. Radiology 212: 615–36
14. Schoepf UJ, Becker CR, Obuchowski NA et al. (2001) Multislice computed tomography as a screening tool for colon cancer, lung cancer and coronary artery disease. Eur Radiol 11: 1975–85
15. Schoepf UJ, Bruening R, Konschitzky H et al. (2000) Pulmonary embolism: comprehensive diagnosis by using electron-beam CT for detection of emboli and assessment of pulmonary blood flow. Radiology 217: 693–700
16. Schoepf UJ, Das M, Schneider AC et al. (2002) Computer-aided detection (CAD) of segmental and subsegmental pulmonary emboli on 1-mm multidetector row CT (MDCT) studies. Radiology 225(P): 384
17. Schoepf UJ, Helmberger T, Holzknecht N et al. (2000) Segmental and subsegmental pulmonary arteries: Evaluation with electron-beam versus spiral CT. Radiology 214: 433–9
18. Schoepf UJ, Holzknecht N, Helmberger TK et al. (2002) Subsegmental pulmonary emboli: Improved detection with thin-Collimation multidetector-row spiral CT. Radiology 222: 483–90
19. Wormanns D, Fiebich M, Saidi M, Diederich S, Heindel W (2002) Automatic detection of pulmonary nodules at spiral CT: clinical application of a computer-aided diagnosis system. Eur Radiol 12: 1052–7

9 Role of CT Angiography in the Management of Thromboembolic Disease

M. Remy-Jardin, N. Bouaziz, P.-Y. Brillet, J. Remy

Introduction

Pulmonary embolism (PE) is a common condition with considerable morbidity and mortality [1]. Prompt and accurate diagnosis is important because the mortality of untreated pulmonary embolism is high and serious complications can occur with its treatment, long-term anticoagulation [2]. Because there are no specific signs or symptoms of this condition, the diagnosis relies on imaging tests. In the early 1990s, the introduction of spiral computed tomography (CT) technology dramatically modified the evaluation of pulmonary arteries, enabling a direct insight into endovascular abnormalities and thus a direct depiction of endoluminal clots. Successive technological advances have reinforced its diagnostic impact, explaining why this imaging tool is now included in the non-invasive diagnostic algorithms proposed in routine clinical practice. The purpose of this article is to focus on multislice spiral CT angiography in the management of thromboembolic disease.

Imaging Technique

In the early 1990s, single-slice spiral CT made it possible to image central and segmental arteries, but this new technique was limited by the time needed to survey the region of interest, i.e., 30 s, obviously too long for dyspneic patients, and the collimation available, i.e., 5 mm, was only compatible with the search for central PE. This first step was followed by the introduction of faster scanning techniques secondary to the availability of pitch values of greater than 1 and subsecond scanning. These techniques, often referred to as thin-collimation single-slice CT, allowed one to obtain a uniform opacification of pulmonary vessels down to 2–3 mm in diameter, and to analyze the peripheral pulmonary circulation with more anatomical details than those available with conventional studies [3, 4]. The introduction of multislice CT has allowed even thinner section collimation to be used (1.0 to 1.25 mm), providing improved image quality while solving a great deal of the difficulties encountered with single-slice spiral CT scanning of the pulmonary circulation [5, 6] (Fig. 1).

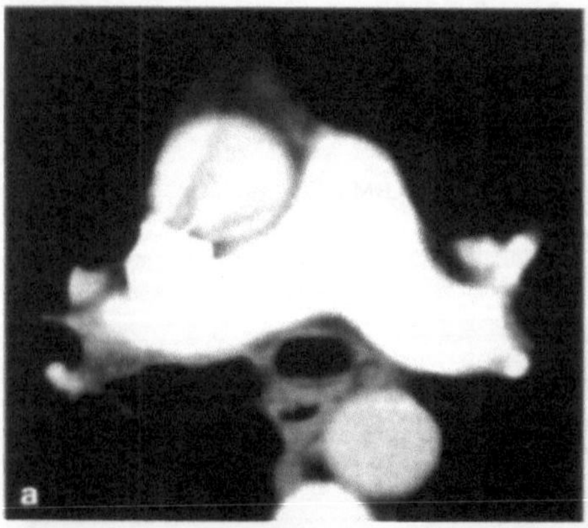

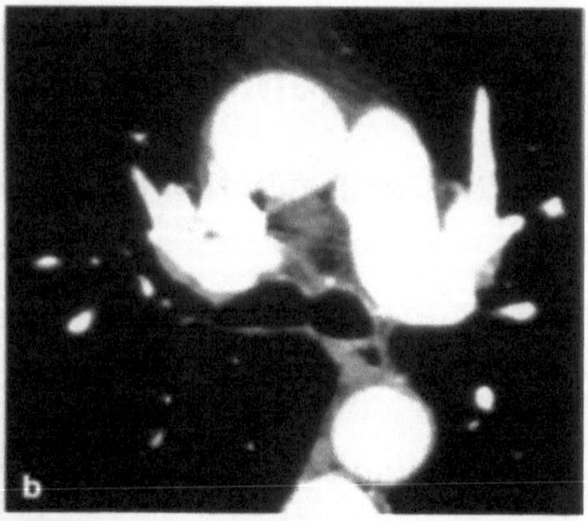

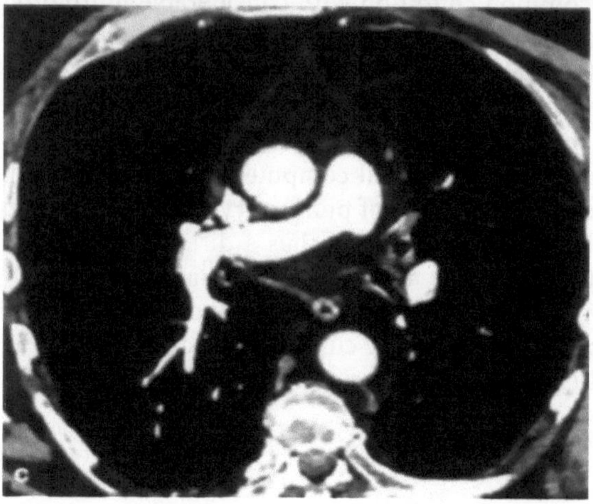

Fig. 1a–c. Impact of spiral CT technology on image quality. **a** Single slice spiral CT angiogram obtained in 1991 with a 5-mm collimation and a pitch of 1 (thickness of reconstructed scans: 6.57 mm). **b** Single slice spiral CT angiogram obtained in 1998 with a 2-mm collimation and a pitch of 2 (thickness of reconstructed scans: 2.65 mm). **c** Multislice spiral CT angiogram obtained in 2000 with a 4 x 1 mm collimation and a pitch of 2 (thickness of reconstructed scans: 1.25 mm). Note the dramatic improvement in spatial resolution enabling analysis of pulmonary arteries down to the subsegmental level on multislice spiral CT scans

Acquisition Protocols

The choice of the optimal imaging protocol depends on the equipment at hand as 4- to 16-row detector scanners are currently available. The concurrent availability of subsecond rotation times together with acquisition of multiple sections during one rotation has made it possible to scan the entire thorax with thin-collimation protocols, often referred to as high-resolution protocols, in the majority of patients (Fig. 2). The breath-hold duration necessary for such an acquisition depends on the number of sections acquired per rotation, ranging from 20 s with a 4-row detector scanner to 8 s with a 16-row detector scanner, while selecting the highest pitch value recommended by the manufacturer, i.e. 1.5 to 2.0. Depending on the scanner used, the thinnest collimation for multislice spiral CT acquisitions ranges from 0.5 to 1 mm, enabling one to provide the most detailed display of the pulmonary arteries [5, 7, 8]. Because a long breath-hold period may not be possible for severely dyspneic patients, a high-speed protocol can be proposed as an alternative to the high-resolution protocol previously described. Such an option requires widening the collimation, ranging from 2.5 mm on 4-row detector scanners to 1.5 mm on 16-row detector scanners. Consequently, the scanning time can be shortened to 5 seconds on the most recent scanners, enabling considerable reduction in respiratory motion artefacts.

Injection Protocols

For each examination, data acquisition is obtained during administration of contrast material. The injection parameters do not differ from those described for single-slice CT, based on the administration of a bolus of iodinated contrast medium using an automatic injector. Different protocols of contrast material administration have been reported, either low-concentration-high-volume or high-concentration-low-volume protocols, resulting in a compromise between the quality of vascular enhancement and the total amount of iodine injected [9]. The particularities of contrast material administration with multislice CT deal with the more frequent use of bolus triggering software programs. These programs allow precise timing of scanning, especially useful for patients with right heart failure and/or pulmonary hypertension, and reduction of the dose of contrast medium administered during the examination [10] (Fig. 3). Nevertheless, an

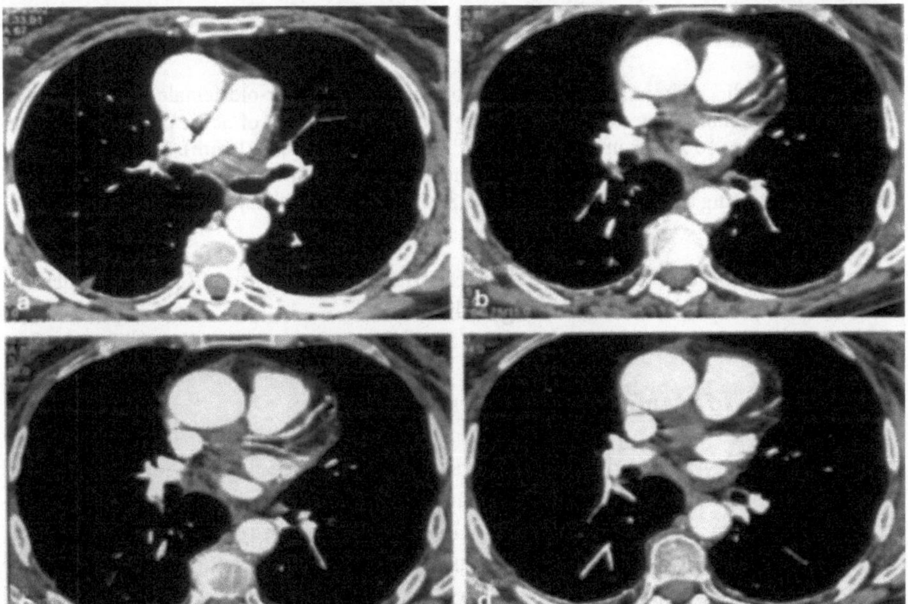

Fig. 2a–d. Multislice spiral CT examination obtained in a 46-year-old female with chronic obstructive pulmonary disease presenting with acute onset of dyspnea (collimation: 16 x 0.75 mm; thickness of reconstructed scans: 1 mm). Presence of multiple, small-sized endoluminal clots on both sides, responsible for partial filling defects at the level of several peripheral pulmonary arteries

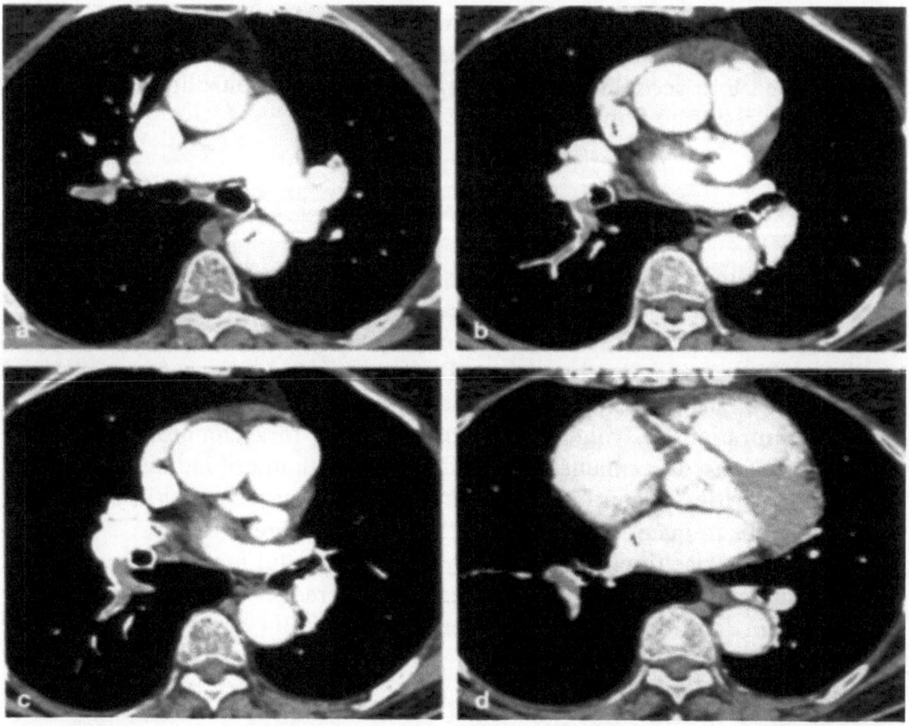

Fig. 3a–d. Multislice spiral CT examination obtained in a 77-year-old female with a previous history of pulmonary hypertension and a high clinical suspicion of acute pulmonary embolism (collimation: 16 x 0.75 mm; thickness of reconstructed scans: 1 mm). Note the excellent degree of vascular enhancement following the administration of 80 mL of a 24% iodinated contrast agent using a bolus triggering software program (start delay: 18 s) on **a–d.**

empiric selection of a 20-s start delay remains adapted to most CT examinations, as previously experienced with single-slice CT.

Optimization of Scanning Parameters

Spiral CT uses X-rays, and under the pressure of the radiological community and the general public, the current trend is to optimize the dose and image quality so that the dose is as low as possible but still consistent with required image quality. Strategies for reduction of the dose delivered during CT examinations include thorough protocol optimization and use of technique charts for patient-based determination of mAs/rotation.

The easiest way to reduce dose is to select the scanning parameters according to the patient's morphotype, adjusting the kilovoltage and milliamperage accordingly. As a consequence, current spiral CT examinations can be obtained at lower doses than those commonly delivered in the past decade, thus contradicting the usual criticism about the dose delivered during a spiral CT angiographic examination. For patients of less than 70 kg, it is currently recommended to use a low kilovoltage, i.e., 120 kV, whereas higher kilovoltage settings, i.e., 140 kV, are chosen for obese patients. With the introduction of multislice CT, kilovoltage settings as low as 80 or 100 kV can be used for contrast-enhanced examinations of the thorax, especially in very slim patients, enabling a reduction by a factor of 2–3 of the dose delivered compared with the selection of 120 kV. An additional positive effect of such a scanning protocol is the increased contrast, thus enabling the reduction of the volume or concentration of the contrast material administered to the patients.

In addition to this approach, the manufacturers have developed on-line tube current modulation systems which allows one to adapt the dose delivered according to the attenuation of the tissues scanned. Adaptive dose modulation allows for further dose reduction by some 10–30%, depending on the shape of the examined body area [11]. Combination of these new tools should be recommended for pregnant patients for whom the risk of venous thromboembolism is increased by a factor of 5 over that of a non-pregnant woman of similar age [12]. In a recent study, Winer–Muram et al. have showed that the average foetal radiation dose with helical CT is less than that with ventilation-perfusion lung scanning during all trimesters, thus concluding that pregnacy should not preclude use of helical CT for the diagnosis of PE [13]. Following technological advances in multislice CT technology, the use of ECG-gated spiral CT acquisitions will allow the radiologists to further decrease the dose delivered during spiral CT angiograms of the pulmonary circulation, delivering the full dose of the examinations exclusively during the diastole.

Impact of Multisclice CT Technology on Image Quality

Initial experience with multislice CT indicates that this method will further refine the diagnostic approach of PE by means of an obvious improvement in image quality. Three recent studies have evaluated the benefit of multislice CT on the detection of acute PE. The first study compared single-slice CT (3 mm collimation) to multislice CT (2.5 mm collimation), and led to the conclusion that multislice CT improved the conspicuity of peripheral arteries and the identification of peripheral filling defects [7]. Improvement was attributed to the thinner collimation, faster scanning and more homogeneous contrast enhancement available with multislice CT. The second study assessed the influence of reconstructed slice thickness on the detection of subsegmental PE [8]. Following a 4 x 1 mm collimation acquisition, use of the 1-mm section width yielded an average increase of 40% when compared with the use of 3-mm-thick sections and of 14% when compared with the use of 2-mm-thick sections. The benefit was more substantial for vessels with an oblique course to the scan plane (i.e., the middle lobe and lingula pulmonary arteries). Diagnostic confidence, interobserver agreement and reproductibility of findings were increased and the number of indeterminate results was decreased. The third study evaluated the impact of multislice CT on image quality and diagnostic value for PE compared to single-slice CT in patients with underlying respiratory disease [6]. The overall quality of CT scans was significantly higher using multislice CT, particularly for subsegmental arteries. This was related to a higher spatial resolution along the longitudinal axis of the patient and to a decrease of respiratory and cardiac motion artefacts. It should be noted that the improvement in spatial and temporal resolution observed with multislice CT did not lead to unusually high rates of positive angiograms, in particular of isolated subsegmental PE.

Imaging of Deep Venous Thrombosis

Combined CT venography and pulmonary angiography is a diagnostic test that screens for pulmonary embolism and deep venous thrombosis (DVT) using a single contrast medium infusion. This technique has been proposed as a cost-effective means for excluding lower-extremity venous thrombosis in patients undergoing CT pulmonary angiography [14]. Key advantages allow that no additional contrast media need to be injected to evaluate both the pulmonary vessels and the deep venous system. However, such a combined approach provides additional radiation exposure to the patients and requires including recent recommendations on low-dose scanning, especially for younger female patients [15].

Conclusion

Multiple data support the concept that single-slice and multislice CT have fundamentally modified the diagnostic approach of patients with suspected pulmonary embolism. Although the definitive role of spiral CT angiography in the diagnostic algorithm has yet to be determined, it is clear that CT angiography has numerous advantages compared to other diagnostic tests. Bearing in mind that an effective diagnostic strategy should be as flexible as possible in order to be applied in every clinical setting, the role of spiral CT angiography in the diagnostic algorithm has to be considered among several practical parameters, such as the experience of the attending physician, degree of severity of the patient's clinical condition, the availability of diagnostic equipment and specific logistics.

References

1. Moser KM (1990) State of the art: venous thromboembolism. Am Rev Respir Dis 414: 235–249
2. Carnasos G, Stewart R, Cluff L (1974) Drug-induced illness leading to hospitalization. JAMA 228:713–717
3. Remy-Jardin M, Remy J, Artaud D et al. (1997) Peripheral pulmonary arteries: optimization of the spiral CT acquisition protocol. Radiology 204: 157–163
4. Remy-Jardin M, Baghaie F, Bonnel F, Masson P, Duhamel A, Remy J (2000) Thoracic helical CT: influence of subsecond scan time and thin collimation on evaluation of peripheral pulmonary arteries. Eur Radiol 10:1297–1303

5. Ghaye B, Szapiro D, Mastora I et al. (2001) Peripheral pulmonary arteries: how far in the lung does multi-detector row spiral CT allow analysis? Radiology 219: 629–636
6. Remy-Jardin M, Tillie-Leblond I, Szapiro D et al. (2002) CT angiography of pulmonary embolism in patients with underlying respiratory disease: impact of multislice CT on image quality and negative predictive value. Eur Radiol 12: 1971–1978
7. Raptopoulos V, Boiselle PM (2001) Multidetector row spiral CT pulmonary angiography: comparison with single-detector row spiral CT. Radiology 221:606–613
8. Schoepf UJ, Holzknecht N, Helmberger TK et al. (2002) Subsegmental pulmonary emboli: improved detection with thin-collimation multi-detector row spiral CT. Radiology 222:483–490
9. Remy-Jardin M, Remy J, Mayo J, Muller NL (2001) Acute pulmonary embolism. In CT angiography of the chest. Lippincott Williams & Wilkins Philadelphia, USA, p 51–66
10. Kirchner J, Kickuth R, Laufer U, Noack M, Liermann (2000) Optimized enhancement in helical CT: experiences with a real-time bolus tracking system in 628 patients. Clin Radiol 55:368–373
11. Mastora I, Remy-Jardin M, Suess C, Scherf C, Guillot JP, Remy J (2001) Dose reduction in spiral CT angiography of the thoracic outlet syndrome by anatomically adapted tube current modulation. Eur Radiol 11: 590–596
12. (1986) Prevention of venous thrombosis and pulmonary embolism. NIH Consensus Development. JAMA 256: 744–749
13. Winer-Muram HT, Boone JM, Brown HL, Jennings SG, Mabie WC, Lombardo GT (2002) Pulmonary embolism in pregnant patients: fetal radiation dose with helical CT. Radiology 224: 487–492
14. Loud P, Grossman CD, Klippenstein DL, Ray CE (1998) Combined CT venography and pulmonary angiography: a new diagnostic method for suspected thromboembolic disease. AJR 170: 951–954
15. Rademaker J, Griesshaber V, Hidajat N, Oestmann JW, Felix R (2001) Combined CT pulmonary angiography and venography for diagnosis of pulmonary embolism and deep venous thrombosis: radiation dose. J Thorac Imaging 16: 297–299

IV Contrast/CT-Angiography

10 Contrast Injection Techniques and CT Scan Timing

K.T. Bae

Introduction

With dramatically shorter image acquisition times for multidetector row CT, optimization of contrast enhancement and scan timing has become increasingly crucial. Among many interacting factors involved in contrast enhancement, contrast injection rate, injection duration, and injection bolus shaping are key factors determining the temporal pattern of contrast enhancement. A high injection rate provides intense arterial contrast enhancement and is preferred in CT angiography and dual-phase CT applications. Injection bolus shaping with an exponential injection method may be used to generate a uniform prolonged contrast enhancement.

The time to peak aortic enhancement is closely associated with injection duration and circulation time. To optimize contrast enhancement timing during a scan, particularly for patients with slow cardiac output, scan delay should be determined individually by test-bolus or bolus-tracking techniques. Scan delay computed from the time to peak test-bolus contrast enhancement may be too early for multidetector row CT, requiring an additional delay. Contrast arrival time measured from the bolus-tracking method may be integrated with the injection duration to predict peak enhancement time. The scan delay is estimated such that the time to peak aortic enhancement is appropriately allocated within the scan duration. With the advance of increasingly fast CT scanners, the injection for CT angiography may become shorter, and scan timing strategy for CT angiography may ultimately resemble that of MR angiography in that scan delay is estimated by integrating contrast arrival, injection duration, and scan duration.

Contrast Injection Rate

In our previous study [1], we have shown that increasing only the rate of contrast medium injection with constant volume and iodine concentration elevates the magnitude of peak enhancement, shortens the duration of peak enhancement, and leads to an early occurrence of peak enhancement. This shortened but elevated peak enhancement is highly desirable in a fast arterial CT scan, e.g., multidetector row CT angiography study, whereas a longer injection is preferred for a long-duration CT scan.

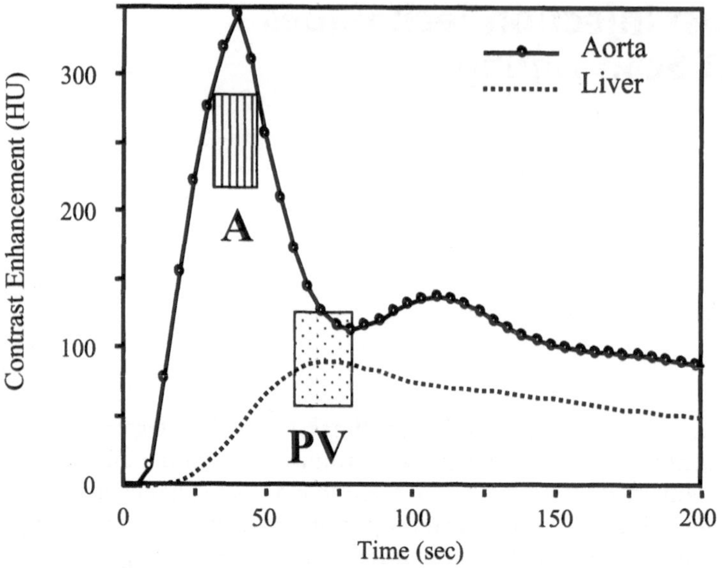

Fig. 1. Simulated aortic and hepatic contrast enhancement curves in a human model with a high contrast injection rate. Aortic (*solid line*) and hepatic (*dashed line*) contrast enhancement curves are simulated using a physiologically based compartment model (body weight 150 lbs and height 5′8″), subject to a high injection rate protocol (150 mL of 320 mgI/ml contrast medium injected at 5 ml/s) [9]. With an increase in injection rate, not only the magnitude of arterial enhancement increases, but also the arterial (*A*) and venous (*PV*) phases of enhancement separate more temporally. This distinct phase separation is beneficial to dual-phase scans of the liver, pancreas, and kidney

The increase in the magnitude of peak enhancement is different in the aorta and in visceral organs. The increase in the aorta is nearly proportional to the increase in injection rate. In contradistinction, the rate of increase in the magnitude of peak hepatic enhancement is much more gradual and apparent only at relatively low injection rates. With an increase in injection rate, not only the magnitude of arterial enhancement increases, but also the arterial and venous phases of enhancement separate more temporally (Fig. 1). This distinct phase separation is beneficial to dual-phase scans of the liver, pancreas, and kidney, because CT images enhanced optimally at each contrast enhancement phase may improve the detection and characterization of lesions.

Contrast Injection Bolus Shaping

The shape of injecting contrast bolus can be tailored to achieve a desired enhancement pattern. The most commonly used contrast bolus shape is a uniphasic injection, i.e., a constant rate for the duration of the injection. With this injection, the arterial time-enhancement response progressively increases and peaks shortly after the completion of the injection, followed by relatively rapid decline in enhancement. This enhancement pattern is referred to as hump enhancement

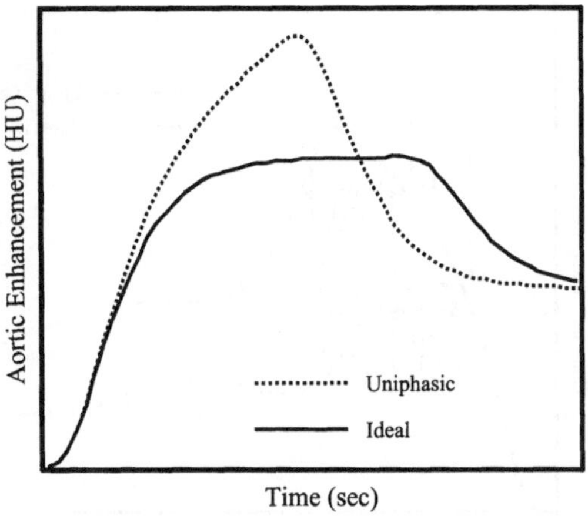

Fig. 2. Simulated aortic contrast enhancement curves in a human model with uniphasic and exponential-decay injections. Uniphasic (*dashed line*) and exponential-decay (*solid line*) injections were simulated with the same amount of contrast medium. For the uniphasic injection, a rate of 3 ml/s was used and the injection duration was 53 s. For the exponential-decay injection, an initial rate of 3 ml/s was used with a 0.01 exponential-decay coefficient. Uniform, prolonged contrast enhancement was achieved with the exponential-decay injection

without a true plateau peak enhancement. The second commonly used injection bolus shape is a biphasic injection, i.e., a fast constant-rate injection followed by a slow constant-rate injection. This injection technique was widely used before the advent of spiral CT when a prolonged enhancement was desired to match a long and slow CT examination. A biphasic injection typically results in a double-peaked arterial contrast enhancement pattern. Fleischmann et al. [2] reported that a biphasic injection designed individually from a test injection improves the uniformity of contrast enhancement with less interindividual variability.

The third injection bolus shaping method is an exponential-decay injection [3]. This injection bolus shape was derived from a physiologically based pharmacokinetic model that predicts that a multiphasic injection bolus with exponentially decreasing rate provides the most uniform vascular enhancement (Fig. 2). Uniform enhancement is useful for the purpose of image processing and display because some 3-D postprocessing techniques are based on a threshold CT attenuation value [4]. Non-uniform enhancement can result in artifactual findings such as filling defects and perceived stenoses [5, 6]. Uniform enhancement is also crucial to achieve a steady-state plasma concentration of iodinated contrast medium during image acquisition for a CT brain perfusion study [7]. Finally, uniform enhancement during image acquisition may alleviate a rigorous image-timing process that is required to synchronize imaging and peak contrast enhancement as in uniphasic injection technique.

Injection Duration

When imaging time is very short, one may be tempted to use a short and very fast injection to achieve a desired arterial enhancement level during image acquisition. This scheme would always work if no limitation existed on the rate of injection we can use. In practice, however, the upper limit of injection rate is frequently limited to 5 ml/s. With this rate, injection of 320 mgI/ml contrast medium for 15 s in a 75-kg individual rate may reach barely over 100 HU peak

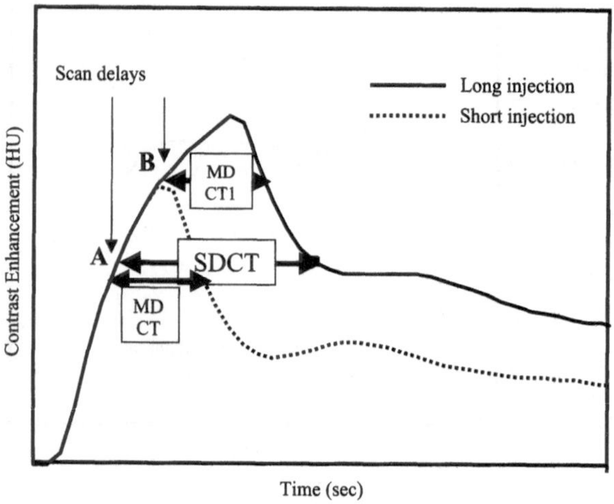

Fig. 3. Simulated aortic contrast enhancement curves in a human model with long and short contrast injections. With a slow CT scan (*SDCT* single-detector row CT), a long injection is preferred to maintain a good enhancement during image acquisition. One may be tempted to use a short injection for a fast scan (*MDCT* multidetector row CT), but then the enhancement may not be sufficiently high. A preferred approach for MDCT scan is keeping the injection duration long but increasing the scan delay from *A* to *B* (*MDCT1*) to acquire image during maximal contrast enhancement

aortic enhancement. This degree of enhancement is not sufficient in most CT applications. Since the injection rate cannot be increased further, in order to generate higher arterial enhancement, the injection duration should be increased. The amount of iodine within the central blood volume increases cumulatively with injection duration, resulting in elevation of peak enhancement. One may use contrast medium of a higher concentration to increase the delivery of iodine mass at a constant injection rate, but again there is a practical limitation on how high the concentration of contrast media can be.

Injection duration is closely related to the magnitude and time to peak enhancement [8]. Injection duration should be prolonged for a long CT scan to maintain good enhancement throughout image acquisition. Too long an injection duration results in wasting contrast medium and in generating unwanted tissue and venous contrast enhancement, but too short an injection duration leads to insufficiently enhanced CT images. There are many factors involved in determining optimal injection duration, such as desired level of enhancement, body size, vessel or organ of interest, contrast concentration, and injection rate [9]. For single-detector row CT angiography, the injection duration is usually set to be the same as the scan duration, but with dramatically reduced scan duration in multidetector row CT, this rule of thumb is no longer applicable. Regardless of scan speed, injection should be sufficiently long to achieve a good enhancement. Injection duration should be kept more or less the same even with a very fast CT scan (Fig. 3). On the other hand, injection duration should be increased further when a longer scan is required.

Our recent study [8] demonstrated that the time to peak aortic enhancement is closely associated with the injection duration and the circulation time. For injection duration shorter than the peak time of a test bolus (T_{TEST}), the time to peak aortic enhancement increases very gradually with injection duration. For injection duration longer than the time T_{TEST}, the aortic enhancement peaks shortly after the end of the injection period, representing the maximal accumulation of contrast medium within the central blood volume compartment. For a typical clinical application, in which an antecubital vein is used as the injection site, we need to also consider a measurement delay time, (called the bolus transfer time [T_{BT}]), from the injection site to the aorta, for the calculation of time to peak aortic enhancement from the start of injection. T_{BT} is slightly shorter than the contrast arrival time. A close relationship between T_{BT} and contrast arrival time (T_{ARR}) was also demonstrated by their similar temporal response to reduced cardiac outputs [10]. T_{BT} and T_{ARR} demonstrated a near identical degree of increase with progressively reduced cardiac outputs. Furthermore, T_{BT} and T_{ARR} will be reduced with faster contrast injection that will facilitate shortening of the contrast travel time.

Scan Timing

CT scanning speed has dramatically increased with multidetector row CT. Because of a fast image acquisition, proper selection of scan timing is critical to optimize contrast enhancement. Improperly-timed scanning may result in reduced contrast enhancement, unwanted venous and background tissue enhancement, and, in some cases, artifacts. Three commonly used approaches for scan timing are a fixed empiric delay, test bolus, and bolus tracking. A fixed delay approach may be adequate for many routine chest and abdominal CT applications. The main advantage of this approach is that it is simple and easy to use; but with this approach, it is difficult to adjust the scan delay, taking into consideration individual patient variations and different contrast medium injection protocols. This is a critical drawback, particularly in optimizing contrast enhancement for dedicated CT angiography applications. With multidetector row CT, because of its shorter scan duration, a fixed delay that is used for routine chest and abdominal CT examinations on single-detector row CT should be increased by 5–15 s to avoid scanning too early (see Fig. 3).

The test-bolus approach is based on injecting a test bolus prior to a full bolus of contrast medium. The test bolus consists of a small amount of contrast medium injected rapidly, usually at the same rate as the full bolus in CT angiography. Immediately following the test-bolus injection, multiple sequential images are acquired at a fixed scan level and a time-enhancement curve is obtained by measuring the enhancement within a region of interest (ROI) chosen over the aorta at that level. The time to peak contrast enhancement of this test-bolus injection (T_{TEST}) is measured and used to calculate the scan delay for the full-bolus injection. T_{TEST}, which is related to the circulation time, helps adjust for individual variations in scan timing. Scan delay (T_{DELAY}) in CT angiography is commonly selected at the time to peak test-bolus contrast enhancement (T_{TEST}) in single-detector CT. However, this exact approach may result in scanning too early in multidetector row CT, again because of shorter scan duration, requiring an additional delay. Although this additional delay depends on the vessels or scan direction, 8–10 s appears adequate in most CT angiography applications (see Fig. 3).

The test-bolus method requires two separate contrast injections and involves additional radiation and examination time. A preferred and more practical approach is the bolus-tracking method. This method begins with placing an ROI on a vessel or organ of interest on a precontrast reference image. While a full bolus of contrast medium is injected, contrast enhancement within the ROI is monitored with serial low-dose, stationary scans. When the enhancement exceeds a predetermined threshold, e.g., 50 or 100 HU, CT scan is triggered. With an additional trigger delay of 2–8 s, CT scan starts. The bolus-tracking method is a robust technique and may be the best available approach for determining scan delay for CT angiography. However, just as an additional delay is required in the test-bolus method, there are two fuzzy factors involved in the bolus-tracking method to estimate the scan delay. It is uncertain what threshold value for the trigger is appropriate and what additional trigger delay should be used. An alternative strategy for determining a scan delay is to use a relatively low threshold value, 30–50 HU, in the bolus-tracking method just to detect the contrast arrival. This contrast arrival time is integrated with the injection duration to predict peak enhancement time. The scan delay is estimated by appropriately timing the center of the scan with the time to peak aortic enhancement [8].

Summary

With dramatically shorter image acquisition times for multidetector row CT, optimization of contrast enhancement and scan timing has become increasingly crucial. Among many interacting factors involved in contrast enhancement, contrast injection rate, injection duration, and injection bolus shaping are key factors determining the temporal pattern of contrast enhancement. A high injection rate provides intense arterial contrast enhancement and is preferred in CT angiography and dual-phase CT applications. Injection bolus shaping with an exponential-decay injection method may be used to generate a uniform prolonged contrast enhancement.

The time to peak aortic enhancement is closely associated with injection duration and circulation time. To optimize contrast enhancement timing during a scan, particularly for patients with slow cardiac output, scan delay should be determined individually by test-bolus or bolus-tracking techniques. Scan delay computed from the time to peak test-bolus contrast enhancement may be too early for multidetector row CT, requiring an additional delay. Contrast arrival time measured from the bolus-tracking method may be integrated with the injection duration to predict peak enhancement time. The scan delay is estimated such that the time to peak aortic enhancement is appropriately allocated within the scan duration.

In the future, a fully automated system of determining optimal contrast enhancement and scanning may be developed by integrating various injection and scanning parameters and bolus-tracking techniques. This will eliminate the need for a test-bolus injection and the use of intuition to figure out complex relationship between pharmacokinetic and imaging parameters.

References

1. Bae KT, Heiken JP, Brink JA (1998) Aortic and hepatic peak enhancement at CT: effect of contrast medium injection rate – pharmacokinetic analysis and experimental porcine model. Radiology 206:455–64
2. Fleischmann D, Rubin GD, Bankier AA, Hittmair K (2000) Improved uniformity of aortic enhancement with customized contrast medium injection protocols at CT angiography. Radiology 214:363–71
3. Bae KT, Tran HQ, Heiken JP (2000) Multiphasic injection method for uniform prolonged vascular enhancement at CT angiography: pharmacokinetic analysis and experimental porcine model. Radiology 216:872–80
4. Rubin GD, Paik DS, Johnston PC, Napel S (1998) Measurement of the aorta and its branches with helical CT. Radiology 206:823–9
5. Funabashi N, Kobayashi Y, Perlroth M, Rubin GD (2003) Coronary artery: quantitative evaluation of normal diameter determined with electron-beam CT compared with cine coronary angiography initial experience. Radiology 226:263–71
6. Hsu RM (2002) Computed tomographic angiography: conceptual review of injection and acquisition parameters with a brief overview of rendering technique. Appl Radiology, June (supplement):33–39
7. Eastwood JD, Lev MH, Provenzale JM (2003) Perfusion CT with iodinated contrast material. AJR Am J Roentgenol 180:3–12
8. Bae KT (2003) Peak contrast enhancement in CT and MR angiography: when does it occur and why? Radiology 227(3):809–816
9. Bae KT, Heiken JP, Brink JA (1998) Aortic and hepatic contrast medium enhancement at CT. Part I. Prediction with a computer model. Radiology 207:647–55
10. Bae KT, Heiken JP, Brink JA (1998) Aortic and hepatic contrast medium enhancement at CT. Part II. Effect of reduced cardiac output in a porcine model. Radiology 207:657–62

11 Contrast Medium Injection in MSCT: Present Status and Future Perspectives

R. Passariello, C. Catalano, F. Venditti, M. Danti

Introduction

In the past years, we have assisted with several technical developments which have totally changed the performances of computed tomography (CT) equipment. Starting from the early 1970s, the scan time was several minutes, the reconstruction time was almost 1 min, the minimum slice thickness was more than 1 cm, the matrix was limited and the contrast resolution was poor. By the late 1990s and the year 2000, there were dramatic improvements in terms of speed of acquisition and reconstruction with a reduction in slice thickness to less than 1 mm and a significant increase in spatial resolution. These technical improvements also meant the possibility to perform new types of studies with CT previously not possible, such as high-resolution dynamic evaluation of parenchymal organs and lesions and non-invasive angiographies.

The faster acquisition has also determined an increase in velocity of contrast media (cm) administration: drip infusion has been substituted by bolus injection with power injectors [1]. At the same time, contrast agent has to be injected at faster flow rates and, most importantly, the timing of cm is strictly related to the heart rate of the patient and his cardiac output. Already with the latest sequential scanners, the circulation time and, as a consequence, the delay time, could be toughly calculated knowing the heart rate of the patient [2].

After the introduction of spiral CT, the mode of cm administration again changed. It is evident that the best contrast enhancement is obtained when the maximum concentration of iodine in the scanned volume is reached during the effective acquisition temporal window. To reach the best contrast enhancement, several different modes of injection have been proposed. These are either uniphasic or biphasic [3,12]. Nevertheless, none of them has provided a prolonged optimal vascular enhancement, to obtain which a mode of injection tailored for each patient was needed, as shown by Fleischmann et al. [4]. Although the customized administration of contrast agent appears the most efficacious, it is rarely utilized in clinical practice, being complicated and making the examination more prolonged. In multislice spiral CT, the temporal window for cm administration has been further reduced by about eight times relative to single-slice spiral CT, with 1 s gantry rotation time.

The contrast enhancement in all CT examinations, but significantly more in spiral CT, depends upon several factors: the amount of contrast agent, the injection flow rate, the synchronization with scanning, the type of vascularization of organs and lesions, the contrast to noise ratio and, finally, the type of contrast medium and its main features (osmolarity, viscosity, vascular persistence and iodine concentration).

The amount of cm administered has a limited and relative significance in arterial enhancement. The enhancement in the venous and parenchymatous phases is determined by the amount of cm administered. Therefore, if a multislice CT arterial study has to be performed, there is no need to administer large amounts of cm; the overall quantity can be easily calculated according to the patient circulation time and imaging window. If a CT study in a venous-delayed phase must be performed, larger quantities of cm must be injected to obtain sufficient venous enhancement in order also to avoid and limit excessive dilution of the contrast agent.

The correct injection flow rate is crucial to obtain good arterial enhancement but has a limited importance regarding the parenchymatous and venous enhancement. Nevertheless, in consideration of the limited acquisition temporal window, a compromise has to be made between the amount of cm administered and the flow rate. Therefore, a high flow rate has to be utilized, particularly when a fast scanning protocol (4 x 5-mm collimation thickness) is applied [5].

In order to obtain an excellent arterial enhancement, the cm administration has to be correctly synchronized with scanning: in consideration of the short scanning time, the possibility of timing errors is significantly higher than with single-slice spiral CT. The method used for determination of the delay time of single-slice spiral CT can be applied to multislice spiral CT (although they appear more useful in the latter) not only in angiographic studies but also in the assessment of parenchymal organs. A correct synchronization is crucial not only for lesion detection but also for characterization. In fact, the type of vascularization can be well demonstrated, particularly if correct timing is utilized.

Iodine Concentration of Contrast Medium

The type of cm utilized appears also important in multislice spiral CT. The osmolarity and viscosity of cm have a limited significance for arterial, venous, and parenchymatous enhancement, although they may determine variations in flow rate. In all CT angiography (CTA) examinations we perform in our institution, the contrast material was warmed to 37 °C before injection, in order to reduce viscosity.

Although there have been several attempts to prepare contrast agents with a prolonged vascular persistence, similar to intravascular cm for magnetic resonance imaging (MRI), the increased scanning speed reduces the need to increase intravascular persistence. A cm feature that is gaining increased importance in multislice spiral CT is the iodine concentration. In fact, the limited temporal window may be overcome by a high iodine concentration, particularly in the arterial phase of the study.

In our institution, we performed a study comparison of CTA of the peripheral arteries. We used three contrast agents with different iodine concentrations (400 mg I/ml, 350 mg I/ml and 300 mg I/ml) and administered a standard dose of iodine (40 g I/examination) corresponding to 100 ml of 400 mg I/ml, 113 of 350 mg I/ml and 133 of 300 mg I/ml. In all subjects, contrast administration was immediately followed by the injection of 30 ml of saline in order to flush the column of contrast agent throughout the peripheral vessels. Previous studies on magnetic resonance showed the importance of flushing saline bolus after contrast injection that significantly shorten the first appearance time of cm as well as the time to maximal signal intensity (SI) and increased the slope of SI [6,7]. Moreover, the flushing volumes wash out effects of the contrast within veins at the injection site and allow real utilization of the entire amount of contrast media we inject. Signal intensity was calculated using standard ROIs positioned at six arterial segments from the celiac trunk to the distal trifurcation vessels. Although the same amount of iodine was utilized, there was a significant increase in attenuation values in the arterial proportional to the concentration of I/ml. The increase of attenuation values (but overall of the distal vessels' visibility and enhancement) in the visual analysis has been significant using a cm with 400 mg I/ml.

In order to determine the importance of the parameter flow of iodine (mg I/s), in a sond phase of our study, we kept the flow rate constant at 3.5 ml/s. For this group we found significant differences in the comparison between 300 mg I/ml and 400 mg I/ml, with the exception of the subpopliteal district; therefore measured values in the group injected with 300 mg I/ml cm were statistically lower than in the other groups. Significant results have also been demonstrated of the correlation of 400 mg I/ml vs. with all the others groups (Dunnett Test $p = 0.02$) (Fig. 1).

All manufacturers of cm are now evaluating the possibility of developing a cm with even higher concentration, which may be particularly useful in the case of a

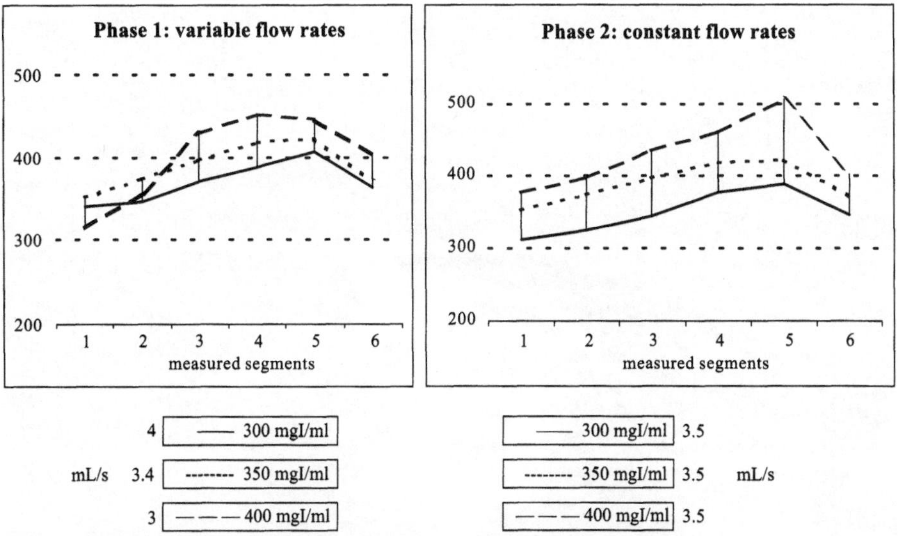

Fig. 1. High versus low iodine contrast agents in MSCTA (Measured segments: *1* aorta, *2* common iliac artery, *3* common femoral artery, *4* superficial femoral artery, *5* popliteal artery, *6* one among the trifurcation vessels)

short scanning time during which a high concentration of iodine must be rapidly reached.

Another experimental study was performed in our institution on a pig model, in order to evaluate the possibility of injecting a contrast agent with a significantly higher iodine concentration (500 mg I/ml) and to compare it with a commercially available contrast agent, with a clinically used concentration (350 mg I/ml). The dose of iodine was 0.5 g I/kg, the flow rate was 3 ml/s with an injection duration time of 23–26 s for 500 mg I/ml cm and of 33–38 s for 350 mg I/ml cm.

In six pigs we evaluated the abdominal vascularization (three injected with 500 mg I/ml and three with 350 mgI/ml), in the remaining two we studied the carotid arterial enhancement. All quantitative analyses were performed positioning a standard ROI (3 mm in diameter) in the aorta, the IVC, the portal vein, the hepatic artery and the carotid artery. In all arterial segments the enhancement was significantly higher when using the 500 mg I/ml contrast agent.

Also for depiction and characterization of hypervascular hepatic lesions such as HCC nodules, recent studies have demonstrated that the use of higher concentrations of iodine cm led to a significantly higher tumor-to-liver contrast and, therefore, to a better detection of hypervascular nodules [8] (Fig. 2).

An important aspect in multidetector-row spiral CT is the flow rate to be utilized. In general, we may say that it depends on the scanned volume and scanning time. Therefore, we must distinguish between examinations of single organs with the purpose of performing tissue characterization, functional studies, and examinations of large volumes, particularly of vascular structures using a thin-slice collimation. In the first case, a higher flow rate (5–6 ml/s) has to be utilized

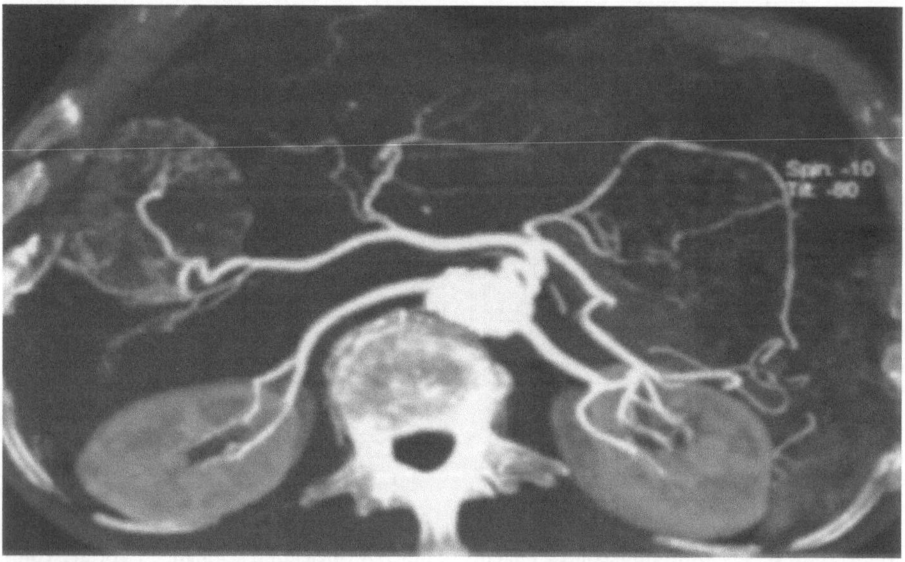

Fig. 2. MSCTA of an hypervascular HCC nodule

in order to administer a consistent amount of cm during the short scanning time. In the case of prolonged acquisition, the flow rate can be reduced (3–4 ml/s) without affecting the overall amount administered.

CT Angiography (CTA)

The target for research on CTA today is to reach the maximal arterial iodine concentration within such short scanning time [4]. In multislice spiral CTA, the amount of contrast agent may vary according to the scanning volumes and time. If a small volume (intracranial circulation, carotid arteries) is studied, a limited amount of cm can be utilized and injected at a high flow rate. The same injection protocol can be applied also when assessing the pulmonary vasculature in cases of suspected pulmonary embolism [9]. In all of these examples, multislice spiral CT allows a reduction in the overall amount of IV cm of at least 35% but even greater in most cases. When large volumes must be scanned, the amount of IV cm must necessarily be increased, although still limited relative to single-slice spiral CT.

Particularly when a limited volume is studied and the scanning time is short, it is advisable to avoid too early or delayed studies, to perform a test bolus sequence or to find a method for determination of bolus arrival. By performing a test bolus, the possibility of errors is limited to a small percentage.

In an our recent study, we optimized the X-ray dose of CTA in the evaluation of peripheral arterial obstructive disease, performing the examinations at low dose with a reduction of about 60% of the standard custom protocol dose. As is known, CT scans with low dose can reduce the signal-to-noise (S/N) ratio and contrast-to-noise (C/N) ratio of the images. With the possibility of using cm with high iodine concentrations (400 mg I/ml), we achieved an improvement of S/N and C/N in that study and optimal results in detection vascular pathologies with a low dose technique (Fig. 3).

The association of X-ray dose reduction and high iodine concentration contrast media to improve vascular enhancement, may spread assiduous use of CT angiography, in particular for the detection of peripheral arterial obstructive disease.

Body CT

In body CT, the amount of cm relative to single-slice spiral CT can be reduced if a limited volume is scanned. The flow velocity is mainly determined by the slice thickness and is a consequence of the scanning time. If an upper abdomen or thorax study has to be performed using a 5-mm collimation, the flow rate must be high (4–6 ml/s) in order to administer an adequate amount of iodinated contrast agent in a short time. If the acquisition is more prolonged, for instance in the case of thin-slice collimation, the contrast agent can be injected at a slower rate (3 ml/s).

Although experimental data indicate an inverse relationship between hepatic contrast enhancement at CT and patient weight, most radiologists administer a

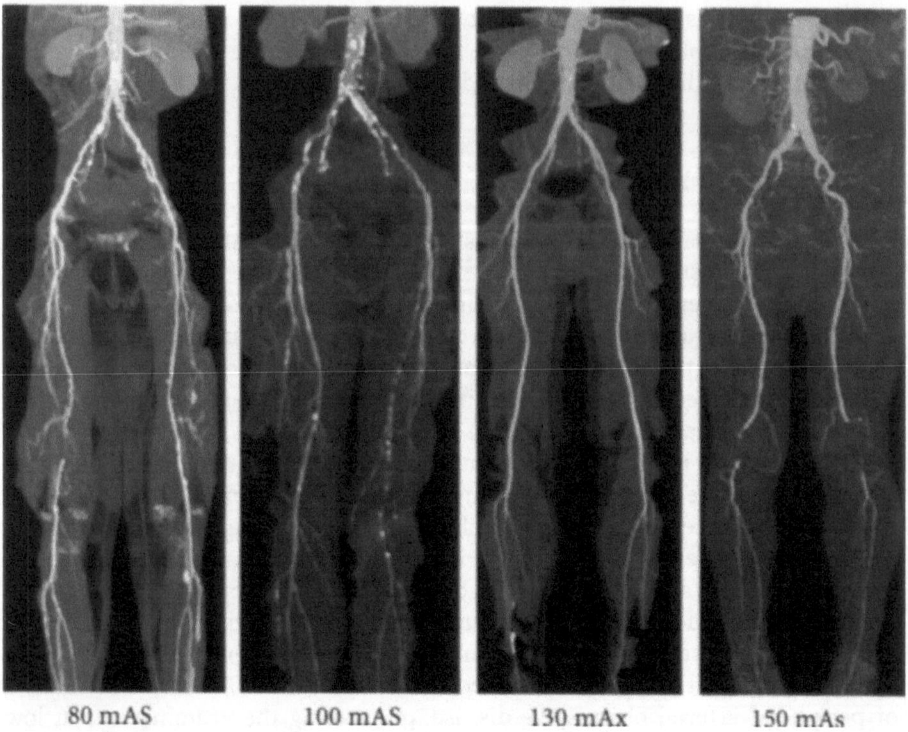

Fig. 3. Comparison of low-dose protocols at MSCTA of peripheral vs. standard arteries: no significant difference is seen either in vascular enhancement, or in detection of stenosis, among the protocols using a higher iodine concentration cm (400 mg I/ml)

uniform dose of cm in all patients. Yamashita et al. have reported better results in performing abdominal CT examinations when the dose of cm is tailored to patient weight [10].

Therefore, the flow rate and, as a consequence, the volume injected, must be modified according to the type of study to be performed and the scanning time and also to the patient's characteristics.

In conclusion, after the introduction of multislice spiral CT, one of the main problems to be solved is the modality of cm administration [11]. The overall quantity, flow rate and type of cm to be utilized still need to be determined. With regard to the cm amount, it seems from this early experience that significantly reduced doses can be utilized relative to single-slice spiral CT, particularly in CTA examinations. Customized protocols may be useful for obtaining a constant and prolonged vascular enhancement, although they may require complicated calculations that are not strictly necessary. The technique of multislice spiral CT is brand new and experimental studies are needed also to determine the best cm to be injected and the modality of administration.

References

1. Passariello R (1985) Angio-CT techniques. Eur J Radiol 5:193–198
2. Passariello R et al. (1980) Automatic contrast medium injector for computer tomography. J Comput Assist Tomogr 4:278–279
3. Heiken JP et al. (1993) Dynamic contrast-enhanced CT of the liver: comparison of contrast medium injection rates and uniphasic and biphasic injection protocols. Radiology 187:327–331.
4. Fleishmann D et al. (1999) Mathematical analysis of arterial enhancement and optimization of bolus geometry for CT angiography using the discrete Fourier transform. J Comput Assist Tomogr 23:474–484
5. Blomey MJ et al. (1997) Bolus dynamics: theoretical and experimental aspects. Br J Radiol; 70:351–359
6. Boos M et al. (2001) Arterial first pass Gadolinium-CM dynamics as a function of several intravenous saline flush and Gd volumes. JMR
7. Mitsuzaki K et al. (1999) Optimal protocol for injection of contrast material at MR Angiography: study of healthy volunteers. Radiology 213:913–918
8. Awai K et al. (2002) Aortic and hepatic enhancement and tumor-to-liver contrast: analysis of the effects of different concentrations of contrast material at multi-detector row helical CT. Radiology 224:757–763
9. Brink JA et al. (1997) Depistion of pulmonary emboli with spiral CT: optimization of display window settings in a porcine model. 204:703–708
10. Yamashita Y et al. (2000) Abdominal helical CT: evaluation of optimal doses of intravenous contrast material-A prospective study. Radiology 216:718–723
11. Luboldt W et al. (1999) effective contrast use in CT angiography and dual-phase hepatic CT performed with a subsecond scanner. Invest Radiol 26:751–750
12. Fleischmann D et al. (2000) Improved uniformity of aortic enhancement with customized contrast medium injection protocols at CT Angiography 214:363–371

12 Multislice CT Angiography of Abdominal Visceral Vessels

G.P. Krestin, F. Cademartiri

Introduction

The gold standard for the study of abdominal vessels is conventional digital subtraction angiography (DSA). The development of non-invasive modalities for the visualization of vessels has been one of the challenges of the latest technical developments in vascular imaging. Computed tomography (CT), and magnetic resonance (MR) have been used for the assessment of vascular diseases in the past decade.

Spiral CT technology markedly improved the possibilities for the application in vascular imaging. The possibility to scan a continuous volume of data during one breath-hold, and to reconstruct overlapping slices at independent z-axis position, determined an increased consistency of the dataset. This resulted in an improved capability of visualization of structures running in axial and irregular planes, such as renal arteries and the branches of the celiac trunk and superior mesenteric artery. Hence, spiral CT has become a widely used non-invasive tool for the study of diseases of the abdominal aorta and its main branches.

Multislice CT (MSCT) determined a consistent improvement in the performance compared to single detector spiral CT scanners [1]. Performance of MSCT is related to the multiple rows of detectors and to the increased gantry rotation speed. Multislice CT technology combines therefore high in-plane and through-plane spatial resolution, with high temporal resolution [1].

A new generation of MSCT scanners, able to image up to 16 slices simultaneously, with a gantry rotation time of 500 ms, and 0.75 mm collimation, has been recently introduced (Sensation 16: Siemens Medical Solutions, Forchheim, Germany). These technical improvements further increase the potential of MSCT angiography for the study of smaller vessels or for an accurate evaluation of vessel lesions. Scan time and spatial resolution are no longer determining parameters, and motion artefacts from pulsation, peristalsis and possibly breathing, only modestly influence the resulting images.

Large abdominal vessels, like abdominal aorta or iliac arteries, have been studied since the beginning of spiral CT imaging. The orientation along the z-axis, and the large diameter determined ideal conditions for good imaging. The possibility of evaluation of smaller vessels suffered from low spatial resolution both in-plane and through-plane. Multislice CT reduced these limitations, with a concomitant increase in diagnostic performance. The further improvement of spatial and temporal resolution introduced by 16-row MSCT scanners allows the

Table 1. Indications for MSCT angiography in abdominal CTA

Splancnic arteries	Renal arteries	Iliac arteries and runoff
Chronic mesenteric ischaemia	Suspected renal artery stenosis	Aneurysms and dissections
Acute thrombo-embolism	Renal donor evaluation and renal graft follow-up	Atherosclerotic occlusion' (claudicatio)
Aneurysms and dissections	Preoperative roadmapping	Acute thrombo-embolism
Neoplastic encasement	Stent planning and follow-up	Preoperative roadmapping
Preoperative liver transplant evaluation		
Postoperative assessment of vascular liver transplant complications		

integration of this technology for routine evaluation of abdominal visceral vessels in all clinical settings. Most of the branches of the abdominal aorta can be easily evaluated with MSCT as a primary diagnostic tool, in roadmapping for surgical procedures and for follow up after vascular interventions.

Methods

The most common indications for MS-CTA of abdominal visceral arteries are summarized in Table 1.

Patient Preparation

No preparation is needed for patients undergoing abdominal MSCT angiography. In some cases, when information about small-bowel or retroperitoneal space are needed, water can be administered orally (10 min before) in order to visualize the bowel loops.

Four-Row and 16-Row MSCT Angiography Protocol

The scan and reconstruction protocols for 4-row and 16-row MSCT are similar in concept (Table 2). They differ mainly by their spatial resolution (from 1 to 0.75 mm collimation). Speed of rotation is the same (500 ms). The sub-millimetric resolution and the shorter scan time determine also a reduction in the total volume of contrast material required for 16-row scanners (from 140 to 100 ml). Technical problems have been solved in order to reduce the artefacts due to cone-beam projection in the new generation of 16-row MSCT scanners. A dedicated reconstruction algorithm affecting image preprocessing preserves image quality without significant distortions.

Table 2. MSCT angiography abdominal scan protocols

Parameters	SSCT[a]	4-MSCT[b]	16-MSCT[c]
Scan			
Detectors	1	4	16
Collimation	3 mm	1 mm	0.75 mm
Feed/rotation (nPitch)[d]	4.5–6 mm (1.5–2.0)	4–6 mm (1–1.5)	12–18 (1–1.5)
Rotation time	1–0.75 s	0.5 s	0.5 s
KV/mAs	120/130	120/130	120/130
Reconstruction			
Effective slice width	3 mm	1–1.25 mm	0.75–1.0 mm
FOV[e]	300 mm	300 mm	300 mm
Increment	1 mm	0.7 mm	0.4–0.6 mm
Filter	Medium smooth	Medium smooth	Medium smooth
Contrast material			
Access	Antecubital	Antecubital	Antecubital
Volume	140 ml	140 ml	100 ml
Rate	3.0–3.5 ml/s	3.5–4.0 ml/s	4.0–5.0 ml/s
Iodine concentration	>320 mg I/ml	>320 mg I/ml	>320 mg I/ml
Injection time	40–46.7 s	35–40 s	20–25 s
Scan time for 30 cm	37.5–66.7 s	37.5–25 s	12.5–7.9 s

[a] *SSCT* single slice CT;
[b] *4-MSCT* 4-row multislice CT;
[c] *16-MSCT* 16-row multislice CT;
[e] *FOV* field of view;
[d] *nPitch* nor[a]*SSCT* sinmalized pitch.

Contrast Material Administration

The optimization of contrast material administration is mandatory to obtain the best results from the angiographic scan [2] (see Table 2). For this purpose, a high injection rate and a power injector should be used compatibly with the size of the IV access and of the chosen vein. To reduce the amount of contrast material needed to preserve image quality, a saline chaser (by means of a double head injector) can be administered in bolus just after the main bolus to flush the contrast material still present in the veins of the arm and in the right heart. With this technique up to 40% of contrast material volume can be spared [2].

Scan time affects the injection parameters and in particular the volume of contrast material. In fact, a 16-row MSCT scan of the entire abdomen can last less than 10 s, and a study of the renal arteries less than 3 s. Therefore the amount of contrast media that needs to be injected can be very low. To reduce the volume of contrast material while maintaining a good peak of attenuation in the vessels, accurate bolus timing techniques should be applied [2]. Our experience with the 16-row MSCT scanner (Sensation 16, Siemens Medical Solutions, Forchheim,

Germany) suggests that a bolus tracking technique (CARE bolus, Siemens Medical Solutions, Forchheim, Germany) provides more reliable and homogeneous results regardless of the patients' characteristics (e.g. body weight, cardiac ejection fraction, heart rate). With bolus tracking a region of interest (ROI) is positioned inside the aorta at the proximal end of the vascular territory to be studied. A threshold is set for the ROI at 100–150 HU above the baseline attenuation level. Contrast material administration and a low-dose monitoring scan series are started at the same time and when the attenuation level in the ROI reaches the threshold value, the scan is automatically triggered.

Post-Processing

The reconstructed images are usually sent to a stand-alone workstation (Leonardo – Siemens Medical Solutions, Forchheim, Germany) for multiplanar and three-dimensional post-Processing. In our experience, conventional film reporting cannot be performed with a multislice dataset because of the large number of images and the constant need of tools to exploit information. The operator performs multiplanar reconstructions (MPR), multiple intensity projections (MIP), and Volume Rendering (VR) reconstructions in order to visualize the configuration and the patency of abdominal vessels. Multiplanar reconstructions are suitable for every application but can be suboptimal in the case of kinking structures. Therefore a curved planar reconstruction (CPR) can be applied in order to stretch the lumen into one plane. The advantage of this technique is that it excludes most of the overlapping structures from the plane of interest, but it can heavily modify spatial relationships between the vessels and surroundings.

The variable anatomy and patient characteristics need tailored planes and reconstruction parameters. For instance, when heavy calcifications are present, an MIP algorithm will be applied with thinner slabs in the coronal and sagittal planes. This will reduce masking of the lumen by calcifications.

Volume rendering is an algorithm that relies on different opacity curves in order to represent different tissues, and shading to create the 3-D effect on the two-dimensional image. It can be useful to enclose the information into one or few images, and can be helpful in the diagnostic phase at the level of the superior mesenteric artery and celiac trunk to better understand the modified vascular anatomy at this level [3, 4]. Volume rendering has also proved to be superior to MIP and suitable for the detection and evaluation of renal arteries [5].

In selected cases, the reconstruction can be focused to the celiac trunk and its branches and on the superior mesenteric artery and its branches. Manual segmentation is generally not necessary, unless interposing and/or overlapping structures limit the field of view. Stenosis can be quantified following the common angiographic criteria, or introducing more parameters such as two orthogonal diameters or the area of the vessel (measured on an orthogonal section plane).

Applications

Conventional DSA is the gold standard for the detection of vascular diseases of the abdomen, but it suffers from several drawbacks. In fact, it is invasive, costly, time-consuming and uncomfortable. Moreover, the extravascular/extrinsic etiology of vascular diseases can be missed.

With single detector spiral CT angiography (CTA) a robust and reliable tool for non-invasive vascular abdominal imaging was introduced. At the beginning, several issues limited the potential of CTA. In particular, the long scan time needed when thin collimation protocols where applied did not allow performing CTA angiographic studies of the entire abdomen within one breath-hold. Therefore, to scan the entire abdomen with the purpose of CTA, a relatively thick collimation (3 mm) and high pitch (pitch 2) were used. If the scan was performed to image renal arteries only, a protocol with 1–2 mm collimation and pitch of 2 was used. All these protocols suffered from the long scan time that needed a large volume of intravenous contrast material (120–150 ml) and/or a lower injection rate to increase injection time (2–3 ml/s).

Even with these limitations, single-detector CTA already played an important role in management of abdominal aortic aneurysms (diagnosis, stent roadmapping and follow-up, acute settings). Until recently, the branches of the abdominal aorta, however, were studied mainly with conventional digital subtraction angiography.

With four-row MSCT, several limitations of the previous generation of spiral CT scanners have been overcome. In particular, the scan speed has improved, allowing scanning of the entire volume within one breath-hold, using thin collimation (1–1.25 mm). These improvements are related to the gantry rotation time of 500 ms, and to the increased number of detector arrays (up to four).

Splanchnic Arteries

MSCT angiography has already demonstrated its potential in abdominal visceral applications. The mesenteric arteries have been evaluated successfully with MSCT angiography [3, 4, 6–8]. The advantages of MSCT allow performing a quick and non-invasive approach to patients with suspected chronic mesenteric ischaemia (Fig. 1) [4, 9, 10].

Both arterial and venous anatomy and patency can be assessed as well as extra-vascular information, which is important for differential diagnosis. Pancreatic arterial and venous neoplastic involvement can be assessed providing differential criteria in the management of patients with pancreatic cancer (Fig. 2) [11, 12].

The good performance of MSCT angiography in the preoperative road mapping and in the postoperative management of patients undergoing liver transplantation has been already reported [13, 14].

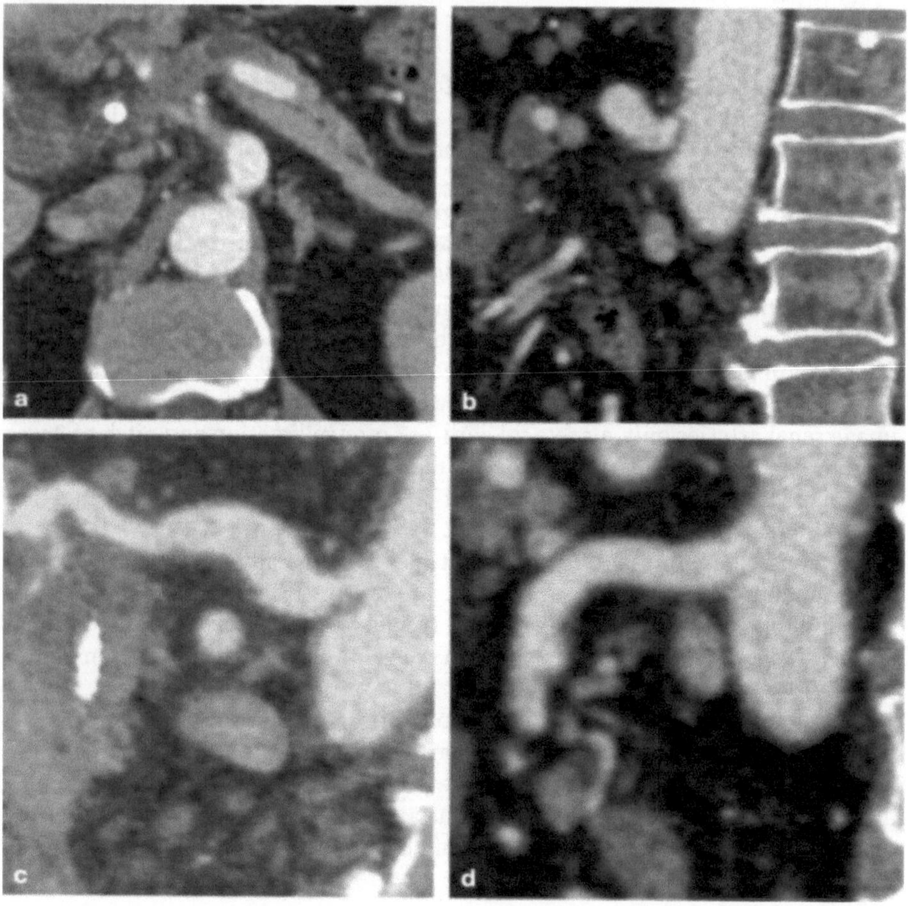

Fig. 1a–h. Example of aterosclerotic disease of the celiaco-mesenteric axes. Stenosis of the celiac trunk with post-stenostic dilatation, displayed in axial, sagittal and curved plane (**a**, **b** and **c**). The superior mesenteric artery appears patent (**d**, **e** and **f**) even if wall abnormalities are present (**f** – *arrow*). Volume rendering reconstructions with thick slab make it possible, to visualise easily the problem at the level of the celiac trunk (**g** and **h**).

Renal Arteries

With single-slice spiral CT angiography overall sensitivity and specificity for assessment of stenoses of grade 0 (none), grade 1 (1–49%), grade 2 (51–99%), and grade 3 (occlusion) were reported as 97 and 100%; 92 and 98%; 96 and 96%; and 100 and 100%, respectively [15]. Good agreement was reported between spiral CT angiographic and DSA findings (K = 0.9) [15]. In another study, sensitivity and specificity were 88 and 98%, respectively, for the detection of stenosis [16]. No series are currently available with MSCT, but further improvement in the results can be expected. Good performance of MSCT in the evaluation of renal stents was reported, and confidence in image interpretation as well as the

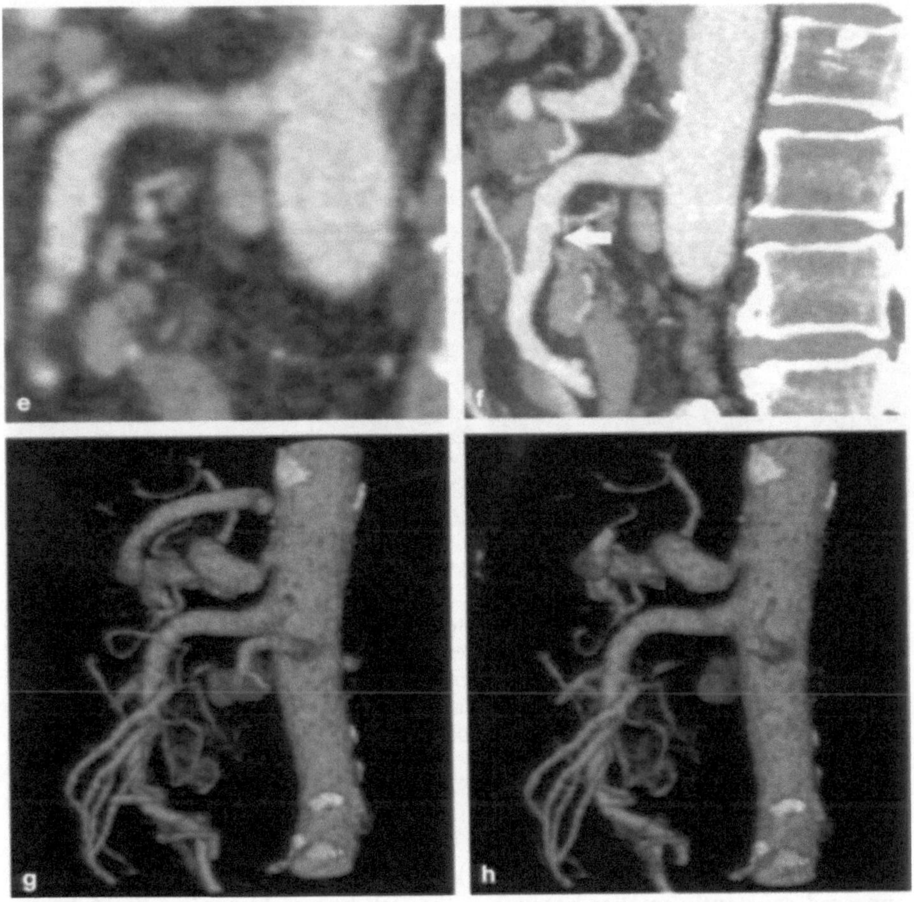

Fig. 1a–h. Continued

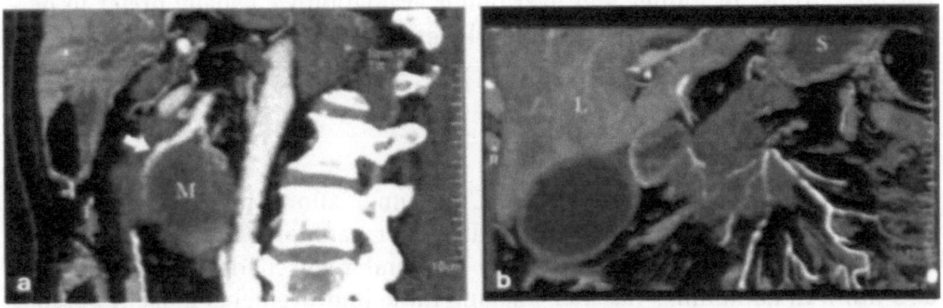

Fig. 2a,b. Example of abdominal vascular encasement. The superior mesenteric artery is encased in a pancreatic mass (*m*). In both the sagittal and coronal plane (**a** and **b**), the walls and the diameter of the superior mesenteric artery appear progressively and irregularly reducing

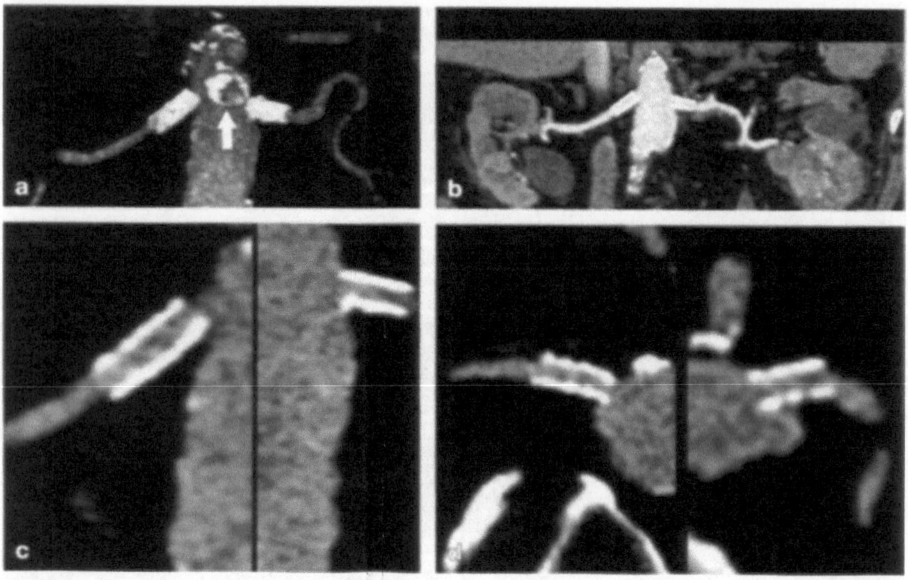

Fig. 3a–d. Example of bilateral renal stent. A stent graft was positioned at the origin of renal arteries on both sides (**a**). In the 3-D volume rendering frontal reconstructions the concentric calcification of the origin of the superior mesenteric artery is also evident (**a** *arrow*). The curved planar reconstruction in the coronal plane shows both renal arteries in their entire pathway (**b**). Focused coronal (**c**) and axial oblique (**d**) reformats allow assessment of the patency of the stents with more accuracy

patency evaluation was optimal (Fig. 3) [17]. However, the lumen of the stents appeared constantly smaller because of the well-known blooming effect due to the hyperattenuation of the stent material [17].

Donor Evaluation

For the purpose of kidney and liver donor evaluation we usually prefer to perform MR angiography, mainly for ethical reasons.

Advantages of 16-Row MSCT

The newer generation of 16-row MSCT scanner allows faster scanning with increased temporal and spatial resolution, by means of more detector arrays, shorter gantry rotation time (e.g. 500 ms) and reduced detector width (e.g. 0.75 mm). In abdominal vascular imaging these improvements make it possible to display stents with higher accuracy, to assess lesions in even smaller vessels, to image patients with low compliance (trauma or acute), to perform isotropic imaging with multiplanar and three-dimensional volume rendering reconstruction, to reduce the amount of intravenous contrast material and to perform plaque imaging. These features are under validation, and preliminary experiences suggest good results. The capability to visualize small vessels increases the need for advanced tools to exploit the potential of the technique. Previously, conventional abdominal CT scan was reported using plain films because of the low number of images per scan. Presently, the amount of information entailed in an abdominal MSCT angiography performed with a 16-row scanner is far more detailed and accurate. Therefore workstation reporting is mandatory in order to fully exploit the information. In addition, the observer (e.g., the radiologist) must be able to use all the available tools for volume navigation (e.g., MPR, MIP, volume rendering) to obtain faster and more accurate diagnostic information. The availability of vessel tracking tools, easy and friendly post-processing workstations and dedicated personnel allow these requirements to be fulfilled for a comprehensive diagnostic approach.

Conclusion

CTA with MSCT technology provides fast motion-free imaging with high resolution and reduced volume of intravenous contrast material. More vessels can be analyzed, however, optimized postprocessing techniques play a major role in order to fully exploit the information contained in the dataset.

A few limitations remain. CTA offers a non-dynamic visualization of the arterial circulation (major diagnostic advantage of conventional DSA) at an increased radiation exposure. Optimization of acquisition protocols and introduction of automated X-ray modulation algorithms will reduce the amount of radiation exposure, keeping image quality unaffected for diagnostic purposes.

Acknowledgements. We thank Rolf Raaijmakers for help in the collection and handling of the imaging material.

References

1. Hu H, He HD, Foley WD, Fox SH (2000) Four multidetector-row helical CT: image quality and volume coverage speed. Radiology 215:55–62
2. Cademartiri F, van der Lugt A, Luccichenti G, Pavone P, Krestin GP (2002) Parameters affecting bolus geometry in CTA: a review. J Comput Assist Tomogr 26:598–607
3. Horton KM, Fishman EK (2000) 3-D CT angiography of the celiac and superior mesenteric arteries with multidetector CT data sets: preliminary observations. Abdom Imaging 25:523–5
4. Horton KM, Fishman EK (2002) Volume-rendered 3D CT of the mesenteric vasculature: normal anatomy, anatomic variants, and pathologic conditions. Radiographics 22:161–72
5. Johnson PT, Halpern EJ, Kuszyk BS et al. (1999) Renal artery stenosis: CT angiography–comparison of real-time volume-rendering and maximum intensity projection algorithms. Radiology 211:337–43
6. Raptopoulos V, Steer ML, Sheiman RG, Vrachliotis TG, Gougoutas CA, Movson JS (1997) The use of helical CT and CT angiography to predict vascular involvement from pancreatic cancer: correlation with findings at surgery. AJR Am J Roentgenol 168:971–7

7. Zeman RK, Davros WJ, Berman P et al. (1994) Three-dimensional models of the abdominal vasculature based on helical CT: usefulness in patients with pancreatic neoplasms. AJR Am J Roentgenol 162:1425–9
8. Laghi A, Iannaccone R, Catalano C, Passariello R (2001) Multislice spiral computed tomography angiography of mesenteric arteries. Lancet 358:638–9
9. Cognet F, Salem DB, Dranssart M et al. (2002) Chronic mesenteric ischemia: imaging and percutaneous treatment. Radiographics 22:863–79; discussion 879–80
10. Horton KM, Fishman EK (2001) Multi-detector row CT of mesenteric ischemia: can it be done? Radiographics 21:1463–73
11. Horton KM, Fishman EK (2002) Multidetector CT angiography of pancreatic carcinoma: part I, evaluation of arterial involvement. AJR Am J Roentgenol 178:827–31
12. Horton KM, Fishman EK (2002) Multidetector CT angiography of pancreatic carcinoma: part 2, evaluation of venous involvement. AJR Am J Roentgenol 178:833–6
13. Katyal S, Oliver JH, 3rd, Buck DG, Federle MP (2000) Detection of vascular complications after liver transplantation: early experience in multislice CT angiography with volume rendering. AJR Am J Roentgenol 175:1735–9
14. Brancatelli G, Katyal S, Federle MP, Fontes P (2002) Three-dimensional multislice helical computed tomography with the volume rendering technique in the detection of vascular complications after liver transplantation. Transplantation 73:237–42
15. Kaatee R, Beek FJ, de Lange EE et al. (1997) Renal artery stenosis: detection and quantification with spiral CT angiography versus optimized digital subtraction angiography. Radiology 205:121–7
16. Beregi JP, Elkohen M, Deklunder G, Artaud D, Coullet JM, Wattinne L (1996) Helical CT angiography compared with arteriography in the detection of renal artery stenosis. AJR Am J Roentgenol 167:495–501
17. Behar JV, Nelson RC, Zidar JP, DeLong DM, Smith TP (2002) Thin-section multidetector CT angiography of renal artery stents. AJR Am J Roentgenol 178:1155–9

V Cardio CT

13 Algorithms and Clinical Application of Multislice Cardiac CT

B. M. Ohnesorge, U. J. Schöpf, K. Nieman, C. R. Becker, T. G. Flohr

Introduction

Cardiac imaging is a demanding application for any non-invasive imaging modality. On the one hand, high temporal resolution is needed to virtually freeze the cardiac motion and to avoid motion artifacts in the images. On the other hand, sufficient spatial resolution – at best sub-millimeter – is required to adequately visualize small and complex anatomical structures like the coronary arteries. The complete heart volume has to be examined within one short breath-hold time to avoid breathing artifacts and to limit the amount of contrast agent if necessary. In 1984, Electron Beam CT (EBCT) has been introduced as a non-invasive imaging modality for the diagnosis of coronary artery disease [1–4]. The temporal resolution of 100 ms allows for motion-free imaging of the cardiac anatomy in the diastolic heart phase even at higher heart rates. Due to the restriction to non-spiral scanning in ECG-synchronized cardiac investigations, a single breath-hold scan of the heart requires slice widths not smaller than 3 mm. The resulting transverse resolution is limited and not adequate for 3D visualization of the coronary arteries. With the advent of sub-second rotation combined with prospective ECG triggering or retrospective ECG gating, mechanical single-slice spiral-CT systems with superior general image quality have been used for cardiac imaging [4, 5]. Since 1999, 4-slice CT systems, which have the potential to overcome the drawbacks of single-slice cardiac CT-scanning, have been used to establish ECG-triggered or ECG-gated multislice CT examinations of the heart and the coronary arteries in clinical use [6–10]. Due to the increased scan speed with four simultaneously acquired slices, coverage of the entire heart volume with thin slices within one breath-hold became feasible. The improved transverse resolution allowed for high-resolution CT imaging of the heart and the coronary arteries [11–14]. First clinical studies have demonstrated the potential of multislice CT to differentiate and classify lipid, fibrous and calcified coronary plaques [15]. Despite all promising advances, some challenges and limitations with respect to motion artifacts in patients with higher heart rates, limited spatial resolution and long breath-hold times remain for 4-slice cardiac CT [12]. In 2001, a new generation of multislice CT systems with simultaneous acquisition of up to 16 slices was introduced [16, 17]. With sub-millimeter slice collimation and gantry rotation times shorter than 0.5 s, spatial resolution and temporal resolution are improved, while examination times are considerably reduced.

In this chapter, we present the technology principles and clinical applications of multislice CT in cardiac imaging and we will discuss the technology advances and improved clinical performance of state-of-the-art 16-slice CT equipment (SOMATOM Sensation 16, Siemens, Germany) compared to 4-slice CT scanners (SOMATOM Sensation 4, Siemens, Germany).

Technology Principles

Technology Overview

CT acquisition of the heart should be performed in a single and short breath-hold scan with high temporal resolution to eliminate cardiac motion and high, isotropic spatial resolution (i.e. sub-millimeter) at the same time to adequately visualize small and complex cardio-thoracic anatomy and the coronary arteries.

In 1984, Electron Beam CT (EBCT) was introduced as the first cross-sectional non-invasive imaging modality that could visualize the cardiac anatomy and the coronary arteries [1]. With presently available EBCT scanners motion-free visualization of the cardiac anatomy is possible in the diastolic phase of the cardiac cycle also at higher heart rates based on a temporal resolution of 100 ms [2]. The heart anatomy can be acquired in a single breath-hold of 30–40 s with slice width of 3 mm that, however, limits the diagnostic accuracy of coronary artery visualization [3]. In 1998, mechanical spiral CT systems with simultaneous acquisition of 4 detector slices and a minimum rotation time of 500 ms were introduced [6, 7, 10] that provided a substantial performance increase over the single- and dual-slice spiral CT systems that had been available until then. These multislice CT scanners can cover larger scan volumes with slice width down to 1.0 mm and thus provide higher spatial resolution for improved visualization of small and complex anatomy and vasculature.

Different detector configurations are in use that enable simultaneous collimation of four slices with different slice widths. In the »fixed array« detector design detector rows with equal spacing are used, the so called »adaptive array« detector design consists of less detector rows with different size that become wider towards the outer area of the detector (Fig. 1). In both concepts the thinnest slices result from collimation of the inner four detector rows and thicker slices are generated by electronic combination of adjacent detector rows.

Higher temporal resolution compared to older mechanical spiral CT scanners is provided by faster rotation speed with rotation time down to 500 ms combined with specialized reconstruction algorithms [10]. Meanwhile, 8- and 10-slice CT scanners are being used that provide further improved volume coverage with about 1 mm slice width and 500 ms rotation time [18]. First 16-slice CT scanners were introduced in early 2002; they provide faster rotation time of 420 ms and sub-millimeter detector collimation for routine volume imaging [16, 17]. All 16-slice CT scanners available today are based on the »adaptive array« detector design. In the example given (SOMATOM Sensation 16, Siemens, Germany, see Fig. 1) the 16 central rows define sub-millimeter detector collimation (i.e. 0.75 mm), the outer four detector rows on both sides define 1.5 mm colli-

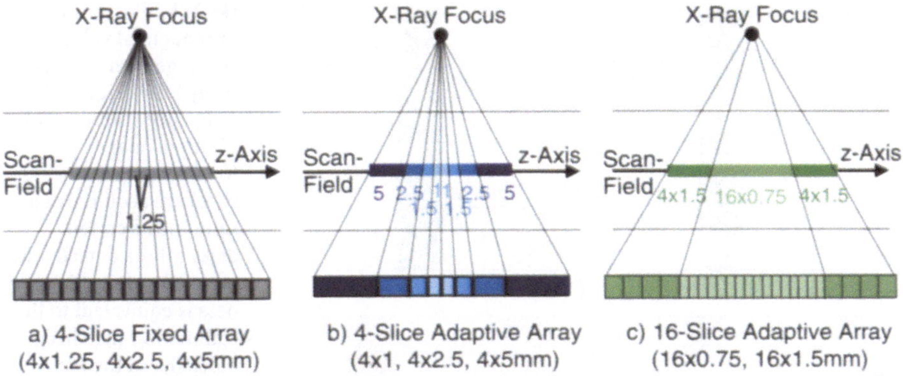

Fig. 1a–c. Equally spaced detector elements build the fixed array detector (FAD) for a 4-slice system (**a**). Different 4-slice collimation settings (4×1.25, 4×2.5, 4×3.75, 4×5 mm) are produced by electronical combination of adjacent elements. Differently sized detector elements build the adaptive array detector (AAD) for a 4-slice system (**b**). Different 4-slice collimation settings (4×2.5, 4×5 mm) are produced by electronical combination of adjacent elements. For 4×1 mm collimation partial shielding of the elements with width 1.5 mm is required. Partial illumination of the inner two detector elements allows for 2×0.5 mm collimation for high-resolution scanning. Latest 16-slice CT scanners are also based on the adaptive array detector (AAD) design with differently sized detector elements (**c**). 16-slice collimation settings 16×0.75 mm and 16×1.5 mm are produced by equally spaced 16×0.75 mm detector elements in the center, 8 additional 1.5 mm detector elements (4 on each side) and electronical combination of adjacent elements

mated slice width. By appropriate combination of the signals of the individual detector rows, either 12 or 16 slices with 0.75 mm or 1.5 mm collimated slice width can be acquired simultaneously. The combination of fast rotation time and multislice acquisition with sub-millimeter spatial resolution has shown to be of particular importance for improved cardiac image quality [17, 19–21].

Motion artifacts that are caused by cardiac pulsation can be minimized in high-resolution CT studies of the heart via scanning or reconstructing scan projection data at a time point with the least cardiac motion, i.e. in the diastolic phase of the heart cycle. The heart phases can be determined from a simultaneously recorded ECG signal. Two different ECG synchronization techniques are most commonly employed for cardiac CT scanning, prospective ECG triggering and retrospective ECG gating.

ECG-Triggered Multislice CT Imaging

Prospective ECG triggering has long been used in conjunction with electron beam CT (EBCT) and single-slice spiral CT [1–4]. A trigger signal is derived from the patient's ECG based on a prospective estimation of the present RR interval and the scan is started at a defined time point after a detected R wave, usually during diastole. Multislice CT allows simultaneous acquisition of several slices in one heartbeat with a cycle time that usually allows scanning in every other

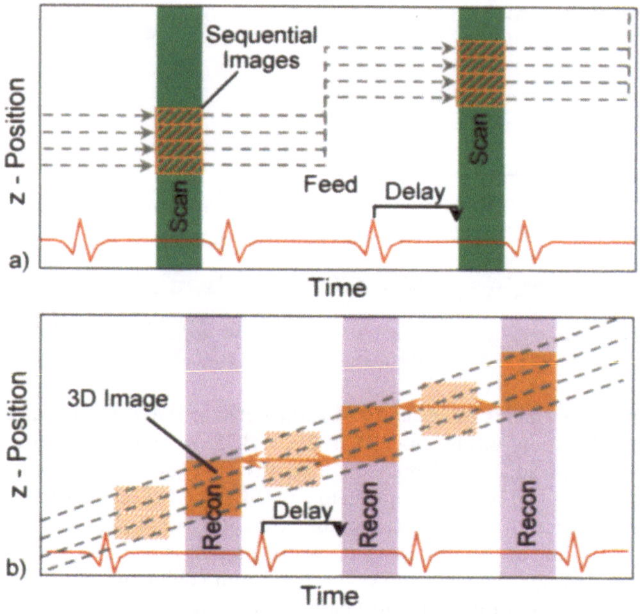

Fig. 2a,b. Illustration of sequential volume coverage with prospectively ECG-triggered multislice scanning (**a**). Multiple images (one image per detector slice) are acquired at a time with a certain delay after a detected R wave. The slice thickness is equivalent to the collimation (hatched blocks) and the temporal resolution equals half the rotation time. Due to the limitation of the scan cycle time to about 1 s, a scan can be acquired every other heart cycle for usual heart rates. A scan with continuous table feed and continuous exposure is acquired for retrospectively ECG-gated multislice spiral scanning (**b**). Stacks of overlapping images can be reconstructed with a temporal resolution of half the rotation time in every cardiac cycle. Continuous 3D images can be reconstructed in different phases of the cardiac cycle by selection of the data ranges with certain phase relations to the R waves

heartbeat (Fig. 2a). Thus shorter breath-hold times are present compared to single-slice scanners and respiratory artifacts can be widely eliminated. To achieve best possible temporal resolution scan data is only acquired during a partial scanner rotation (≈ 2/3 of a rotation with 240–260° projection data) that covers the minimum amount of data required for image reconstruction. Conventional partial scan reconstruction based on fan beam projection data results in a temporal resolution that equals the acquisition time of the partial scan. Optimized temporal resolution can be achieved with parallel beam-based »half-scan« reconstruction algorithms that provide a temporal resolution of half the rotation time in a center area of the scan field of view (250 ms for 500 ms rotation time and 210 ms for 420 ms rotation time) [6, 7, 10, 16]. Thus, prospective ECG triggering is also the most dose-efficient way of ECG-synchronized scanning as only the very minimum of scan data needed for image reconstruction is acquired. However, usually only rather thick slice collimation (3 mm with EBCT, 2.5–3 mm with 4-, 8-, and 16-slice CT) is being used for prospectively triggered acquisition within a reasonably short single breath-hold. Thus, resulting data sets are often not suitable for 3D reconstruction of small cardiac anatomy. Also prospectively ECG-triggered technique greatly depends on a regular heart rate of the patient and is bound to result in misregistration in the presence of arrhythmia.

ECG-Gated Multislice CT Scanning and Image Reconstruction

Retrospective ECG gating overcomes the limitations of prospective ECG triggering with regard to scan time and spatial resolution and can provide higher consistence of image quality for examination of patients with changing heart rate during the scan. This approach requires multislice spiral scanning with slow table motion and simultaneous recording of the ECG trace that is used for retrospective assignment of scan data and heart motion [8–10]. Phase-consistent coverage of the heart requires a highly overlapping spiral scan with a spiral table feed adapted to the heart rate in order to avoid gaps between image stacks that are reconstructed in consecutive heart cycles. These image stacks are reconstructed at the exact same phase of the heart cycle and cover the entire heart and adjacent anatomy in the considered scan range (Fig. 2b). Images are reconstructed in every heart beat and faster scan coverage is possible as compared to prospective ECG triggering. Moreover, the continuous spiral acquisition enables reconstruction of overlapping image slices and thus a longitudinal spatial resolution about 20% below the slice-width can be achieved (e.g., 2.5 mm for 3.0 mm slices, 1.0 mm for 1.25 mm slices, 0.8 mm for 1.0 mm slices and 0.6 mm for 0.75 mm slices). For these reasons, retrospective ECG gating is the preferred method for imaging small cardiac anatomy and the coronary arteries with thin slices and high spatial resolution in short single breath-hold times.

In every heart beat fan beam data of a partial rotation (usually 240–260°) is utilized for image reconstruction that provides a temporal resolution equivalent to half of the rotation time in a centered region of interest (250 ms for 500 ms rotation time and 210 ms for 420 ms rotation time). A multislice spiral interpolation between the projections of adjacent detector rows is used in order to compensate for table movement and to provide a well-defined slice sensitivity profile and images free of spiral movement artifacts. The temporal resolution can be improved by using scan data from more than one heart cycle for reconstruction of an image (»segmented reconstruction«) [9, 22, 23] (Fig. 3). The partial scan data set for reconstruction of one image then consists of projection sectors from multiple consecutive heart cycles. Depending on the relation of rotation time and patient heart rate a temporal resolution between rotation-time/2 and rotation-time/2 M is present (M equals the number of projection sectors and the number of used heart cycles) (Fig. 4). Despite theoretically better temporal resolution, »segmented« reconstruction algorithms do not regularly provide superior image quality for display of small cardiac anatomy as the algorithms are very sensitive to changing heart rates. Therefore, segmented reconstruction and in particular the use of data from more than two heart beats per image is often not practical.

Recent publications [16] have demonstrated that cone-beam reconstruction algorithms become mandatory for general purpose CT scanning with eight and more slices to avoid severe cone-beam artifacts. The severity of cone-beam induced artifacts depends on the number of simultaneously acquired slices, on the width of one collimated slice and on the distance of an object from the center of rotation. Cone-beam artifacts are most pronounced at high contrast structures. Typical sources of cone-beam artifacts are the ribs or the pelvic bones. Since the

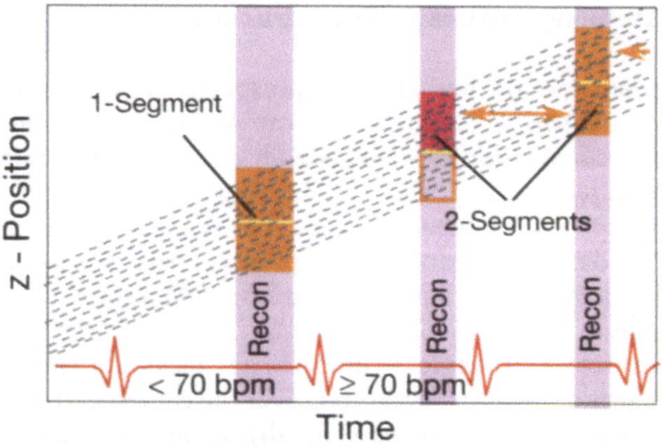

Fig. 3. Schematic illustration of an adaptive segmented image reconstruction approach for ECG-gated 16-slice spiral CT scanning. *Dashed lines* are used to indicate the z positions of the detector slices, which continuously and linearly change position relative to the patient with constant spiral feed. The ECG signal is simultaneously recorded during scan acquisition and is displayed at the bottom of the diagram. At heart rates below a certain threshold, one segment of consecutive multislice spiral data is used for image reconstruction. At higher heart rates, two sub-segments from adjacent heart cycles contribute to the partial scan data segment. In each cardiac cycle, a stack of images is reconstructed at different z positions covering a small sub-volume of the heart, which is indicated as a *box*. The combination of sub-volumes from all heart cycles during the scan provides a continuous 3D data set of the entire heart

heart is usually sufficiently centered and does not contain large high contrast structures, cone-beam artifacts are still negligible for today's 16-slice CT scanners [20, 21]. If a computational expensive cone-beam reconstruction is not required for ECG-gated cardiac scanning, the available computational power of the CT system can be used to speed up image reconstruction. Cardiac CT scanning with more than 16 collimated slices, however, will require advanced cardiac cone-beam algorithms in future CT systems [24].

Usually the diastolic phase of the cardiac cycle is chosen for image reconstruction of cardiac and coronary morphology, however, due to the highly overlapping

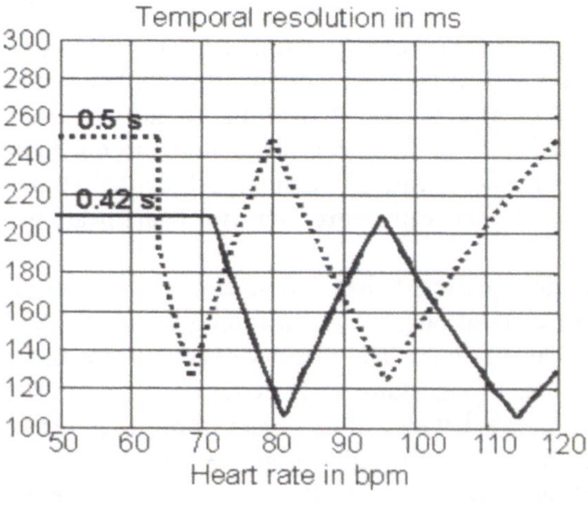

Fig. 4. Temporal resolution as a function of the heart rate for the adaptive segmented reconstruction approach using 0.5 s and 0.42 s gantry rotation time. If data from two consecutive heart cycles is used for image reconstruction the temporal resolution strongly depends on heart rate. For 0.42 s rotation time, the temporal resolution reaches its optimum of 105 ms at 81 bpm. Thus clinically robust image quality can be achieved also in patients with higher heart rates, i.e., in patients with stable sinus rhythm and heart rates in the range 75–85 bpm

scan acquisition, image data can be reconstructed for each x-, y- and z-position within the scanned volume over the entire course of the cardiac cycle. This allows for retrospective selection of reconstruction points that provide best image quality in an individual patient and for anatomy with special motion patterns [25, 26]. To improve image quality in the presence of arrhythmia, the reconstruction interval individual image stacks can be discarded or arbitrarily shifted within the cardiac cycle, so that reconstruction always coincides with the same interval during diastole at each level of the cardiac volume. Beside the morphology information that is derived from image reconstruction in diastole, additional reconstructions of the same scan data set in different phases of the cardiac cycle (see Fig. 2b) enable analysis of basic cardiac function parameters such as end-diastolic volume, end-systolic volume and ejection fraction.

Relatively high radiation exposure is involved with retrospectively ECG-gated imaging of the heart because of continuous X-ray exposure and overlapping data acquisition at low-spiral table feed. All data can be used for image reconstruction in different cardiac phases but only if a very limited interval (i.e. diastolic phase) in the cardiac cycle is targeted during reconstruction a significant portion of the acquired data and radiation exposure is redundant. A high potential for exposure reduction during ECG-gated spiral scanning is offered by an on-line reduction of the tube output in each cardiac cycle during phases that are of less importance for ECG-gated reconstruction (»ECG-pulsing«) [10]. In this approach, the nominal tube output is only applied during the diastolic phases of the cardiac cycle that are likely to be reconstructed. In the rest of the cardiac cycle, the tube output is reduced. Depending on the heart rate, an overall exposure saving of 30–50% can be achieved without compromising on image quality [27].

A special technique for ECG-gated spiral scanning with increased volume coverage for cardio-thoracic application has been introduced for 4-slice CT scanners [28]. It allows for suppression of cardiac pulsation owing to reconstruction with a temporal resolution that equals half the rotation time and to ECG gating that eliminates scan data acquired during the systolic phase with its rapid heart motion. Latest 16-slice CT scanners equipped with this protocol can provide motion-free coverage of the entire thoracic anatomy with sub-millimeter slices within a single breath-hold. However, cone-beam reconstruction techniques may be required for this application as also high-contrast thoracic anatomy located in the periphery of the scan field of view is of interest for diagnosis [29].

Performance Evaluation with Phantom Studies

The performance of 4-slice CT scanners in comparison to a new 16-slice CT scanner (SOMATOM Sensation 4 and Sensation 16, Siemens, Forchheim, Germany) with respect to cardiac imaging has been evaluated with computer simulation studies and phantom measurements. The results demonstrate the advancements of 16-slice CT scanners in scan speed and spatial resolution.

The achievable spatial resolution with usual high-resolution cardiac scan protocols is demonstrated with a z-resolution phantom (Fig. 5). The z-resolution

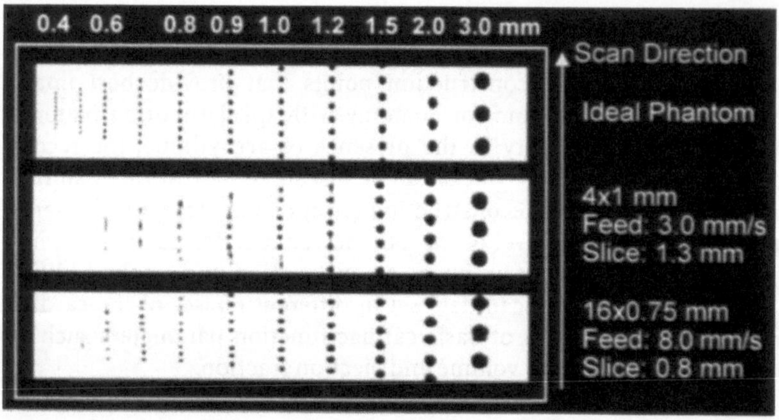

Fig. 5. Investigation of the spatial resolution in the scan direction for cardiac CT examinations with 4- and 16-slice CT with a resting longitudinal resolution phantom. The phantom includes air-filled spheres with 0.4 to 3.0 mm diameter that can be examined with MPR cuts along the scan direction. A maximum longitudinal resolution of 0.8–1.0 mm can be achieved with 4-slice CT using 4×1mm collimation, 1.3 mm slice-width, 0.6 mm image increment and 3 mm/s table feed. 16-slice CT provides up to 0.6 mm longitudinal resolution based on 16×0.75 mm collimation, 0.8 mm slice-width, 0.4 mm image increment and 8.0 mm/s table feed

phantom consists of a Lucite plate with rows of cylindrical holes of different diameters in the transverse direction. The 4-slice CT scanner with 4×1mm collimation, 0.5 s rotation speed and 3 mm/s table feed (pitch 0.375) can resolve structures of 1.0 mm in size using 1.3 mm reconstructed slice-width and 0.5 mm image increment. With 16-slice CT technology and sub-millimeter collimation the spatial resolution is improved with higher scan speed at the same time. Based on 16×0.75 mm collimation, 0.42 s rotation speed and 8.0 mm/s table feed (pitch 0.28), 0.6 mm small objects can be delineated using 0.8 mm reconstructed slice-width and 0.4 mm image increment.

A computer model of an anthropomorphic heart phantom demonstrates the clinical relevance of the increased spatial resolution with 16-slice CT acquisition (Fig. 6). The model includes contrast-enhanced coronary arteries containing stents and atherosclerotic plaques of known dimensions and categories. With 16-slice CT scan data can be reconstructed with different slice-width for optimization of the trade-off between spatial resolution and signal-to-noise ratio for a certain clinical application. For 16×0.75 mm collimation, slices with a thinnest possible slice-width of 0.8 mm can be generated thus allowing for substantially improved visualization of coronary artery lumen compared to 4-slice CT.

Clinical Imaging Protocols

The optimal scan technique to be used for a certain application very much depends on the requirements by means of spatial and contrast resolution of the considered application. Prospective ECG triggering can be readily used for con-

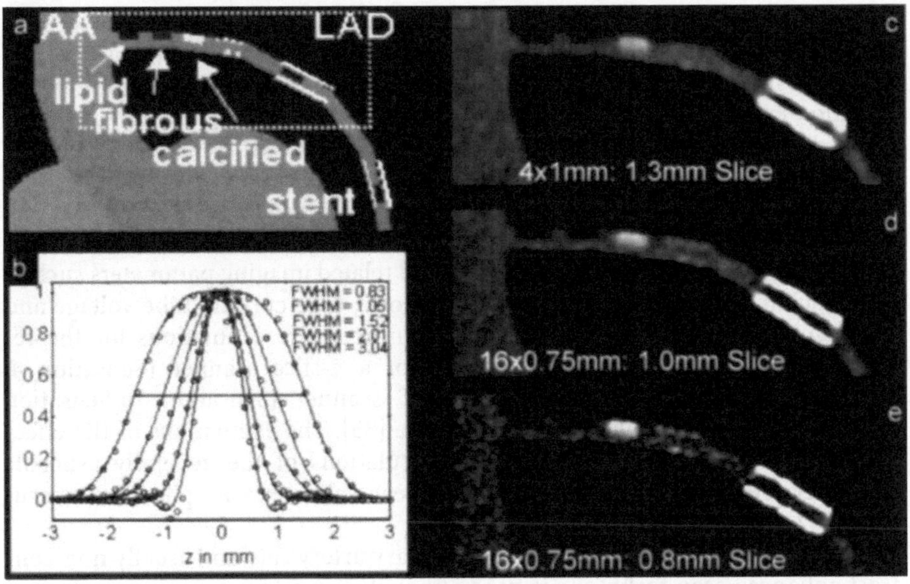

Fig. 6a–e. An anthropomorphic numerical heart and coronary artery phantom was used to evaluate the influence of spatial resolution and slice-width on visualization of coronary artery lumen and coronary plaque. The contrast enhanced left coronary artery segments (enhancement 250 HU) contain plaques with different properties and a stent in the proximal left coronary artery descending (LAD): lipid plaque 30 HU, fibrous plaque 80 HU, calcified plaque 500 HU and a stent with 50% in-stent lumen narrowing caused by a lesion with 30 HU (**a**). 16-slice CT with 16×0.75 mm collimation allows for retrospective reconstruction of different slice-thicknesses between 0.8 mm and 3.0 mm (**b**). The phantom was reconstructed with 1.3 mm (**c**), 1.0 mm (**d**) and 0.8 mm (**e**) slice-width and the proximal LAD was displayed with multiplanar reformations. Differentiation of the lesions and visualization of in-stent lumen is possible with slice-width ≤1.0 mm

trast-enhanced imaging of great vessel morphology within limited scan ranges and for non-contrast enhanced detection of coronary calcification with low radiation exposure. Nevertheless, retrospective ECG gating has shown to be useful for quantification of coronary calcium with improved reproducibility due to coverage with overlapping slices and shorter scan times [30]. Contrast-enhanced visualization of small cardiac morphology and the coronary arteries with best possible spatial and temporal resolution as well as long range coverage of the cardio-thoracic vasculature is only feasible with retrospectively ECG-gated scan acquisition. With 4-slice CT scanners and retrospectively ECG-gated spiral scanning a true 3-dimensional data set of the cardiac and coronary anatomy can be acquired with 0.6×0.6 mm in-plane resolution and 1.0 mm longitudinal resolution based on 4×1mm slice collimation. A 10–12 cm scan range can be covered in a 30–40 s breath-hold time. Technology advances to 8-slice CT scanners can reduce breath-hold times to 20–25 s. Recent 16-slice CT scanners provide improved longitudinal resolution via sub-millimeter slice-collimation (0.75 mm) and improved in-plane spatial resolution of 0.5×0.5 mm. Despite thinner slice collimation, breath-hold times are reduced to 15–20 s for covering a 12 cm scan range via simultaneous acquisition of 12 or all 16 detector slices.

Diagnostically sufficient image quality has to be provided at the minimum radiation exposure possible. Therefore, scan protocols have to be developed for different applications with optimized ratio of image quality, spatial resolution and limitation of radiation exposure. Various publications are available that discuss the radiation exposure of multislice CT in cardiac application [31, 32]. Partially, great disagreement of dose values can be found that is mainly due to lack of standardization of used protocols and related imaging parameters such as slice-thickness, in-plane resolution, image noise, tube current, tube voltage and scan ranges. Below we summarize radiation exposure estimations for the recommended and standardized protocols of a 4-slice scanner (Sensation 4, Siemens, Germany) and of a 16-slice CT scanner (Sensation 16/Sensation Cardiac, Siemens, Germany) currently in use [33]. The estimations of the effective patient dose values are based on calculations of the generally available computer program WinDose [34] that has been validated with phantom measurements [35] (Table 1).

For detection and quantification of coronary artery calcium, usually non-contrast enhanced scan technique is used although accurate measurement of coronary calcium is also feasible based on a thin-slice CT angiography protocol [36]. For intravenous coronary CT angiography contrast media injection must be carefully tailored by either using a test bolus or automatic bolus triggering technique. Since scan times for imaging of the heart on modern 4-, 8- or 16-slice CT scanners range from 15 to 40 s, 80 to 150 ml contrast media at injection rates between 3 to 5 ml/s is needed to maintain homogenous vascular contrast throughout the scan. Saline chasing has proven mandatory for reduction of contrast media needed for high and consistent vascular enhancement and for avoiding streak artifacts, which frequently arise from dense contrast material in the superior vena cava and the right atrium and sometimes interfere with the evaluation especially of the right coronary artery. Techniques for contrast bolus optimization have been developed in the past [37] but have not been widely used since reasonable results could be obtained by adapting single-slice CT strategies for contrast administration to dual- and 4-slice CT. However, the introduction of ever-faster CT acquisition techniques now requires careful custom tailoring of the bolus for achieving adequate and consistent contrast media attenuation within the cardiovascular system.

Clinical Application

Quantification of Coronary Calcification

Electron Beam CT scanning (EBCT) has been established as a non-invasive imaging modality for the detection and quantification of coronary calcium by using the Agatston-scoring algorithm [2]. With EBCT scanning, typically 3 mm thick slices are acquired contiguously with prospective ECG triggering in mid-diastole and an exposition time of 100 ms per slice. An effective exposure of about

Table 1

	ECG-Trigger (Ca-Score)		ECG-Gating (Ca-Score)			ECG-Gating (High-Resolution)		
	4-Slice CT	16-Slice CT	4-Slice CT	16-Slice CT		4-Slice CT	16-Slice CT	
Scan range [mm]	120	120	120	120	120	100	100	100
Collimation [mm]	4×2.5	12×1.5	4×2.5	12×1.5	16×1.5	4×1	12×0.75	16×0.75
Slice-Width [mm]	3.0	3.0	3.0	3.0	3.0	1.3	0.75/1.0	0.75/1.0
Rotation Time [ms]	500	420	500	420	420	420	420	420
Table Feed	10 mm/scan	18 mm/scan	7.5 mm/s	13.2 mm/s	16 mm/s	3 mm/s	6.6 mm/s	8 mm/s
kv/mA	120/100	120/100	120/100	120/100	120/100	120/300	120/370	120/370
$CTDI_w$ [mGy]	2.74	2.16	10.1	9.54	10.5	36.0	42.0	43.3
Eff. Dose [mSv], Male/Female (ECG-Pulsing)	0.54/0.76	0.45/0.65	1.9/2.8	1.9/2.7	2.2/3.1	5.7/8.5	6.8/10.1	7.1/10.5
Eff. Dose [mSv], Male/Female (ECG-Pulsing)	n.a.	n.a.	1.0–1.4/ 1.4–2.0	1.0–1.4/ 1.4–1.9	1.1–1.5/ 1.5–2.2	2.9–4.0/ 4.2–5.9	3.4–4.8/ 5.1–7.1	3.6–5.0/ 5.3–7.4

0.9 mSv was reported for this protocol [38]. A known limitation of coronary artery calcium scoring with EBCT is the high interscan variability associated with this test [39]. This high variability has limited the use of coronary artery calcium measurements for tracking the progression of atherosclerosis e.g. under statin (lipid-lowering) therapy, which may become a potentially powerful future application of this technique [40].

Since the introduction sub-second rotation imaging of coronary artery calcium has also been evaluated with single-slice [4] and dual-slice mechanical spiral CT [41]. Due to increased imaging performance in terms of temporal resolution and volume coverage multislice CT can be expected to allow for coronary calcium quantification with substantially higher accuracy and better performance than mechanical single-and dual-slice CT [30, 38]. Optimal acquisition techniques have to be developed and Ca-scoring data acquired with multislice CT need careful clinical evaluation and comparison to EBCT.

Both, ECG-triggered sequential and ECG-gated spiral scanning can be used as acquisition technique. Scan data is acquired without contrast enhancement in cranio-caudal direction from the caudal part of the pulmonary artery trunk to the apex of the heart (≈12 cm scan range). 3 mm slice-width is routinely used for EBCT scanning as it represents the thinnest slice-width that allows for a single breath-hold scan. 2.5–3.0 mm slice width is usually being used with 4-, 8- and 16-slice CT scanners as the closest match to the standard EBCT protocols. A tube voltage of 120 kV is recommended as it provides the best relation of contrast-to-noise ratio and radiation exposure. For most multislice CT scanners 100 mA tube current is used to achieve sufficient signal-to-noise levels to detect small calcified lesions. The tube current may be increased for obese patients (e.g. to 150 mA) to maintain a diagnostic signal-to-noise level at the expense of increased radiation exposure.

ECG-triggered scanning allows for covering the scan volume in 20–25 s with 4-slice CT scanners and in 10–15 s with 8- and 16-slice CT scanners. Depending on the scanner used slice collimation varies between 2.5 and 3 mm. Depending on the used mA effective patient dose varies between 0.5 and 0.7 mSv for male and between 0.6 and 0.9 mSv for female patients (see also Table 1). Every scan covers a sub-volume that consists of several adjacent slices and thus the probability of interscan misregistration caused by heart movement in the z-direction is reduced and higher detection accuracy may be expected compared to ECG-triggered single-slice acquisition. Comparative studies of EBCT and prospectively ECG-triggered multislice CT could demonstrate good agreement with the measurements in phantom experiments [30] and high correlation in patient studies [38,42]. However, a high mean inter-examination variability of 22–32% comparable to the inter-examination variability of 2 consecutive EBCT examinations is being observed with prospectively ECG-triggered multislice CT due to the presence of motion artifacts and misregistration in between the sequential slices.

ECG-gated spiral scanning provides shorter breath-hold times as compared to ECG-triggered scanning as well as more consistent volume coverage based on overlapping slices. 12 cm scan range can be completed in 15–20 s with 4-slice CT and in 6–10 s with 8- and 16-slice CT. The spiral interpolation algorithms generate 3 mm thick slices (full width at half maximum) based on a slice collimation of 2.5 mm for 4- and 8-slice CT scanners and 1.25–1.5 mm for 16-slice CT scanners (see also Table 1). Optimal detection accuracy of small calcified lesions might be achieved with 16-slice scanners via reconstruction of 3 mm thick slices based on scan acquisition with sub-millimeter collimation [43]. Retrospectively ECG-gated spiral scanning represents the preferred scan technique for minimized inter-examination variability. Recent independent studies found interscan variability of about 10% and even below for repeat 4-slice CT scanning [30, 44, 45] which may be accurate enough to sensitively detect changes in the total atherosclerotic disease burden in patients with and without specific therapy. Interscan variability may be further improved with latest 16-slice CT scanners primarily based on faster rotation time and increased scan speed (Fig. 7). In

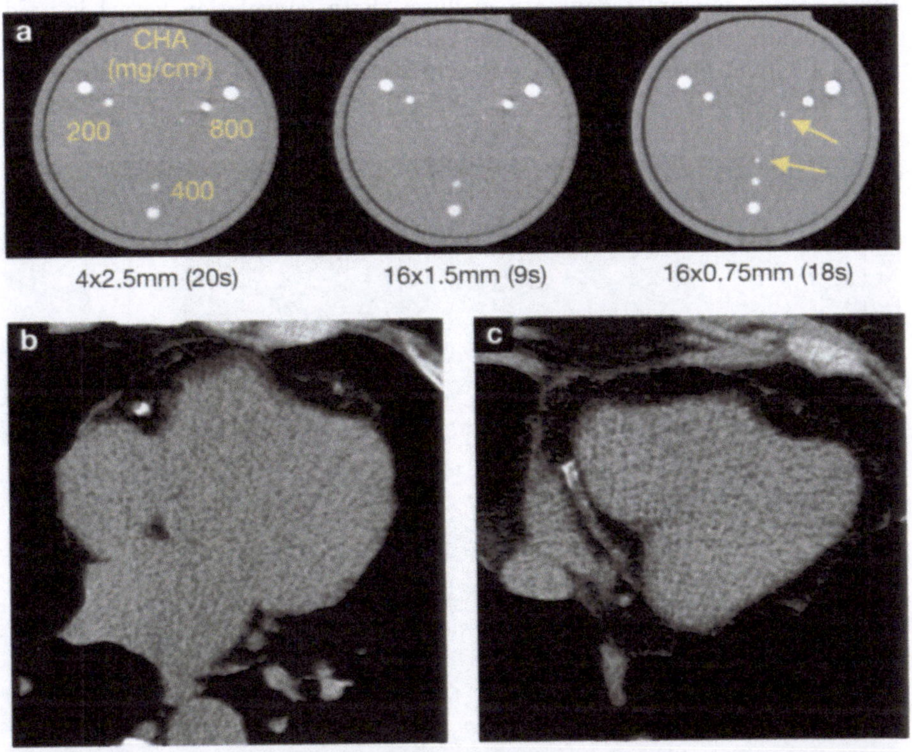

Fig. 7a–c. Different scan protocols for 4- and 16-slice CT were compared in a phantom study to investigate the sensitivity for the detection of small amounts of coronary calcification. The phantom consist of a Lucite cylinder embedded in an anthropomorphic chest phantom with inserts of different concentration of Calcium Hydroxyl Apatite (CHA) and different diameters (200, 400 and 800 mg/cm³ CHA) (**a**). Slices with 3 mm slice-width were reconstructed based on scan data acquired with 133mAs and 4x2.5 mm, 16x1.5 mm and 16x0.75 mm collimation. The smallest calcifications (1 mg mass, arrows) can only be detected with the 16x0.75 mm protocol. A case study performed with 16-slice CT and 16x1.5 mm collimation reveals small calcifications in the middle segment (**b**) and in the distal segment (**c**) of the right coronary artery. (Case study by courtesy of the department of Radiology, Grosshadern Clinic, University of Munich, Germany).

comparison to prospectively ECG-triggered technique, CT acquisition with retrospective ECG gating is associated with higher effective radiation exposure (1.9 mSv for male and 2.8 mSv for female). Frequently, healthy, asymptomatic individuals undergo coronary calcium scoring in the context of primary prevention. Especially in this population, it is imperative to limit radiation dose to a minimum. This can be achieved by properly adapting scan protocols [46], or by using sophisticated technical developments such as ECG-based tube current modulation [27], which can decrease effective radiation exposure of the patient by as much as 50% [27].

The modulation transfer function of the convolution kernel that is used for image reconstruction has high influence on in-plane spatial resolution and signal-to-noise ratio and has thus high influence on quantitative measurements. For coronary calcium scanning a medium sharp convolution kernel is used that provides moderate image noise for low radiation exposure and about 0.6 × 0.6 mm in-plane resolution (50% and 2% values of the modulation transfer function: ρ (50%) ≈ 4.0 cm^{-1}, ρ (2%) ≈ 9.0 cm^{-1}). Edge-enhancement of the con-

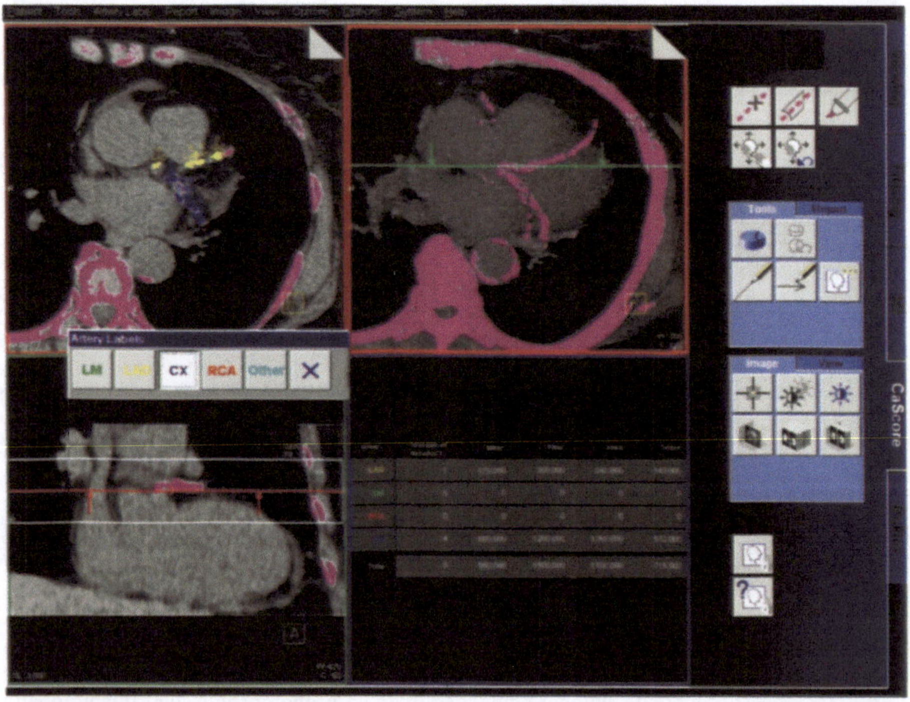

Fig. 8. Presentation of the platform used for quantification of coronary calcification (syngo Calcium Scoring, Siemens, Forchheim, Germany). Lesions exceeding the calcium threshold of 130 HU are identified with 3D-based picking and viewing tools and are assigned to the different coronary arteries LM; LAD, CX and RCA. Coronary calcification are quantified my means of Agatston score, calcium volume and calcium mass. Calibration factors that are pre-determined with phantom measurements and that depend on the scan protocol are the basis for calculation of calcium mass. The quantitative measurements are displayed and reported in table format

volution kernel should be avoided as it may lead to an overestimation of scores and to misleading artifactual lesions at the pericardium close to the coronary arteries.

The most commonly used algorithm for quantification of coronary artery calcium is the traditional semi-quantitative score based on slice by slice analysis of CT images as described by Agatston [2]. Recent studies describe better results for inter-scan and inter- and intra-observer variability with use of quantitative measures as compared to the traditional Agatston scoring method [30, 44, 45]. Advanced software platforms (Fig. 8) allow for assessment of equivalent volume and total calcified plaque burden in terms of absolute calcium mass based on actual scanner-specific calibration factors [44, 47]. This latter technique probably has the greatest potential to increase accuracy, consistency and reproducibility of coronary calcium assessment [47] and thus may replace traditional scoring methods in the near future [48].

Cardiac and Coronary CT Angiography

For non-invasive cardiac and coronary CT angiography high requirements for spatial resolution, low-contrast detachability and temporal resolution have to be fulfilled at the same time. Image quality depends on various patient and scanner parameters and optimization of examination protocols is critical for best balance of imaging parameters and best examination results.

Cardiac and coronary CT imaging with multislice CT requires ECG-gated thin-slice spiral scan protocols with table speed adapted to the heart rate in order to ensure complete phase-consistent coverage of the heart with overlapping image slices. Most multislice CT scanners provide scan protocols with fixed overlapping spiral pitch between 0.30 and 0.375 that enable gap-less volume coverage for heart rate higher than ≈ 40 min^{-1}. The spiral pitch is defined as the table feed per rotation divided by the width all collimated detector slices.

Usually, the cranio-caudal size of the heart to be covered by the scan is in the range 10–12 cm. 4-slice CT scanners with 500 ms rotation time and an individual detector-width of 1.0 mm, cover the entire heart during a 30–40 s breath-hold with reconstructed slice-width of 1.3 mm. With 8-slice CT scanners the breath-hold time can be reduced to 20–25 s without improvement of the spatial or temporal resolution. Recent 16-slice CT scanners provide high-resolution cardiac scan protocols with sub-millimeter slice-collimation (0.75 mm) and in-plane spatial resolution up to 0.5×0.5 mm [49, 50]. The image reconstruction protocols are adapted to the clinical priorities. Usually, slices not thinner than 1.0 mm are reconstructed with 0.6×0.6 mm in-plane resolution to achieve optimal contrast resolution for assessment of coronary narrowing and coronary lesions (Fig. 9). Special algorithms with slice-width down to 0.75 mm and in-plane resolution of 0.5×0.5 mm can be applied for high-resolution reconstruction of small high-contrast structures (e.g. coronary stents and calcified coronary segments) in a limited range (Fig. 10).

Rotation times down to 420 ms and the extended number of slices, up to 16, result in a reduced scan time of 15–20 s (see also Table 1). Thus, 16-slice CT can

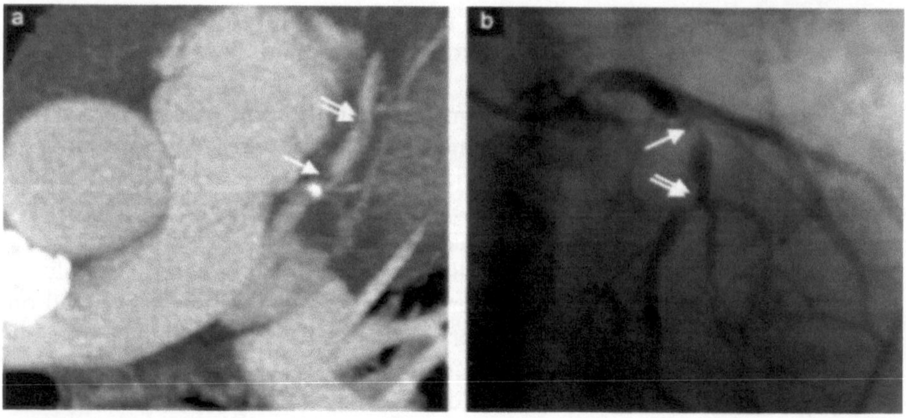

Fig. 9a,b. Coronary CT angiography examination of a patient with suspected coronary artery disease (**a**) using a 16-slice CT scanner with 16×0.75 mm detector collimation and 420 ms rotation speed in correlation to conventional coronary angiography (**b**). Coronary CT angiography reveals high-grade stenosis in the proximal left descending coronary artery near the bifurcation of the first diagonal branch (*arrow*, 90% stenosis) and in the middle segment of the left descending coronary artery next to the bifurcation of the second diagonal branch (*double arrow*, 70% stenosis). Both lesions are confirmed by coronary angiography. (Case by courtesy of Dr. Soo CS, HSC Medical Center, Kuala Lumpur, Malaysia)

also cover larger scan ranges of 18–20 cm with ECG-gated thin-slice spiral scan protocols in a reasonably short breath-hold of 25–30 s that enables high-resolution imaging of most parts of the great thoracic vasculature and coronary bypass grafts over their entire course (Fig. 11).

Optimization of scan protocols by means of radiation exposure is particularly important for contrast-enhanced CT imaging the coronary arteries. Sufficiently high spatial resolution and low-contrast resolution has to be achieved in normal and also in larger patients at the minimal-possible radiation exposure. For tube voltage of 120 kV and 500 ms rotation time tube current of ≈ 300 mA should be used for imaging 4- and 8-slice CT with slice-width of 1.3 mm. The tube current needs to be increased to ≈ 350–400 mA for 16-slice CT with sub-millimeter slice collimation and faster rotation time. Retrospectively, ECG-gated scan acquisition with highly overlapping spiral pitch in a 10 cm scan range requires radiation exposure of about 6–7 mSv for male and about 8–11 mSv for female patients (protocol examples in Table 1). Despite increased tube current and spatial resolution with 16-slice CT scanners, radiation exposure does not considerably increase due to better dose utilization of 16-slice detector geometry [16, 17]. However, radiation exposure increases with reduced spiral pitch and with extension of the scan range. With ECG-gated dose-modulation radiation exposure is reduced by 30–50% depending on heart rate resulting without compromising on image quality in the fully exposed phase of the cardiac cycle. ECG-gated dose modulation reduces radiation exposure to about 3–5 mSv for male and to about 4–8 mSv for female patients and should be used for all patients with a reasonably stable rhythm during the scan.

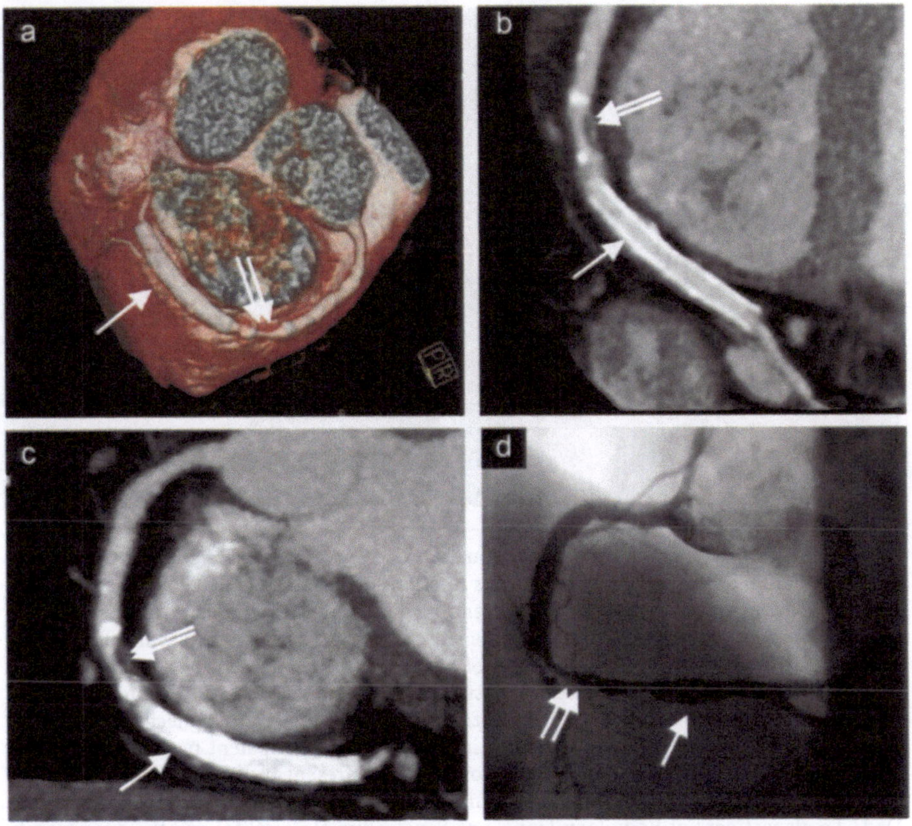

Fig. 10a–d. Coronary CT angiography examination of a patient after PTCA with stent in the distal right coronary artery using a 16-slice CT scanner with 16×0.75 mm detector collimation and 420 ms rotation speed. The patient presented for follow-up examination after the intervention and was examined to rule-out re-stenosis. Coronary CT angiography reveals a patent stent lumen (*arrow*) but calcified and non-calcified atherosclerosic lesions and high-grade lumenal narrowing of about 70% proximal to the stent (*double arrow*). The lumenal narrowing can be readily displayed with 3D-volume rendering technique in combination with cut-planes that remove overlaying anatomy (**a**). Multiplanar reformation allows for visualization of the open in-stent lumen and of the narrowed lumen proximal to the stent (**b**). Additional display of the same anatomy with maximum intensity projection provides clear assessment of the calcified and non-calcified atherosclerotic lesions related to the stenotic lesion (**c**). Conventional angiography confirms the patent stent and the 70% stenosis (**d**) that was successfully dilated in the same session. (Case by courtesy of Dr. Soo CS, HSC Medical Center, Kuala Lumpur, Malaysia)

The overall diagnostic quality of non-invasive cardiac and coronary CT angiography largely depends on choice of the appropriate reconstruction time-point within the cardiac cycle, patient heart rate during the examination and contrast enhancement. The motion pattern of the left heart and the left anterior descending (LAD) and circumflex (CRX) coronary arteries follows the left ventricular

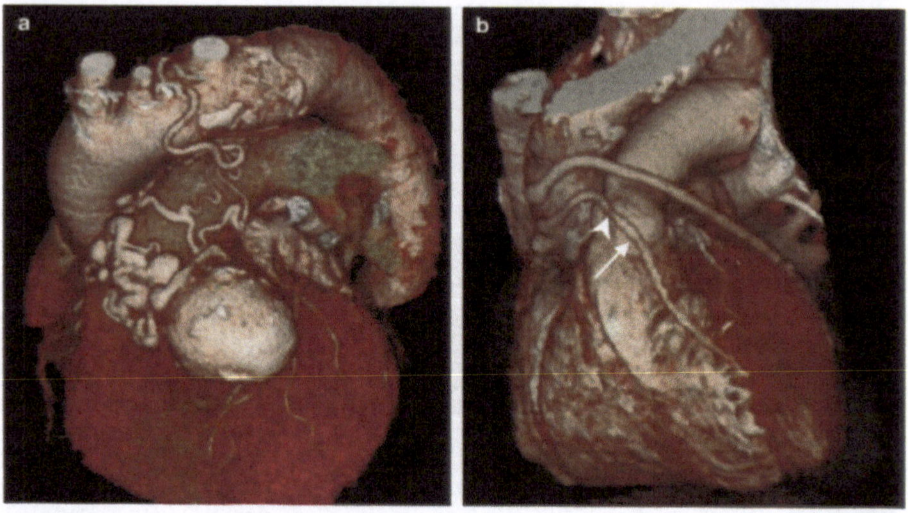

Fig. 11a,b. Coronary CT angiography examination of 2 patients using a 16-slice CT scanner with 16x0.75mm detector collimation, 420ms rotation speed and extended volume coverage of 15cm in order to visualize the heart, the ascending aorta and the pulmonary vessels. The first case demonstrates abnormal anatomy of the left descending coronary artery including multiple fistula (a). Real-time 3D rendering is of advantage for assessment of the complex anatomy conditions. In the second case 3 bypasses to right coronary artery, left coronary artery descending and marginal branch are visualized with 3D volume rendering technique (b). The bypass to the left coronary artery descending (arrow) shows a patent proximal and distal anastomosis. However, a 50% stenosis (arrow head) is present in the proximal part of the bypass. The other 2 bypasses reveal open lumen over the entire course. (Cases by courtesy of Dr. G. Lo, department of Radiology, Hongkong Sanatorium Hospital (**a**) and the departments of Radiology and Cardiology, Rhön-Klinikum Bad Neustadt, Germany (**b**)).

contraction whereas the right coronary artery (RCA) moves synchronous with the right heart, i.e. the right atrium. Because of these different motion patterns, different reconstruction time points over the cardiac cycle can result in optimal display of different cardiac anatomy and different coronary arteries [25, 26]. Most studies agree that patient heart rate is inversely related to image quality at cardiac and coronary CT angiography [12–14, 25, 26] by means of motion artifacts. It has been shown that multislice CT provides best diagnostic accuracy and reliability of results in patients with slow heart rates. Study data based on 4-slice CT with 500 ms fastest rotation time indicates that an upper heart limit to consistently achieve appropriate image quality can be set between 65min^{-1} and 75min^{-1} [25, 26]. At higher heart rates adequate image quality can be achieved in numerous cases but overall results are less consistent and reproducible. For scanners with faster rotation time down to 420 ms robustness of image quality by means of motion is remarkably increased, however, slow heart rates are still required to consistently achieve high-image quality. Thus, it appears recommendable to pharmacologically (i.e. oral administration of beta-blockers) slow down the heart rate of individuals undergoing CT coronary angiography after contraindications to such a regimen have been ruled out. Reliable evaluation of larger cardiac morphology such as the cardiac chambers and the great vessels is possible also in patients that present with higher heart rates during the scan although some image artifacts may be present.

The reliability of multislice cardiac and coronary CT angiography in patients with arrhythmias is limited. However, misinterpretations of the ECG signal can be partially compensated by retrospective editing of the ECG-trace. Persistent irregular heart rates, such as in patients with atrial fibrillation, can result in inter-slice discontinuities and reduced interpretability of coronary segments but the assessment of the greater cardiac morphology such as the ventricles and atria usually remains possible.

Presence of severe calcification represents a limitation of CT coronary imaging because beam hardening and partial volume effects can completely obscure the coronary lumen and do not allow for assessment of the integrity of the coronary lumen. Related to similar effects, metal objects such as stents, surgical clips and sternal wires can also obscure the evaluation of underlying structures. Use of the thinnest possible slice-width reduces partial-volume artifacts and improves assessibility of calcified coronary segments. Additionally, dedicated filtering could be beneficial to the imaging of calcified vessels.

Optimization of contrast media injection protocols for cardiac and coronary CT angiography is aimed at providing homogenous enhancement within the entire course of the coronary arteries in order to facilitate density-threshold dependent 2D and 3D visualization. Optimal contrast attenuation within the vessel is high enough to allow for lesion detection but not as high as to obscure calcified coronary artery wall lesions with higher Hounsfield Unit (HU) attenuation (i.e. >350 HU). With 4-slice CT ($\approx$ 40 s scan time) this is achieved in the majority of patients with 140 ml of 300 mg/ml iodinated contrast material injected at a flow rate of 3.5 ml/s. Owing to increased acquisition speed with 16-slice CT ($\approx$ 20 s scan time) the amount of contrast media can be reduced to 80–100 ml, delivered at an injection rate of 3–4 ml/s. Use of saline chasing technique (e.g. with a bolus of 50 ml of saline injected immediately after the iodine bolus) may be helpful for better contrast bolus utilization and for reducing streak artifacts arising from dense contrast material in the superior vena cava and the right heart.

Evaluation of Cardiac Function

Beside the diagnosis of cardiac and coronary morphology, evaluation and quantification of cardiac function provides important information for the assessment of cardiac and coronary diseases. In addition to image reconstruction in the diastolic phase of the cardiac cycle for assessment of morphology ECG-gated multislice spiral CT can provide additional 3D reconstructions in different heart phases based on the same scan data. Thus, the diagnosis of cardiac and coronary morphology and also of basic cardiac function parameters such as left and right ventricular ejection fraction and end-diastolic and end-systolic volume can be derived from a single contrast-enhanced ECG-gated spiral examination with thin-section acquisition.

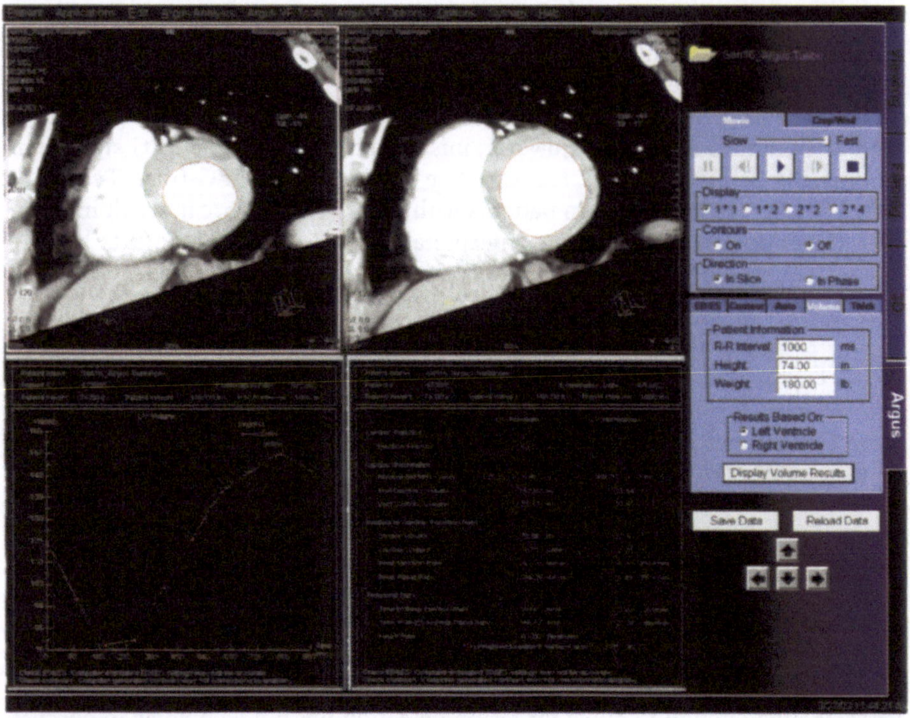

Fig. 12. CT angiographic examination of a patient with an occlusion of the left descending coronary artery using a 16-slice CT scanner with 16×0.75 mm detector collimation and 420 ms rotation speed. In addition to reconstruction of the coronary artery tree, ECG-gated spiral image reconstruction was performed in 10 different time points during the cardiac cycle with a distance of 10% of the RR-interval to provide input data for cardiac function evaluation. End-diastolic volume and end-systolic volume of the left ventricle as well as ejection fraction can be readily assessed based on short axis and long axis multiplanar reformations with 5 mm thickness that are loaded into a dedicated functional evaluation software (syngo Argus, Siemens, Germany). (Case by courtesy of the department of Radiology, Tübingen University, Germany)

First study results [51] show that basic cardiac-function parameters derived with 4-slice CT correlate well with the gold-standard techniques MRI and coronary angiography based on a standardized heart-phase selection for end-diastolic and end-systolic CT reconstruction and semi-automated evaluation tools (Fig. 12).

Although dose is being significantly reduced during end-diastole and systole with ECG-controlled tube current modulation sufficient contrast resolution can still be obtained for functional evaluation. Use of multiplanar reformations in short and long heart axis with thickness of 5–8 mm enables appropriate delineation of the ventricle wall in both end-diastolic and end-systolic reconstruction. Automated direct 3D reconstruction of oblique planes in pre-defined views such as short and long heart axis and in multiple phases of the cardiac cycle will enable a more efficient workflow for cardiac function analysis in the future.

Rapid cardiac motion during the systolic phase of the cardiac cycle can cause motion artifacts in the end-systolic reconstructions. However, correct delineation of the ventricle walls is usually still possible with sufficient accuracy. Latest 16-slice CT scanners have the potential to further improve the accuracy of cardiac function measurement as compared to 4- and 8-slice CT scanners based on increased gantry rotation speed from 0.5 s to 0.42 s with a best possible temporal resolution of 105 ms. More advanced analysis of cardiac function such as quantitative wall motion analysis does require temporal resolution consistently better than 100 ms. At this point even faster gantry rotation speed will be needed in combination with new segmented reconstruction algorithms for retrospective improvement of temporal resolution at the expense of reduced spatial resolution in the longitudinal direction.

Cardio-Thoracic Imaging

Thoracic CT studies are frequently degraded by motion artifacts caused by transmitted cardiac pulsation. Typical diagnostic pitfalls caused by transmitted cardiac pulsation are false-positive findings of aortic dissection and distortion of paracardiac lung segments. Suppression of cardiac pulsation artifacts improves image quality in CT studies of the thorax including the heart. Important indications are the planning and follow up of surgical procedures, diagnosis or exclusion of aortic dissection and aortic aneurisms, detection of pulmonary embolism, assessment of congenital heart and vessel disease and early detection and reliable diagnosis of paracardiac lung nodules.

Prospectively ECG-triggered and retrospectively ECG-gated protocols have been successfully applied to suppress cardiac pulsation in thoracic studies. With 4-slice CT, ECG-triggered or ECG-gated thin-slice scanning of the thorax is usually not possible within a single breath-hold but can be used for re-scanning the part of the thorax where most pulsation is present. With the substantial performance increase of 16-slice CT retrospectively ECG-gated coverage of the thorax is feasible in a single breath-hold and with a single contrast-injection (Fig. 13). Thus, this technique has now the potential to be used as a standard technique for multislice spiral examination of the lung and thoracic vasculature, such as the thoracic aorta, where cardiac pulsation may degrade image quality. As a future step ECG-gated thoracic imaging may become possible even with submillimeter resolution owing to 16-slice CT in combination with specialized ECG-gated cone-beam reconstruction techniques that enable faster volume coverage [29].

Future Perspective

Further CT technology enhancements are required for accurate and consistent diagnosis of cardiac and coronary diseases including the detection and quantification of coronary lumenal narrowing and coronary atherosclerotic lesions. Detection and quantification of coronary stenosis with the ability to differentiate

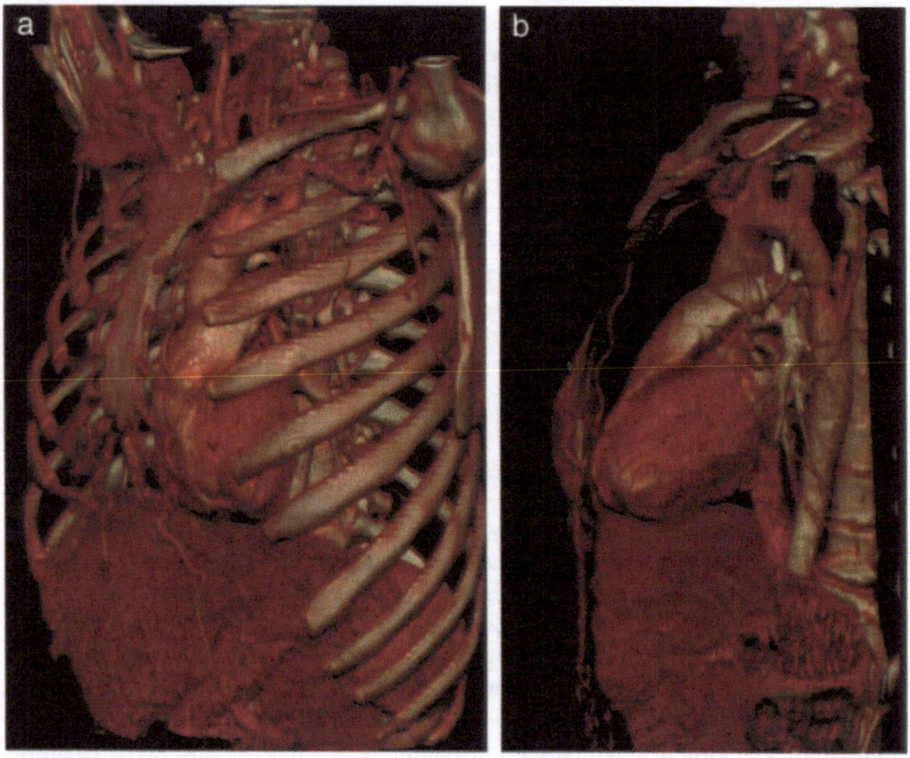

Fig. 13a,b. ECG-gated examination of the thoracic aorta in a 30 s breath-hold using a 16-slice CT scanner with 16×0.75 mm detector collimation and 420 ms rotation speed. The thoracic vasculature is displayed with 3D-volume rendering technique. Based on ECG-gated reconstruction that suppresses cardiac pulsation the entire thoracic aorta can be evaluated free of pulsation artifacts. (Case by courtesy of the department of Radiology, Cleveland Clinic Foundation, USA)

10–20% vessel lumen change represents a viable future goal for cardiac CT imaging. Consequently, a goal of future CT systems is to achieve a spatial resolution in all three dimensions (isotropic) of 0.4–0.5 mm for visualization of the main coronary vessels and 0.3 mm or better for smaller branches. Recent study data indicate that a heart-rate-independent temporal resolution of 100 ms or less allows for elimination of motion artifacts in phases of the cardiac cycle with limited cardiac motion and usual heart rate (approximately up to 100 min^{-1}) [52]. For motion-free imaging at very high heart rates and in phases with rapid cardiac motion for analysis of cardiac function a temporal resolution of 50 ms or less might be required [53]. Scan acquisition within a single and short breath-hold time is mandatory for minimized contrast medium injection and to avoid respiratory artifacts. Breath-hold times of 15 s or less are appropriate for stable patients but breath-hold times of 10 s or less are advisable for less stable emergency patients. Ideally, all data of the complete heart anatomy would be acquired within a single heart cycle or less without patient movement. All these requirements related to spatial resolution, temporal resolution and scan time have to be achieved without substantial increase of radiation exposure that should not exceed the amount of invasive diagnostic coronary angiography.

The very short acquisition times of EBCT down to 50 ms combined with prospectively ECG-triggered scanning enable motion-free imaging of the coronary arteries for patients with moderate and higher heart rates and stable sinus rhythm. However, the restrictions in spatial resolution and contrast-to-noise ratio as well as rather long breath-hold times limit the ability of EBCT today to visualize all main coronary artery segments and non-calcified atherosclerotic plaques. New EBCT detectors are under evaluation that allow for simultaneous acquisition of two 1.5 mm slices and increased in-plane spatial resolution via finer structuring of the elements of the fixed detector ring. With these detectors the heart can be scanned with 1.5 mm slices in a 30–40 s breath-hold. Further increased spatial resolution in the longitudinal axis and breath-hold times of <20 s can be achieved if EBCT systems with multiple stationary detector rings would become available that provide simultaneous ECG-synchronized acquisition of about 12 or more slices with less than 1 mm collimation per slice. Such EBCT-based multislice detector concepts would require fundamental changes in the scanner hardware, substantial upgrade of the electron beam power, as well as new cone-beam reconstruction algorithms. Thus, EBCT technology might improve in the future if the described technology challenges can be overcome with high development efforts.

The temporal resolution of current multislice CT scanners needs to be improved to provide motion-free and robust coronary imaging also for moderate and high heart rates. Increased temporal resolution can be achieved by segmented reconstruction techniques using two or more segments from consecutive heart cycles for reconstruction. Latest 16-slice scanners achieve 0.42 s rotation time and a best temporal resolution of 105 ms by using two-segment reconstruction [20, 21]. However, segmented reconstruction can improve temporal resolution only in a limited range of heart rates and at the expense of blurring artifacts in the presence of heart rate changes. Further increased rotation speed is the most favorable approach to increase temporal resolution. For example, 0.3 s rotation time can produce a consistent temporal resolution of 150 ms for all heart rates that may be able to provide motion-free data in patients with low and moderate heart rate (presumably up to 80 min^{-1}), thereby reducing the number of patients that require heart rate controlling medication. Obviously, significant development efforts will be needed to handle the increase of mechanical forces and the increased data transmission rates. Rotation times of less than 0.2 s that would be needed to provide temporal resolution of less than 100 ms, independent of heart rate, appear to be beyond today's technical limits. Concepts with multiple tubes and detectors have been described already in 1975. Theoretically, such approaches would allow for temporal resolution better than 100 ms with mechanical CT without significantly increased rotation speed if the substantial system design challenges can be overcome. Thinner slices are technically feasible but require a higher radiation dose to maintain a high contrast-to-noise and more detector-slices to maintain a short scan time (<20 s). As a complement to further increased spatial resolution advanced beam-hardening and metal artifact

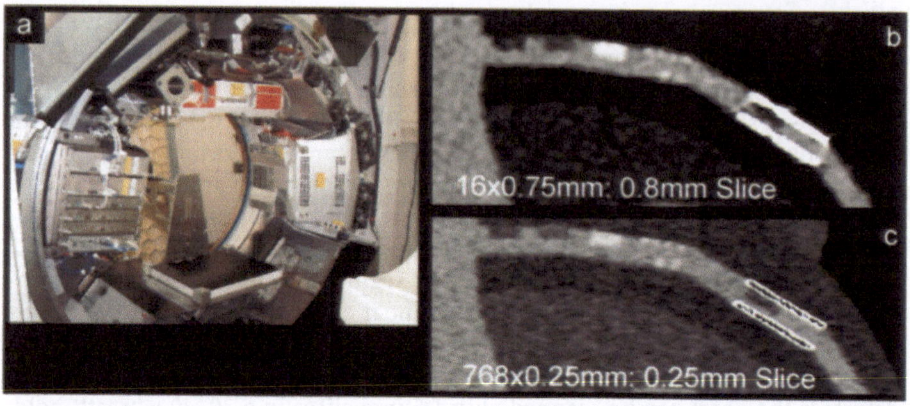

Fig. 14a–c. The anthropomorphic heart and coronary artery phantom displayed in Fig. 6 was used to compare the maximum possible spatial resolution of 16-slice CT with future area detector CT systems (**a**) that may provide detector pixel sizes below 0.5 mm. Such systems may be able to cover the heart in a single scanner rotation with isotropic resolution of 0.25 mm. Extremely high spatial resolution can improve visualization of in-stent lumen and small coronary segments compared to 16-slice CT (**b**) but do not necessarily provide improved delineation of non-calcified coronary lesions due to compromised signal-to-noise ratio (**c**)

reduction algorithms can be developed that improve imaging of calcified and stented coronary vessels, which to date are restricted to cerebral and bone imaging.

The ultimate CT-scanner should cover the entire coronary anatomy in a single heart beat without movement of the table. This can be achieved with area detectors that cover about 120 mm scan range with at least 0.5 mm spatial resolution (Fig. 14). Area detector technology and related new cone-beam reconstruction techniques are in research, that can provide in-plane and through-plane spatial resolution of 0.2 mm. With these CT scanners imaging of high-resolution morphology as well as dynamic and functional information via repeated scanning of the same scan range may be possible. The application potential of such technology is being evaluated with first experimental systems using phantom models and post mortem hearts. Initial experience shows that today's flat panel detector technology is yet too limited in low contrast resolution and the high radiation dose that is needed to provide adequate signal-to-noise ratio even for high contrast studies is unacceptable for use in human subjects. Due to the intrinsic slow decay times of flat panel detectors available today only slow rotation times ≥10 s are possible (Fig. 14) at the present time.

Latest multislice CT scanners also allow combining 16-slice CT with PET cameras. These systems may allow for a clinical combination of cardiac CT imaging and cardiac PET scans in a single examination and subsequent fusion of the information on cardiac morphology and myocardial function and metabolism (Fig. 15). The clinical potential of these scanners is currently under evaluation and first study data can be expected in the near future.

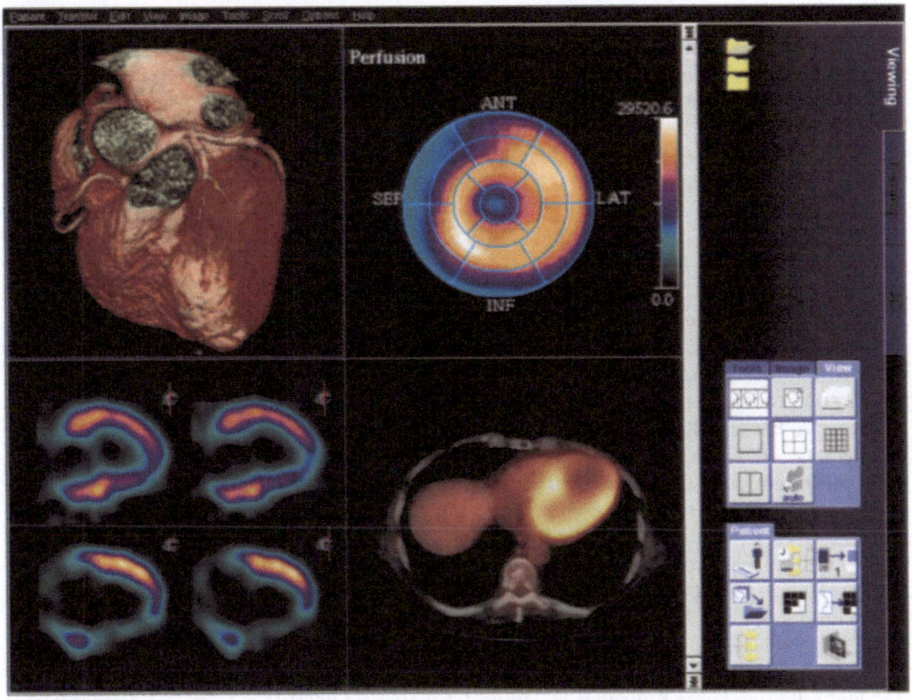

Fig. 15. CT/PET examination of a patient with a known occlusion of the left descending coronary artery and history of myocardial infarction (biograph Sensation 16, Siemens, USA/Germany). The 3D-volume rendering reconstruction of the ECG-gated 16-slice CT scan reveals the occluded coronary vessel and a related infarct scar. The PET scan demonstrates a perfusion defect and necrotic myocardium at the anterior wall. (Case by courtesy of the department of Radiology of the Tübingen University, Germany and the department of Nuclear Medicine of the Technical University of Munich, Germany)

References

1. Boyd DP, Lipton MJ (1982) Cardiac computed tomography. Proceedings of the IEEE 71: 298–307
2. Agatston AS, Janowitz WR, Hildner FJ, Zusmer NR, Viamonte M, Detrano R (1990) Quantification of coronary artery calcium using ultrafast computed tomography. JACC 15: 827–832
3. Achenbach S, Moshage W, Ropers D, Nössen J, Daniel WG (1998) Value of electron-beam computed tomography for the non-invasive detection of high-grade coronary artery stenoses and occlusions. N Engl J Med 339: 1964–1971
4. Becker CR, Jakobs TF, Aydemir S et al. (2000) Helical and single-slice conventional CT versus electron beam ct for the quantification of coronary artery calcification. AJR 174: 543–547
5. Bahner ML, Böse J, Lutz A, Wallschläger H, Regn J, van Kaick G (1999) Retrospectively ECG-gated spiral CT of the heart and lung. Eur Radiol 9: 106–109
6. Ohnesorge B, Flohr T, Schaller S, Klingenbeck-Regn K, Becker CR, Schöpf UJ, Brüning R, Reiser MF (1999) Technische Grundlagen und Anwendungen der Mehrschicht CT. Radiologe 39: 923–931

7. Klingenbeck K, Schaller S, Flohr T, Ohnesorge B, Kopp AF, Baum U (1999) Subsecond multi-slice computed tomography: basics and applications. Eur J Radiol 31: 110–124
8. Ohnesorge B, Flohr T, Becker CR, Kopp AF, Knez A, Baum U, Klingenbeck-Regn K, Reiser MF (2000) Cardiac imaging by means of electrocardiographically gated multisection spiral CT: initial experience. Radiology 217: 564–571
9. Kachelrieß M, Ulzheimer S, Kalender WA (2000) ECG-correlated image reconstruction from subsecond multi-row spiral CT scans of the heart. Med Phys 27: 1881–1902
10. Ohnesorge B, Becker CR, Flohr T, Reiser MF (2002). Multi-Slice CT in Cardiac Imaging – Technical Principles, Clinical Application and Future Developments. Springer Publishing Berlin Heidelberg New York
11. Knez A, Becker CR, Leber A, Ohnesorge B, Reiser MF, Haberl R (2000) Non-invasive assessment of coronary artery stenoses with multidetector helical computed tomography. Circulation 101: e221–e222
12. Niemann K, Oudkerk M, Rensing BJ, van Ooijen P, Munne A, van Geuns RJ, de Feyter P (2001) Coronary angiography with multi-slice computed tomography. Lancet 357: 599–603
13. Knez A, Becker CR, Leber A, Ohnesorge B, Becker A, White C, Haberl R, Reiser MF, Steinbeck G (2002). Usefulness of Multislice Spiral Computed Tomography Angiography for Determination of Coronary Artery Stenoses. Am J Cardiol 88:1191–1194
14. Kopp AF, Schröder S, Küttner A, Baumbach A, Heuschmid M, Georg C, Kuzo R, Ohnesorge B, Karsch K, Claussen CD (2002). High Resolution Multi-Slice Computed Tomography with Retrospective Gating for Angiography in Coronary Arteries: Results in 102 Patients. Eur Heart J 23:1714–1725
15. Schröder S, Kopp AF, Baumbach A, Küttner A, Georg C, Ohnesorge B, Herdeg C, Claussen CD, Karsch KR (2001). Non-Invasive Detection and Evaluation of Atherosclerotic Plaque with Multi-Slice Computed Tomography. JACC 37:1430–1435
16. Flohr T, Stierstorfer K, Bruder H, Simon J, Schaller S (2002) New technical developments in multislice CT, part 1: approaching isotropic resolution with sub-mm 16-slice scanning. Fortschr Röntgenstr 174: 839–845
17. Flohr T, Stierstorfer K, Bruder H, Simon J, Schaller S, Ohnesorge B (2002) New technical developments in multislice ct, part 2: sub-millimeter 16-slice scanning and increased gantry rotation speed for cardiac imaging. RöFo, Fortschr Röntgenstr 174: 1022–1027
18. Funabashi N, Komiyama N, Yanagawa N et al. (2003) Coronary artery patency after metallic stent implantation evaluated by multislice computed tomography. Circulation 107: 147–148
19. Kopp AF, Küttner A, Heuschmid M, Schröder S, Ohnesorge B, Claussen CD (2002) Multidetector-row CT cardiac imaging with 4 and 16 slices for coronary cta and imaging of atherosclerotic plaques. Eu Radiol 12 [Suppl 2]: S17–S24
20. Flohr TG, Küttner A, Bruder H, Stierstorfer K, Halliburton SS, Schaller S, Ohnesorge BM (2003) Performance evaluation of a multi-slice CT system with 16-slice detector and increased gantry rotation speed for isotropic submillimeter imaging of the heart. Herz 28: 7–19
21. Flohr TG, Schöpf UJ, Küttner A, Halliburton SS, Bruder H, Süß C, Schmidt B, Hofmann L, Yucel EK, Schaller S, Ohnesorge BM (2003). Advances in Cardiac Multi-Slice CT-Imaging with 16-Slice CT-Systems. Acad Radiol 10:386–401
22. Flohr T, Ohnesorge B (2001) Heart-rate adaptive optimization of spatial and temporal resolution for ECG-gated multi-slice spiral CT of the heart. J Comp Assist T 25: 907–923
23. Ohnesorge B, Flohr T, Becker CR, Knez A, Schöpf U, Klingenbeck K, Brüning R, Reiser MF (2001). Technical Aspects and Applications of Fast Multislice Cardiac CT. Medical Radiology, Diagnostic Imaging and Radiation Oncology, Multislice CT. Chapter 15:121–130. Springer Verlag Berlin, Heidelberg 2001
24. Bruder H, Flohr TG, Stierstorfer K, Rauscher A, Hölzel A, Schaller S (2002) ECG-Gated Dynamic Cardiac Volume Imaging with CT Area Detectors (Abstract). Radiology 225(P): 310
25. Hong C, Becker,CR, Huber A, Schöpf UJ, Ohnesorge B, Knez A, Brüning R, Reiser MF (2001) ECG-gated reconstructed multi-detector row CT coronary angiography: effect of varying trigger delay on image quality. Radiology 220: 712–717

26. Kopp AF, Schröder S, Küttner A, Heuschmid M, Georg C, Ohnesorge B, Kuzo R, Claussen CD (2001) Coronary arteries: retrospectively ECG-gated multi-detector row CT angiography with selective optimization of the reconstruction window. Radiology 221: 683–688
27. Jakobs T, Becker CR, Ohnesorge B, Flohr T, Schoepf UJ, Reiser MF (2002) Reduction of radiation exposure with ecg-controlled tube current modulation for retrospectively ECG-gated helical scans of the heart. Eur Radiol 12: 1081–1086
28. Flohr T, Prokop M, Schöpf, Kopp A, Becker C, Schaller S, White R, Ohnesorge B (2002) A new ECG-gated multislice spiral CT scan and reconstruction technique with extended volume coverage for cardio-thoracic applications. Eur Radiol 12: 1527–1532
29. Flohr T, Bruder H, Küttner A, Heuschmid M, Schaller S, Ohnesorge BM (2002) ECG-gated spiral scanning of the lung and mediastinal vessels with optimized temporal resolution and cone-correction on a 16-slice CT system: performance evaluation and initial clinical results. Radiology 225(P): 449 (Abstract)
30. Kopp AF, Ohnesorge B, Becker C, Schröder S, Heuschmid M, Küttner A, Kuzo R, Claussen CD (2002) Reproducibility and accuracy of coronary calcium measurement with multidetector-row versus electron beam CT. Radiology 225: 113–119
31. Ulzheimer S, Halliburton SS, McCollough CH, Becker CR, White RD, Kalender WA (2002) Evaluation of image quality and calcium scoring performance in multislice cardiac computed tomography. Radiology 221(P):458 (Abstract)
32. Hunold P, Vogt FM, Schmermund A, Kerkhoff G, Debatin JF, Barkhausen J (2002) Radiation exposure during noninvasive coronary artery imaging: comparison of multislice CT and electron beam CT. Radiology 225: 145–152
33. Schöpf UJ, Becker CR, Ohnesorge BM, Yucel EK (2003) CT of coronary artery disease. Radiology (in press)
34. Kalender WA, Schmidt B, Zankl M, Schmidt M (1999) A PC Program for estimating organ dose and effective dose values in computed tomography. Eur Radiol 9: 555–562
35. Schmidt B, Ulzheimer S, Kalender WA (2001) Dose in multi-slice cardiac CT: assessment of organ effective dose values with Monte Carlo methods. Radiology 221(P): 414 (Abstract)
36. Hong C, Becker CR, Schöpf UJ, Ohnesorge B, Brüning R, Reiser MF (2002) Absolute quantification of coronary calcification in non-contrast and contrast-enhanced multislice CT studies. Radiology 223: 474–480
37. Fleischmann D, Rubin GD, Bankier AA, Hittmair K (2000) Improved uniformity of aortic enhancement with customized contrast medium injection protocols at CT angiography. Radiology 214: 363–371
38. Becker CR, Kleffel T, Crispin A, Knez A, Young Y, Schöpf UJ, Haberl R, Reiser MF (2001) Coronary artery calcium measurement: agreement of multirow detector and electron beam CT. Am J Roentgenol 176: 1295–1298
39. Achenbach S, Ropers D, Mohlenkamp S et al. (2001) Variability of repeated coronary artery calcium measurements by electron beam tomography. Am J Cardiol 87: 210–213
40. Achenbach S, Ropers D, Pohle K et al. (2002) Influence of lipid-lowering therapy on the progression of coronary artery calcification – a prospective study. Circulation 106: 1077–1082
41. Shemesh J, Apter S, Stroh CI et al. (2000) Tracking coronary calcification by using dual-section spiral CT: a 3-year follow-up. Radiology 217: 461–465
42. Daniell A, Friedman J, Berman D et al. (2002) Concordance of Coronary Calcium Estimation between Multi-Detector and Electron Beam CT. Circulation 106 [Suppl II]: 479 (Abstract)
43. Ohnesorge B, Flohr T, Heuschmid M, Becker C (2002) Evaluation of different examination protocols for coronary artery calcium quantification with ECG-gated 16-slice spiral CT. Radiology 225(P): 239 (Abstract)
44. Ohnesorge B, Kopp AF, Fischbach R et al. (2002). Reproducibility of coronary calcium quantification in repeat examinations with retrospectively ECG-gated multislice spiral CT. Eur Radiol 12: 1532–1540
45. Moser K, Bateman T, Case J et al. (2002) The influence of acquisition mode on the reproducibility of coronary artery calcium scores using multi-detector computed tomography (Abstract). Circulation 106 [Suppl II]: II–479

46. Hong C, Bae KT, Pilgram TK et al. (2002) Coronary artery calcium measurement with multi-detector row CT: in vitro assessment of effect of radiation dose. Radiology 225: 901–906
47. Ulzheimer S, Kalender WA (2003) Assessment of calcium scoring performance in cardiac computed tomography. Eur Radiol 13: 484–497
48. Becker CR, Schöpf UJ, Reiser MF (2003) Coronary calcium scoring: medicine and politics. Eur Radiol 13: 445–447
49. Nieman K, Cademartiri F, Lemos PA, et al (2002). Reliable noninvasive coronary angiography with fast submillimeter multislice spiral computed tomography. Circulation 106: 2051–2054
50. Ropers D, Baum U, Pohle K, Anders K, Ulzheimer S, Ohnesorge B, Schlundt C, Bautz W, Daniel WG, Achenbach S (2003). Detection of Coronary Artery Stenoses with Thin-Slice Multi-Detector Row Spiral Computed Tomography and Multiplanar Reconstruction. Circulation 107:664–666
51. Juergens KU, Grude M, Fallenberg EM, Heindel W, Fischbach R (2002) Using ECG-gated multidetector CT to evaluate global left ventricular myocardial function in patients with coronary artery disease. AJR Am J Roentgenol 179: 1545–1550
52. Achenbach S, Ropers D, Holle J et al. (2000) In-plane coronary arterial motion velocity: measurement with electron beam CT. Radiology 216: 457–463
53. Wang Y, Watts R, Mitchell I et al. (2001) Coronary MR angiography: selection of acquisition window of minimal cardiac motion with electrocardiography-triggered navigator cardiac motion prescanning – initial results. Radiology 218: 580–585

14 Cardiac CT: From 4 to 16 Rows

A. F. Kopp, A. Küttner, T. Trabold, M. Heuschmid, S. Schröder,
C.D. Claussen

Introduction

Examination of the function, perfusion, and viability of the heart muscle as well as of the morphology and function of the coronary arteries is of utmost importance in the diagnostic assessment of coronary artery disease. The current gold standard to assess the degree of stenotic artery disease is coronary angiography. In Germany alone, the total number of angiographic procedures rose by 45% from 1995 to 2000, while the fraction of interventional procedures remained almost constantly low at about 30% [1]. Although coronary angiography has become a safe procedure with only a small risk associated [2], the inconvenience for the patient as well as the economic burden have fueled the quest to find an alternative, non-invasive method to visualize and assess coronary arteries. In the last three years mechanical multidetector-row CT (MDCT) systems with simultaneous acquisition of four slices and half second scanner rotation have become widely available [3–5]. Current recommendations to perform non-invasive coronary CT angiography rely on studies performed with this 4-row generation [5–10]. With the recent introduction of 16-row technology, spatial and temporal resolution was significantly improved. This leap in technology will redefine the role of coronary CTA in clinical cardiology.

The present chapter focuses on the technology principles and clinical applications of multislice CT in cardiac imaging and we will discuss the technology advances and improved clinical performance of state-of-the-art 16-slice CT equipment.

Calcium Scoring

Half the coronary deaths and the majority of myocardial infarctions in the United States occur in persons characterized as low or intermediate risk [11]. Electron-beam-computed tomography (EBCT) measurement of coronary arterial calcification in large groups of individuals has provided important epidemiologic statistics regarding the relationship between coronary arterial calcification and coronary events [11, 12]. In contrast to more traditional non-invasive testing methods such as treadmill exercise, stress echocardiography and stress thallium 201, CT can be performed in patients with resting ECG abnormalities or digitalis medications, as well as those unable to exercise [11, 12]. The study of progression and regression of established atherosclerosis and how differences in calcium score over time result in differences in event rates is one of the most interesting clinical applications of calcium scoring [13]. It is conceivable that such serial measurements of calcium score could provide a powerful and much needed predictive tool. Although the current method of calcium scoring reliably detects the presence of calcium deposits, their use in serial studies for tracking the progression of calcification has been hampered by the limited reproducibility of the calcium scores currently in use. The widely used Agatston score based on the peak-density measurement on EBCT yields 28 to 72% interstudy variability [14–17], which jeopardizes the ability to detect any changes within this range. This variability has demanded large changes in an individual patient's calcium score before investigators can be confident of the progression of coronary arterial calcification [14, 18, 19]. Without the ability to measure coronary artery calcification in individuals with reasonable certainty and precision, as well as repeatedly over meaningful time intervals the effect of treatment regimens on the progression of coronary arterial calcification in individual patients cannot be determined.

Spiral multislice CT holds promise to overcome this limitation: Coupling the technique of retrospective gating with nearly isotropic volumetric imaging the reliability of coronary calcium quantification especially for small plaques was found to significantly improve [20]. Using ECG-gated volume coverage with multislice spiral CT and overlapping image reconstruction (2.5 mm collimation, 1 mm increment) an interscan variability of approximately 5–8% can be achieved [21]. With the advent of multislice CT with significantly reduced interstudy variability we can now begin to define the effects of treatment regimens on coronary arterial calcification and to determine whether changes in coronary arterial calcification in individual patients have predictive value for future coronary events. If these differences in calcium score over time result in a difference in event rates, it is conceivable that serial measurements of calcium score by MDCT will provide a powerful and much needed predictive tool [22].

CTA Coronary Angiography for Detection of Stenoses

The imaging protocol for MDCT angiography of the coronary arteries on a 4-row scanner is relatively straightforward. To establish the scan delay time a test bolus of 15 ml CM and 20 ml saline chaser bolus is used. The circulation time is determined by measurements of CT density values in the ascending aorta. Imaging commences at the circulation time plus 3 s [23]. A bolus of 120 ml non-ionic contrast (400 mg I/ml) is injected trough an 18-gauge catheter into an antecubital vein [24]. Usually, the cranio-caudal size of the heart to be covered by the scan is in the range 10–12 cm. 4-slice CT scanners with 500 ms rotation time and an individual detector-width of 1.0 mm cover the entire heart during a 30–40 s breath-hold with reconstructed slice-width of 1.3 mm [25]. For optimal image quality the reconstruction window within the cardiac cycle should be selected individually for each of the three major coronary arteries [26–28] (Fig. 1).

The results of MDCT coronary angiography in the detection and quantification of coronary lesions with 4-row technology obtained so far from different

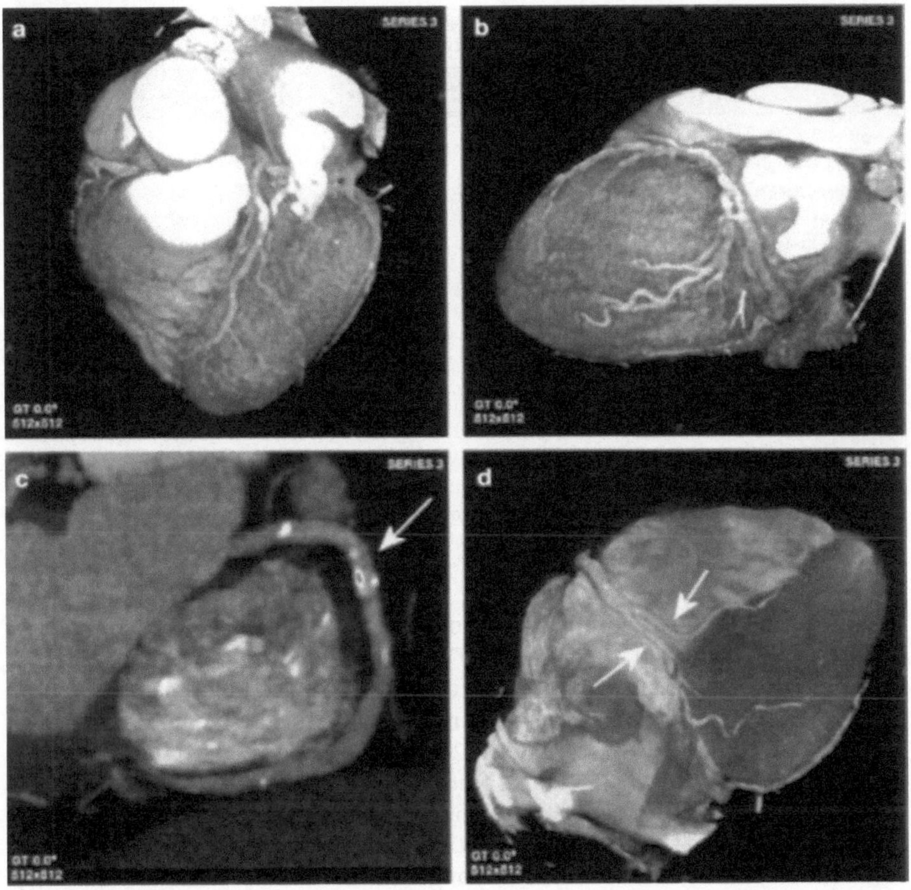

Fig. 1a–d. MDCT angiography with 4-row technology (collimation 4×1 mm, pitch 1.5, 120 cc Imeron 400). **a** Anterior view of left coronary artery with LAD in volume rendering technique. **b** Lateral view of left coronary artery with LAD and circumflex branch. **c** Maximum intensity projection of right coronary artery with calcified plaques (*arrow*). **d** Diaphragmatic surface with posterolateral and interventricular branches of RCA (*arrows*)

centers are encouraging [29, 30] (Table 1): CTA of the coronary arteries yielded a sensitivity of 75–90%, a specificity of 90–95%, a positive predictive value of 0.7–0.9, and a negative predictive value of 0.8–0.9 for detection of hemodynamically significant stenoses in the major segments of the coronary arteries [24]. However, in these studies 20–30% of the proximal arteries could not be adequately evaluated.

True isotropic resolution has not been reached with 4-slice CT systems. Consequently, an increased number of simultaneously acquired slices and sub-millimeter collimation for cardiac applications was the next step on the way towards true isotropic scanning with multislice CT. The 16-row multislice CT scanner Siemens SOMATOM Sensation 16 was introduced in 2002, offering simultaneous

Table 1. Results for 4- and 16-row MDCT angiography (MDCTA) for detection of hemodynamically relevant stenoses. *n* number of patients included in the study

Author	n	Sensitivity [%]	Specificity [%]
4-row MDCTA			
Kopp et al. [46]	102	86	93
Achenbach et al. [47]	64	91	84
Becker et al. [7]	48	82	97
Nieman et al. [10]	31	91	97
Nitatori et al. [48]	18	40	71
Fischbach et al. [49]	27	76	93
Herzog et al. [50]	120	71	92
16-row MDCTA			
Küttner [51, 52]	60	72/98[a]	97/98[a]
Ropers [31]	77	73/92[b]	92/90[b]
Niemann [32]	59	95[c]	86[c]

[a]data for patients with Ca-Score <1000, [b]data for patients with heart rate <60, [c]only vessels with diameter >2 mm included.

acquisition of 16 slices with 0.75 mm or 1.5 mm collimated slice width each. Similar to the 4-slice CT scanner the SOMATOM Sensation 16 has an adaptive array detector. It consists of 24 detector rows, the 16 central ones being 0.75 mm wide in the center of rotation, the 4 outer ones on both sides being 1.5 mm wide. The total z coverage in the iso-center is 24 mm. For CTA of the coronary arteries a collimation of 0.75 mm (13.2 mm/s feed) with a gantry rotation time of 420 ms is used. Spiral scanning with sub-millimeter slices represents an important step on the way towards true isotropic resolution for routine clinical applications. As a consequence, the distinction between longitudinal and in-plane resolution may gradually become a historical remnant, and the traditional axial slice will loose its clinical predominance.

The simultaneous acquisition of 0.75-mm cross-sections yields higher spatial resolution, and at the same time, the overall scan time is substantially shorter than with previous scanners. Improved spatial resolution, through reduction of partial volume effects, improves diagnostic accuracy and potentially reduces the problems caused by calcification, whereas a shorter scan time may improve scan quality through the shorter breathhold duration and, in addition, requires less contrast agent. Finally, the faster rotation (420 ms) compared with previous scanners provides higher temporal resolution. The protocol for obtaining a coronary CTA in our institution was changed accordingly: First, a precontrast scan is performed to determine the total calcium burden of the coronary tree (collimation 1.5 mm, table feed 3.8 mm/rotation, tube current 133 eff. mAs at 120 kV). To determine the circulation time, 20 ml of contrast media (20 ml at 4 ml/s, 400 mg iodine/ml) and a chaser bolus of 20 ml saline is administered in an antecubital vein. By using a dual-head power injector a total of only 80 ml intravenous contrast agent plus a 20 ml chaser bolus is injected (50 ml at 4.0 ml/s, then 30 ml at 2.5 ml/s). CT imaging starts at the diaphragm caudally of all cardiac structures and stops at the aortic root cranial to the coronary ostia. The contrast

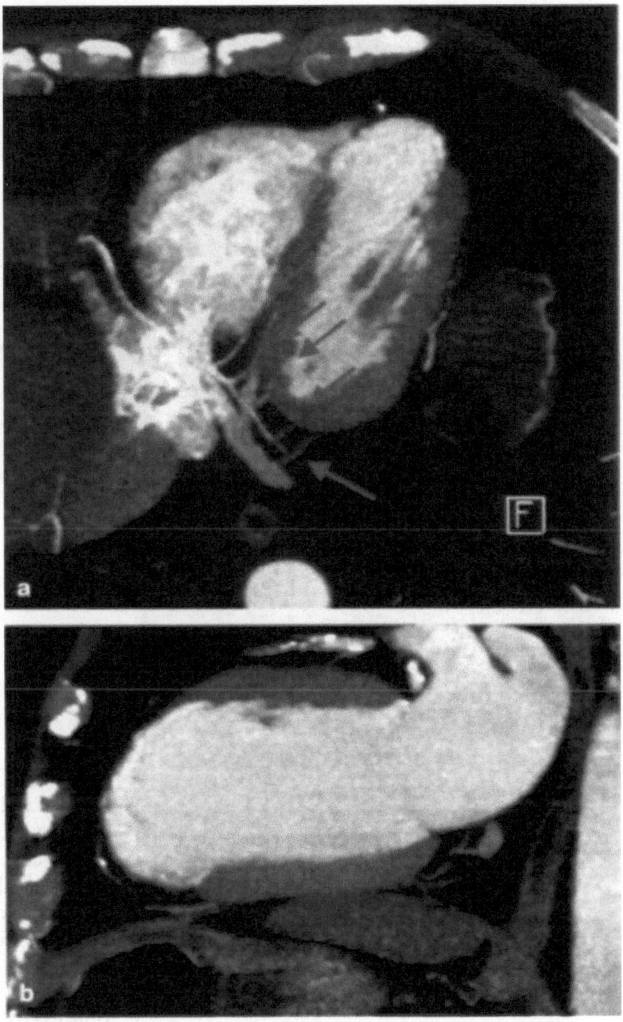

Fig. 2a,b. 66-year-old male patient with known single vessel coronary artery disease. **a** MDCT angiography of the right coronary artery with a 16-row CT-scanner (Somatom Sensation 16, 80 cc Imeron 400). Even subsegmental branches (*arrows*) can be readily delineated. **b** MPR in the long axis depicts aneurysm of left ventricle s/p myocardial infarction

enhanced scan is acquired with a 0.75 mm collimation, a table feed of 3.8 mm/rotation, and a tube current 500 eff. mAs at 140 kV (Fig. 2).

In a first study to assess 16-slice technology for coronary CTA we included a total of 60 consecutive patients referred to our institution for invasive coronary angiography due to suspected coronary artery disease (CAD) or suspected progress of a known CAD. In a total of 763 coronary segments conventional coronary angiography (CCA) detected a total of 75 lesion >50%. MDCT correctly assessed 54 (72%) of these. 21 lesions were missed or incorrectly underestimated (3 lesion missed due to motion artifacts, 9 had severe calcifications and 9 lesions were missed despite sufficient image quality). 21 lesions were overestimated and counted as false positive. Sensitivity was 72%, specificity 97%, the positive

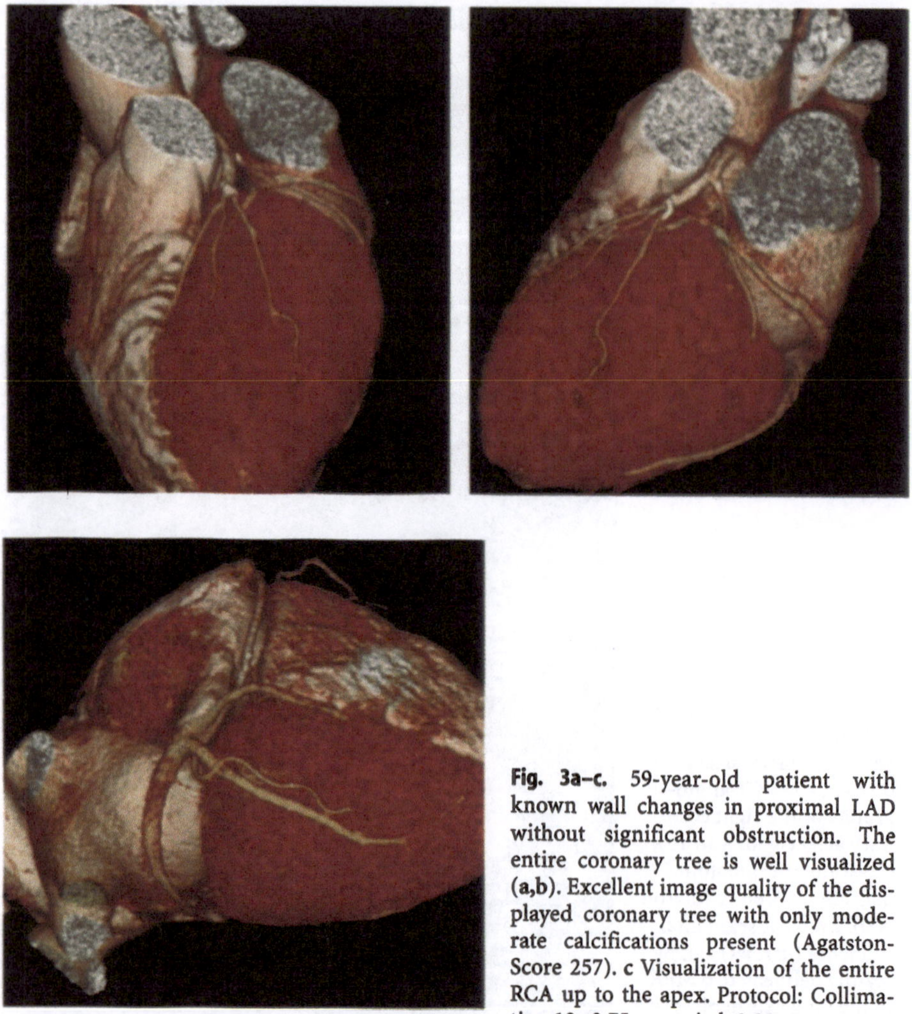

Fig. 3a–c. 59-year-old patient with known wall changes in proximal LAD without significant obstruction. The entire coronary tree is well visualized (**a,b**). Excellent image quality of the displayed coronary tree with only moderate calcifications present (Agatston-Score 257). **c** Visualization of the entire RCA up to the apex. Protocol: Collimation 12×0.75 mm, pitch 0.31

predictive value 72% and the negative predictive value was 97%. However, when limiting the analysis to patients with an arbitrarily chosen threshold of 1000 Agatston Score Equivalent (ASE) (n=46, 14 patients had an ASE >1000) as criteria for severe calcifications, CCA detected a total of 40 lesions >50%. MDCT correctly assessed 39 (95%) of these. One lesion was missed in a marginal branch and 10 lesions were overestimated and counted as false positive. Threshold corrected sensitivity was 98%, specificity 98%, the positive predictive value 80% and the negative predictive value was 100% (Fig. 3).

Similar results were obtained by other groups (see Table 1): Ropers et al. analyzed coronary stenoses in 16-row coronary MDCTA with a reference diameter down to 1.5 mm, thus covering all lesions that may be potential targets for revascularization [31]. Both motion and calcification rendered fewer arteries

(12%) unevaluable than in most previous studies and a high sensitivity (92%) and specificity (93%) for the detection of coronary stenoses was achieved [31]. Nieman et al. [32] demonstrated similar results with a sensitivity, specificity, and negative predictive value of 95, 86 and 97%, respectively, in a comparable patient population using the same 16 slice CT technology. However, their analysis was restricted to the major branches with a vessel size ≥2 mm. Striking about this study was that only 7% of all coronary branches were poorly assessable.

Plaque Imaging

The underlying pathophysiological mechanism of acute coronary syndrome is plaque disruption, subsequent thrombosis and acute myocardial infarction. Direct visualization of epicardial coronary arteries is necessary to assess the focal severity and clinical relevance of these vessel wall alterations. The visualization of plaques has a twofold clinical background. On one hand, obstructive coronary artery disease causing chronic ischemia to the vessel dependent myocardial tissue needs to be assessed to determine an adequate revascularization strategy (condition of stable angina pectoris). On the other hand, precursors of the already mentioned unheralded plaque rupture causing unstable angina, myocardial infarction or sudden death should be assessed to take preventive measures to avoid these acute coronary syndromes. Evidence suggests that atherosclerotic plaque composition and configuration are important predictors of plaque stability. Most ruptures occur in plaques containing a soft, lipid-rich core that is covered by a thin and inflamed cap of fibrous tissue. Small ruptures often remain clinically silent, but more extensive plaque ruptures may cause the onset of unstable angina, myocardial infarction or sudden death. Thus, the reliable non-invasive detection and classification of coronary lesion would constitute an important step forward in risk stratification of patients with known or suspected coronary artery disease. Currently, only highly invasive intravascular ultrasound allows assessment of plaque composition.

Intravascular ultrasound imaging offers several advantages in the evaluation of CAD. First, due to the imaging from inside the vessel, ICUS provides images of the atherosclerotic plaque, not only the lumen. Tomographic orientation of ICUS offers a three-dimensional visualization of the entire circumference of the vessel wall and not just biplanar projections. Also, correct angiographic vessel or stenosis measurements (QCA) requires calibration to correct for radiographic magnification, a potential source for errors. ICUS uses an electronically generated scale, performing direct planimetry. The tomographic perspective of ultrasound enables an assessment of vessels that are difficult to image by angiography, including diffusely diseased segments, ostial or bifurcation stenoses, as well as eccentric plaques.

ICUS consists of a catheter incorporating a miniaturized transducer and a console to reconstruct the images. Ultrasound frequencies between 20 and 50 MHz are used, yielding a practical axial resolution of ≈150 μm. Lateral resolution averages 250 μm. Current catheters range from 2.6 and 3.5 French (0.87 to 1.17 mm) and can be placed through a 6-French guiding catheter. Mechanically rotated devices and multielement electronic arrays are available. Standard techniques for intracoronary catheter delivery are used for intravascular examination. The operator advances or retracts the ICUS device over the wire, recording the data for subsequent analysis. A motorized pullback device is used to withdraw the catheter at a constant speed (0,5 mm/s). Complication rates of an ICUS exam varies from 1 to 3%; transient spasm being the most frequent complication. The complication rate of major dissection or vessel closures is ≈0,5%.

When MDCT was introduced in 1999, soon evidence was found, that even preclinical atheroma and non-calcified plaque tissue could be identified. However, these early results had to be confirmed whether MDCT was really able to correctly assess not only the severity of the lumen loss, but also plaque composition and plaque configuration. Thus, the purpose of one of our first studies was to investigate whether plaque composition as assessed by MDCT was corresponding to the gold standard ICUS. A total of 15 patients that were scheduled for ICUS-guided percutaneous transluminal angioplasty (PTCA) were enrolled in this study. Angiographic exclusion criteria were left main disease, total occlusions and vessel diameter <2 mm and bypass lesions. According to the study protocol, all patients were examined by MDCT within 24 h prior to the coronary intervention. Immediately before the intracoronary intervention, ICUS was performed to analyze the vessel configuration proximal to the target lesion and within the lesion. To ensure that identical plaques were assessed by the different techniques and to allow for precise correlations, landmarks such as the origin or side-branches and the distance to the target lesion were used. The assessed plaque configuration was classified according to the following ICUS criteria published by our group and others:

- Soft plaques: More than 80% of the plaque area is composed of tissue with an echogenity of lower than the echogenity of the surrounding adventitia.
- Intermediate plaques: More than 80% of the plaque area is composed of tissue producing echoes as bright or brighter than those of the surrounding adventitia but without acoustic shadows.
- Calcified plaques: This plaque type involves bright echoes with acoustic shadowing accompanying >90° of the vessel wall circumference.

A total of 34 plaques (RCA n=12, LAD n =22) were analyzed by both methods with respect to lesion configuration. On ICUS, 12 plaques were classified as soft, 5 plaques as intermediate and 17 plaques as calcified (Fig. 4). When comparing these data to MDCT data, the plaques identified by ICUS as soft had a mean densitiy 14±26 HU, those classified as intermediate had a mean density of 91±21 HU and calcified plaques had a mean density 419±194 HU. Calcifications were also found in intermediate plaques, however, only small sprinkles of calcium deposits were found. Interestingly, even with only 34 plaques analyzed, the test for statistical significance was highly positive (Kruskal-Wallis test, $p<0.0001$). Since some patients had up to 5 plaques, plaque density results had to be tested for independence of the patient itself. First, it was tested whether patient groups with either one, two, three, four, or five plaques were significantly different from each other, which was not the case ($p=0.876$). Also the independence of patient group and plaque composition was demonstrated ($p=0.817$). These data suggest

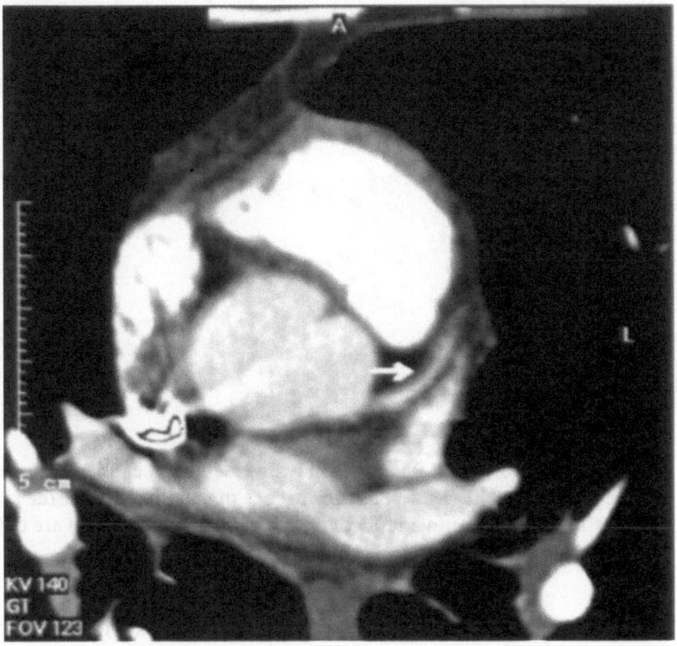

Fig. 4. Non-calcified soft lipid-rich plaque in LAD (*arrow*). The plaque was confirmed at intracoronary ultrasound

that MDCT is capable of differentiation between different plaque compositions. The density measurements performed by MDCT correlated highly with the well established ICUS criteria »soft«, »intermediate« and »calcified«. There was no overlap in the mean density values among the three groups of plaques. Thus, especially soft plaques with presumably lipid-rich core might be identified by density values <50 HU. Intermediate plaques showed a density ranging from 50–119 HU. Lesions with a density >120 HU correlated to calcified plaques in the ICUS study. A more precise view by MDCT on plaque configuration by visualizing lipid cores, fibrous caps or smallest calcified sprinkles was restricted due to limited spatial resolution of 4-row MDCT used in this first study.

In 2002 with the introduction of the 2nd generation of multislice spiral scanners with up to 16 detector rows and a gantry rotation time as low as 420 ms, an improved tool to visualize coronary lesion became available. Next to a possible prognostic factor of plaque visualization, a keen interest remains whether plaque morphology also is a predictor for the assessment of stenosis. To answer this question, a total of 41 patients referred to our institution for conventional coronary angiography (CCA) were also examined by 16-row MDCT. The primary aim of this pilot study was to use 16-row MDCT to analyze different types of plaques and their predominance in high-grade lesions. On the basis of original axial slices, 3D-volume-rendering images as well as thin-sliding maximum-intensity projections, each coronary plaque identified by CCA as a high-grade stenotic lesion or occlusion was assessed. Depending on the identified plaque composition, each plaque was classified in one of 6 groups as follows:

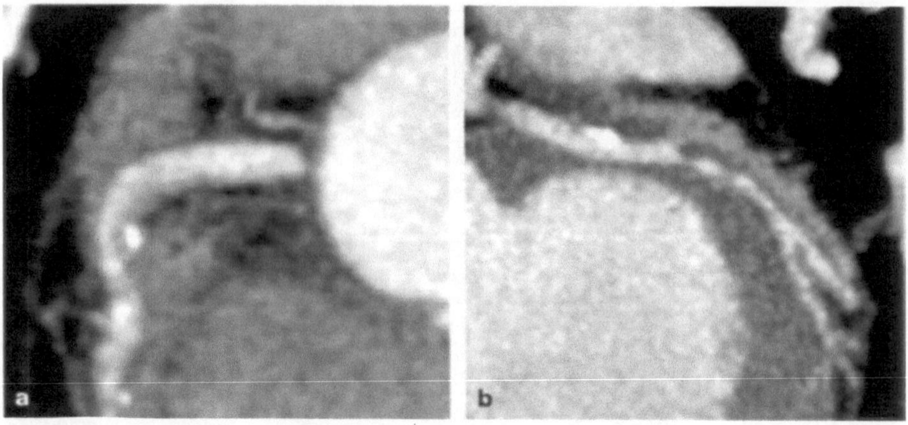

Fig. 5a,b. 58-year-old male patient with two vessel disease (16-row coronary MDCTA). Note the excellent image quality as well as the absence of calcifications at the site of obstruction. High-grade ostial lesion (**a**) and a tandem lesion in proximal RCX (**b**) are to be seen

1. calcified plaque adhered to vessel wall, no vessel obstruction,
2. calcified plaque, CT morphologically complete vessel obstruction,
3. calcified plaque conglomerate,
4. non-calcified plaque,
5. mixed plaque with calcifications predominantly present,
6. mixed plaque with non-calcified tissue predominantly present.

Conventional coronary angiography revealed a total of 49 high grade lesions (>70%) and 20 complete occlusions in a total of 533 coronary artery segments.

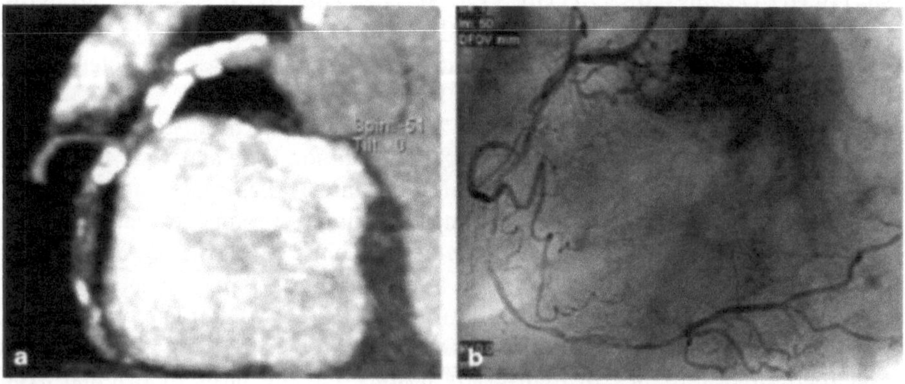

Fig. 6a,b. 71-year-old male patient with tree vessel disease. **a** Prominent calcifications in the proximal RCA causing no significant lumen loss. In the descending RCA a complete vessel occlusion is caused by a mixed plaque with predominantly non-calcified plaque tissue present. **b** Corresponding angiogram

All 69 plaques causing high grade stenosis or complete occlusion could be reliably detected by MDCT (Fig. 5). No plaque was attributed group 1 characteristics. One plaque was attributed group 2 characteristics, six plaques had group 3 characteristics, 20 plaques had group 4 characteristics, 29 plaques were assigned to group 5 and 13 plaques to group 6. Thus, of all high-grade lesions only 9/69 (13%) were caused by calcified plaques. »Soft plaques« (group 4 plaques) caused already 20/69 (29%) high-grade lesions and the majority of all high-grade lesions was caused by mixed plaques 42/69 (61%), of which predominantly calcified plaques accounted for 29/69 (42%) lesions and group 6 (predominantly non-calcified plaques) accounted for 13/69 (19%) lesions. These suggest that a binary decision tree calcified vs. non-calcified plaque tissue is not sufficient to characterize high-grade lesions since both entities are present in the majority of high-grade lesions (Fig. 6).

Function

With ECG-gated MDCT spiral scanning 2D or 3D images can be reconstructed in incrementally shifted heart phases with a temporal resolution of up to 125 ms. With multiplanar reformation, the heart can be displayed in any desired plan, such as the short and long axis. This allows functional analysis in a one-stop shopping approach for every patient undergoing CTA of the coronary arteries (Fig. 7). The ability to obtain functional information from routine contrast-enhanced cardiac examinations on a conventional whole-body CT scanner could obviate the need for an additional study with a second imaging modality. Halliburton et al. evaluated MDCT as a method for volume determination of the left ventricle by comparison to the gold standard, cine magnetic resonance imaging in 15 patients with chronic ischemic heart disease [33]. Measurement of left ventricular volume during end-diastole and end-systole volume with MDCT compared to MRI on a fast gradient system was significantly less for both volumes. However, values for ejection fraction with MDCT and MRI were not statistically different. Similar results were reported by several authors [34, 35] (Fig. 8). The exact determination of left ventricular volume during end-systole seems to be the most critical issue with a temporal resolution of 125 ms. Further improvement in temporal resolution will facilitate functional analysis.

When multiple cardiac phases are extracted, animated movies of the beating heart can be available. However, only limited data is available for the usefulness of the functional assessment of wall motion using MDCT. Mochizuki et al. evaluated post-processing interactive multiplanar animation for the evaluation of wall motion in 15 patients in comparison with conventional left ventriculography [36]. By extracting multiple cardiac phases, interactive animated movies were generated. Extracted cardiac phases ranged from 8 to 11, depending on the patient's heart rate. The interactive animated movies were displayed in 6 planes, the left ventricle was divided into 7 segments according to the AHA classification. Wall motion was visually scored into 3 grades: normal, hypokinesis, and akinesis (severe hypokinesis to dyskinesis). The scores of MDCT and biplane ventriculography agreed in 99 of 105 (94%) segments [36].

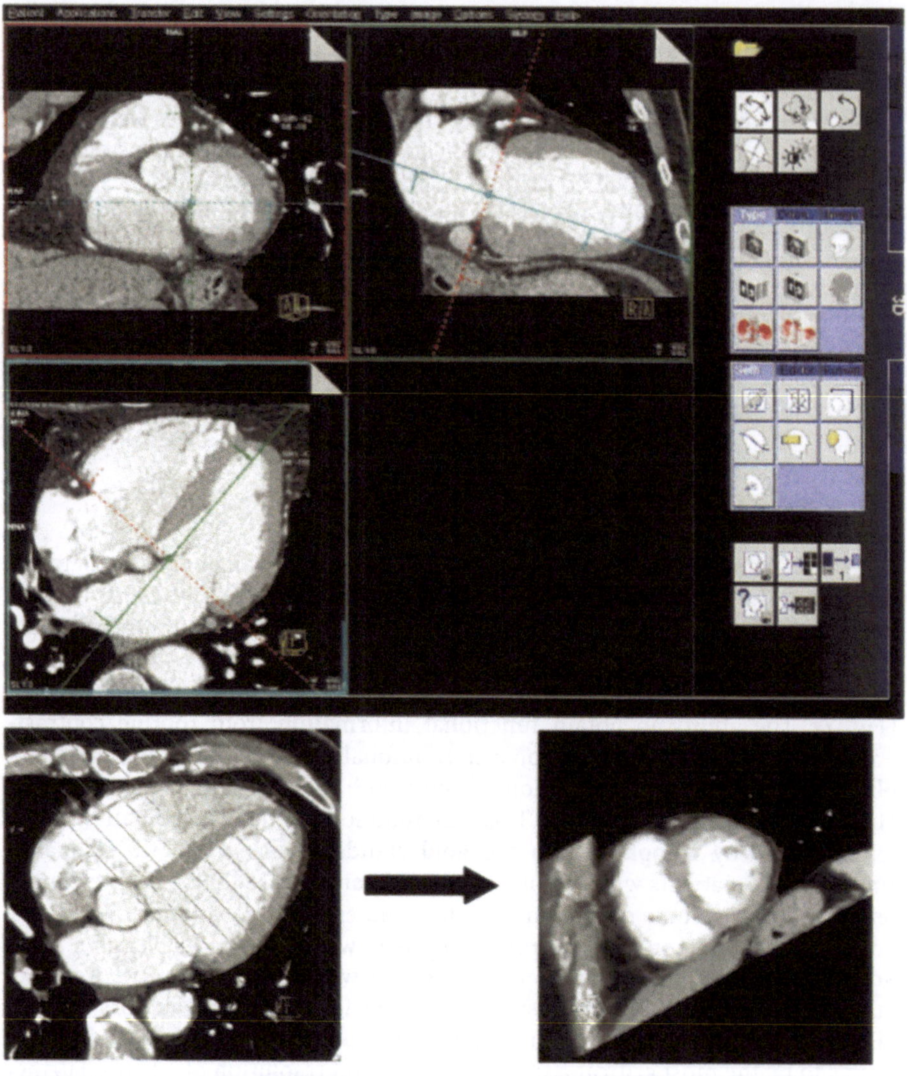

Fig. 7. Reconstruction of MPRs in the long and short axis for functional analysis. This task is facilitated by dedicated software tools

Myocardial Perfusion

Myocardial perfusion defects are often observed as low density in the risk area of acute myocardial infarction on contrast enhancement helical CT [37]. However, the clinical meaning of this perfusion defect has not been elucidated yet. Koyama et al. presented first data on the potential role of CT in 45 patients with acute myocardial infraction in regard to the clinical outcome after successful reperfusion therapy [38]. They visually assessed myocardial perfusion in regard to

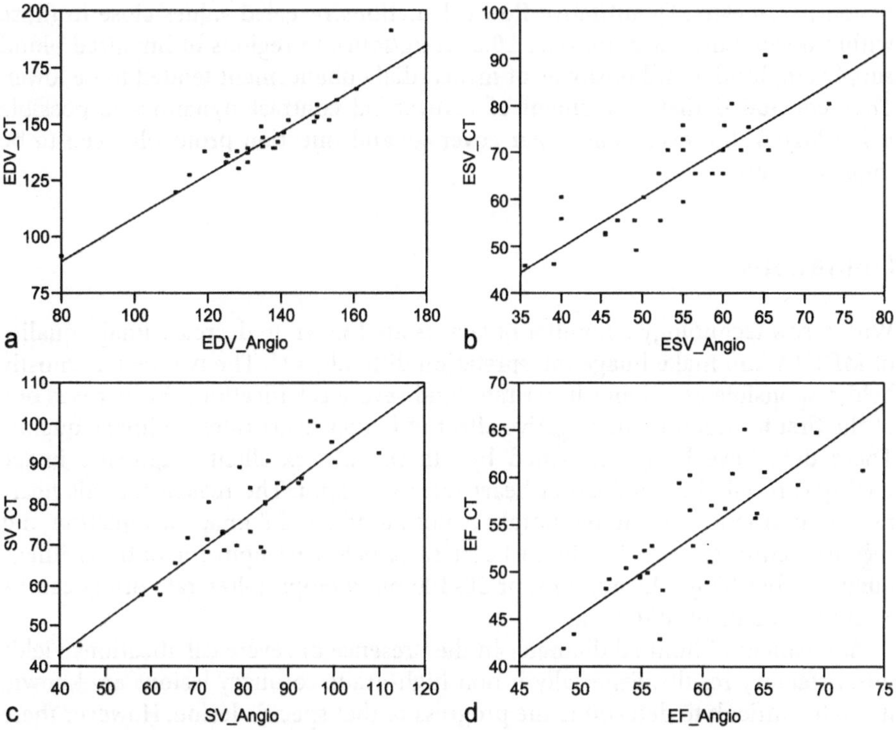

Fig 8a–d. Scatterplot for enddiastolic (**a**) and endsystolic (**b**) volume obtained from conventional angio vs. 4-row MDCT in 30 patients. The calculated stroke volume (**c**) and ejection fraction (**d**) show good correlation of r=0,88 and 0,82 (MDCT vs. ventriculography)

the depth of the perfusion defect. When compared with SPECT, these data corresponded nicely to the non-viable infarct area and its depth allowed to predict the outcome in the chronic phase. Even the volume of the infarcted area could be reliably assessed. In addition to these early perfusion defects, Koyama found that in some patients the perfusion defects disappeared when the CT scan was repeated several minutes later (late enhancement) [39]. In regard to the existence of early perfusion effect and late enhancement, they classified patients with acute myocardial infarction into three groups: group 1 showing no perfusion abnormalities, group 2 showing early perfusion defect and late enhancement, group 3 showing persistent perfusion defect in early and late phase. Koyama concluded that this myocardial perfusion pattern on contrast-enhanced CT might predict clinical outcome of acute myocardial infarction after reperfusion therapy [39].

Assessment of more than one or two time points of enhancement and the calculation of classic myocardial perfusion parameters with MDCT is even more challenging. In a first attempt, Wintersberger et al. analyzed myocardial contrast dynamics using ECG-triggered MDCT in 9 patients [40]. A prospectively ECG-triggered transaxial dynamic scan (4x5 mm) over 35 heart beats was applied to analyze myocardial enhancement patterns with subsequent assessment of perfusion parameters. Quantitative flow calculations revealed values close to those within normal myocardium (0.73±0.20 ml/g/min). In regions of impaired blood supply amplitudes and upslopes of myocardial enhancement tended to be lower. They concluded that assessment of myocardial contrast dynamics is possible using MDCT, however, ventricular coverage and injection protocols need to be improved [40].

Limitations

With 4-row technology a number of factors are known to decrease image quality of MDCTA and make image interpretation difficult [41]. The two factors mostly held responsible are higher heart rates and severe calcifications. Becker was one of the first to describe the negative effect of higher heart rates on image quality. These data have been confirmed by others [42]: excellent diagnostic image quality can only be obtained at heart rates <65 bpm. The reason for this heart rate limitation lies in the temporal resolution of the CT image acquisition and reconstruction system. To obtain heart rates below 65 bpm for optimal image quality either 80 mg Esmolol i.v. or 50–100 mg metoprololtartrate orally can be administered prior to the scan.

Assessment of luminal diameter in the presence of severe calcifications yields unsatisfactory results. Especially if non-high-grade coronary lesions are known, it can be difficult to determine the progress of that specific lesion. However there is only limited published data available that quantifies the amount of calcification critical for image interpretation. In a recent study we included a total of 66 patients with a history of coronary artery for MDCTA. Total calcium score as well as all coronary arteries including distal segments and side branches were assessed in respect of evaluability and the presence of coronary artery lesions or occlusions. Results were then compared to quantitative coronary angiography. Of all patients only 24 (36%) were diagnosed correctly. In the other 42 patients the clinical diagnosis was either not possible or incorrect. Artifacts due to elevated heart rates or severe coronary artery calcification were the main cause of degraded image quality inhibiting correct diagnosis. Analysis of the data suggested a threshold for maximum heart rate and maximum calcification (63 bpm and Agatston score 300, respectively). A second analysis was made using these thresholds. Now 22 out of 24 (91%) patients were correctly diagnosed. This indicates that MDCTA can also be performed in patients with manifest coronary artery disease when selected properly within certain thresholds. Reasonable thresholds might be heart rates >63 bmp and severe calcifications with a total Agatston score >300.

Patient Dose

Despite its undisputed clinical benefits, multislice scanning is often considered to require increased patient dose [43]. Indeed, a certain dose increase compared to single-slice CT is unavoidable due to the physical principles of multislice CT [44].

During ECG-gated spiral imaging of the heart, data are acquired with overlapping spiral pitch and continuous X-ray exposure. Thus, ECG-gated spiral acquisition requires higher patient dose than ECG-triggered sequential acquisition for comparable signal-to-noise ratio. When performing multiple reconstructions in different cardiac phases for optimal image quality of individual vessels, all spiral data are used for image reconstructions and no data is omitted. To obtain the same diagnostic information, multiple sequential acquisitions would have to be performed with repeated injections of contrast material. This would eventually result in the same or even higher X-ray exposure. However, ECG-gated spiral acquisition by prospectively ECG-controlled on-line modulation of the tube output allows reduction of X-ray exposure [45]. By reduction of the tube output during heart phases that are not likely to be targeted by the ECG-gated reconstruction dose savings up to 50% are possible. Dose is further reduced with increased number of simultaneously acquired slices. The collimated dose profile is in general a trapezoid in the axial direction. In the plateau region of the trapezoid, the entire focal spot is seen by the detector. In the penumbra regions, the focal spot is seen by the detector only partially, due to the limitation of the X-ray beam by the pre-patient collimator. With single-slice CT, the entire trapezoidal dose profile can contribute to the detector signal. With multislice CT, only the plateau region of the dose profile may be used to ensure equal signal level for all detector slices. The penumbra region has to be discarded, either by a post-patient collimator or by the intrinsic self-collimation of the multislice detector, and represents »wasted« dose. The relative contribution of the penumbra region increases with decreasing slice width, but it decreases with increasing number of simultaneously acquired slices. The relative dose utilization of the 4-slice CT scanner SOMATOM Volume Zoom is 70% for 4×1 mm collimation and 85% for 4×2.5 mm collimation. The 16-row scanner has an improved dose utilization of 76%/82% for 16×0.75 mm collimation and 85%/89% for 16×1.5 mm collimation, depending on the size of the focal spot (large/small).

Conclusion

The emergence of multidetector-row CT had significant impact on cardiac imaging. Cardiac calcium scoring and CTA of the coronary arteries as well as functional analysis are no longer limited to a dedicated EBCT scanner. Cardiac imaging can now be performed on a standard body MDCT scanner. Even with 4-row technology non-invasive MDCTA provides high diagnostic accuracy in the detection of coronary stenoses. First results obtained with the recently introduced 16-row technology showed further improvement in terms of image quality and diagnostic accuracy. If further studies confirm these first results, 16-row-MDCT could be recommended to act as a gatekeeper prior to cardiac catheterizations. In addition, this new technology holds promise to allow for the non-invasive detection and characterization of coronary atherosclerotic plaques.

References

1. Mannebach H, Hamm C, Horstkotte D (2001) 17th report of performance statistics of heart catheterization laboratories in Germany. Results of a combined survey by the Committee of Clinical Cardiology and the Interventional Cardiology (for ESC) and Angiology Working Groups of the German Society of Cardiology-Cardiovascular Research for the year 2000. Z Kardiol 90: 665–667
2. Kwok BW, Lim TT (2000) Cortical blindness following coronary angiography. Singapore Med J 41: 604–605
3. Kopp AF, Ohnesorge B, Flohr T, Georg C, Schröder S, Küttner A, Martensen J, Claussen CD (2000) Multidetector CT des Herzens: Erste klinische Anwendung einer retrospektiv EKG-gesteuerten Spirale mit optimierter zeitlicher und örtlicher Auflösung zur Darstellung der Herzkranzgefäße. Fortschr Röntgenstr 172: 1–7
4. Sablayrolles JL, Besse F, Giat P (2001) Technical developments in cardiac CT: 2000 update. Rays 26: 3–13
5. Gerber TC, Kuzo RS, Karstaedt N et al. (2002) Current results and new developments of coronary angiography with use of contrast-enhanced computed tomography of the heart. Mayo Clin Proc 77: 55–71
6. Janowitz WR (2001) Current status of mechanical computed tomography in cardiac imaging. Am J Cardiol 88: 35E–8E
7. Becker CR, Ohnesorge BM, Schoepf UJ, Reiser MF (2000) Current development of cardiac imaging with multidetector-row CT. Eur J Radiol 36: 97–103
8. Knez A, Becker C, Ohnesorge B, Haberl R, Reiser M, Steinbeck G (2000) Noninvasive detection of coronary artery stenosis by multislice helical computed tomography. Circulation 101: E221–E222
9. de Feyter PJ, Nieman K (2002) New coronary imaging techniques: what to expect? Heart 87: 195–197
10. Nieman K, Oudkerk M, Rensing BJ, van Ooijen P, Munne A, van Geuns RJ, de Feyter PJ (2001) Coronary angiography with multi-slice computed tomography. Lancet 357: 599–603
11. Wexler L, Brundage B, Crouse J et al. (1996) Coronary artery calcification: pathophysiology, epidemiology, imaging methods, and clinical implications. Circulation 94: 1175–1192
12. Sechtem U (2000) Electron beam computed tomography: on its way into mainstream cardiology? Eur Heart J 21: 87–91
13. Flamm SD (1998) Coronary arterial calcium screening: ready for prime time? Radiology 208: 571–572
14. Devries S, Wolfkiel CJ, Shah V, Chomka E, Rich S (1995) Reproducibility of the measurement of coronary calcium with ultrafast CT. Am J Cardiol 75: 973–975
15. Shields JP, Mielke CH, Rockwood TH, Short RA, Viren FK (1995) Reliability of electron beam computed tomography to detect coronary artery calcification. Am J Card Imaging 9: 62–66
16. Bielak LF, Kaufmann RB, Moll PP, McCollough CH, Schwartz RS, Sheedy PF (1994) Small lesions in the heart identified at electron beam CT: calcification or noise? Radiology 192: 631–636
17. Hernigou A, Challande P, Boudeville JC, Sene V, Grataloup C, Plainfosse MC (1996) Reproducibility of coronary calcification detection with electron-beam computed tomography. Eur Radiol 6: 210–216
18. Wang S, Detrano RC, Secci A, Tang W, Doherty TM, Puentes G, Wong N, Brundage BH (1996) Detection of coronary calcification with electron-beam computed tomography: evaluation of interexamination reproducibility and comparison of three image-acquisition protocols. Am Heart J 132: 550–558
19. Hoeg JM, Feuerstein IM, Tucker EE (1994) Detection and quantification of calcific atherosclerosis by ultrafast computed tomography in children and young adults with homozygous familial hypercholesterolemia. Arterioscler Thromb Vasc Biol 14: 1066–1074

20. Carr JJ, Danitschek JA, Goff DC, Crouse JR, III, D'Agostino R, Chen MY, Burke GL (2001) Coronary artery calcium quantification with retrospectively gated helical CT: protocols and techniques. Int J Card Imaging 17: 213–220
21. Ohnesorge B, Knez A, Becker CR et al (2000) Reproducibility of coronary calcium scoring with EBCT and ECG-gated multi-slice spiral CT. Circulation 102: S405
22. Schoepf UJ, Becker CR, Obuchowski NA et al. (2001) Multi-slice computed tomography as a screening tool for colon cancer, lung cancer and coronary artery disease. Eur Radiol 11: 1975–1985
23. Haberl R, Steinbilger P (2001) New perspectives of non-invasive imaging with cardiac CT. J Clin Basic Cardiol 4: 241–245
24. Kopp AF, Ohnesorge B, Flohr T, Schroeder S, Claussen CD (1999) Multidetector-row CT for the noninvasive detection of high-grade coronary artery stenoses and occlusions: first results. Radiology 213(P): 435
25. Herzog C, Ay M, Engelmann K, Abolmaali N, Dogan S, Diebold T, Vogl TJ (2001) Visualisierungsmodalitäten in der Multidetektor CT-Koronarangiographie des Herzen: Korrelation von axialer, multiplanarer, dreidimensionaler und virtuell endoskopischer Bildgebung mit der invasiven Diagnostik. Fortschr Röntgenstr 173: 341–359
26. Kopp AF, Schröder S, Küttner A et al. (2001) Coronary arteries: retrospectively ECG-gated multi-detector row CT angiography with selective optimization of the image reconstruction window. Radiology 221: 683–688
27. Hong C, Becker CR, Huber A, Schoepf UJ, Ohnesorge B, Knez A, Bruning R, Reiser MF (2001) ECG-gated reconstructed multi-detector row CT coronary angiography: effect of varying trigger delay on image quality. Radiology 220: 712–717
28. Georg C, Kopp AF, Schröder S, Küttner A, Ohnesorge B, Martensen J, Claussen CD (2001) Optimierung des Bild-Rekonstruktionszeitpunktes im RR-Intervall für die Darstellung der Koronararterien mittels Mehrzeilen-Computertomographie. Fortschr Röntgenstr 173: 536–541
29. Knez A, Becker CR, Leber A et al. (2001) Usefulness of multislice spiral computed tomography angiography for determination of coronary artery stenoses. Am J Cardiol 88: 1191–1194
30. Schröder S, Kopp AF, Baumbach A et al. (2001) Non-invasive detection and evaluation of atherosclerotic plaques with multi-slice computed tomography. J Am Coll Cardiol 37: 1430–1435
31. Ropers D, Baum U, Pohle K et al. (2003) Detection of coronary artery stenoses with thin-slice multi-detector row spiral computed tomography and multiplanar reconstruction. Circulation 107: 664–666
32. Nieman K, Cademartiri F, Lemos PA, Raaijmakers R, Pattynama PM, de Feyter PJ (2002) Reliable noninvasive coronary angiography with fast submillimeter multislice spiral computed tomography. Circulation 106: 2051–2054
33. Halliburton S, Petersilka M, Schvartzman P, Obuchowski N, White R (2001) Validation of left ventricular volume and ejection fraction measurement with multi-slice computed tomography: comparison to cine magnetic resonance imaging. Radiology 221(P): 452
34. Wintersperger BJ, Hundt W, Knez A, Thilo C, Huber A, Nikolaou K (2002) Left ventricular systolic function assessed by ECG gated multirow-detector spiral computed tomography (MDCT): Comparison to ventriculography. Eur Radiol 12: S192
35. Juergens KU, Fischbach RM, Grude M, Wichter T, Fallenberg EM, Opitz C, Heindel WL (2002) Evaluation of left ventricular myocardial function by retrospectively ECG-gated multislice spiral CT in comparison to CINE magnetic resonance imaging. Eur Radiol 12: S191
36. Mochizuki T, Higashino H, Kayama Y, Ikezoe J, Shen Y, Matsumoto K (2001) Evaluation of wall motion using multi-detector-row CT: new application of post-processing interactive multi-planar animation of the heart. Radiology 221(P): 413
37. Hilfiker PR, Weishaupt D, Marincek B (2001) Multislice spiral computed tomography of subacute myocardial infarction. Circulation 104: 1083

38. Koyama Y, Matsuoka H, Higashino H, Kawakami H, Sogabe I, Mochizuki T (2001) Myocardial perfusion defect in acute myocardial infarction on enhanced helical CT after successful reperfusion therapy: a prognostic value. Radiology 221(P): 195
39. Koyama Y, Matsuoka H, Higashino H, Kawakami H, Sogabe I, Mochizuki T (2001) Early myocardial perfusion defect and late enhancement on enhancement CT predict clinical outcome in patients with acute myocardial infarction after reperfusion therapy. Radiology 221(P): 196
40. Wintersperger BJ, Ruff J, Becker CR et al. (2002) Assessment of regional myocardial perfusion using multirow-detector computed tomography (MDCT). Eur Radiol 12: S294
41. Kopp AF, Küttner A, Schröder S, Heuschmid M, Claussen CD (2001) New developments in cardiac imaging: the role of MDCT. J Clin Basic Cardiol 4: 253–260
42. Schroeder S, Kopp AF, Kuettner A et al. (2002) Influence of heart rate on vessel visibility in noninvasive coronary angiography using new multislice computed tomography. Experience in 94 patients. Clin Imaging 26: 106–111
43. Cohnen M, Poll L, Puttmann C, Ewen K, Modder U (2001) Radiation exposure in multislice CT of the heart. Fortschr Röntgenstr 173: 295–299
44. Becker CR, Schatz l M, Feist H, Bauml A, Bruning R, Schopf UJ, Reiser MF (1998) Strahlenexposition bei der CT-Untersuchung des Thorax und Abdomens. Vergleich von Einzelschicht-, Spiral- und Elektronenstrahlcomputertomographie. Radiologe 38: 726–729
45. Ohnesorge B, Flohr T, Becker C, Kopp AF, Knez A, Reiser M (2000) Dose evaluation and dose reduction strategies for ECG-gated multi-slice spiral CT of the heart. Radiology 217(P): 487
46. Kopp AF, Schröder S, Küttner A, Ohnesorge B, Heuschmid M, Georg C, Claussen CD (2000) Multidetector-row CT for noninvasive coronary angiography: results in 102 patients. Radiology 217(P): 375
47. Achenbach S, Giesler T, Ropers D et al. (2001) Detection of coronary artery stenoses by contrast-enhanced, retrospectively electrocardiographically-gated, multislice spiral computed tomography. Circulation 103: 2535–2538
48. Nitatori T, Takahasi S, Yokoyama K, Takahara T, Hachiya J (2001) Comparison of the detectability of coronary arterial stenotic lesions by MR angiography and multidetector CT. Radiology 221(P): 200
49. Fischbach RM, Wichter T, Juergens KU et al. (2001) Mehrschicht-Spiral-CT (MSCT) der Koronararterien: Vergleich mit der Koronarangiographie. Fortschr Röntgenstr 173: S26
50. Herzog C, Diebold T, Dogan S, Moritz A, Schaechinger M, Vogl T (2001) Value and limits of multislice-cardiac-CT: a prospective study in over 500 patients. Radiology 221(P): 412
51. Küttner A, Trabold T, Beck T et al. (2003) MDCT-Koronarangiographie unter Verwendung der 420 ms Rotationszeit vs. konventionelle Koronarangiographie: Erste Ergebnisse mit 57 Patienten. Fortschr Röntgenstr 175: S113
52. Schröder S, Kopp AF, Küttner A et al. (2003) Noninvasive coronary angiography with 16- slice detector computed tomography: Initial experience. JACC 41: 467A

15 Imaging of Coronary Atherosclerosis

C. R. Becker

Introduction

Contrast-enhanced CT studies of the coronary arteries were performed first to visualize the vessel lumen and to achieve an angiographic-like presentation of the coronary arteries in combination with three-dimensional postprocessing methods. By its cross-sectional nature, multidetector row CT (MDCT) has the ability not only to visualize the coronary artery lumen but also to demonstrate changes in the coronary artery wall.

MDCT scanners operated with an acquisition mode called retrospective ECG gating. The combination of fast gantry rotation, slow table movement and multi-slice-helical acquisition allows for acquisition of a high number of X-ray-projection data. The ECG trace is recorded simultaneously during the helical scan acquisition. The X-ray projections of the mid-diastolic phase are selected to reconstruct images from the slow-motion diastole phase of the heart.

The redundant radiation occurring during the radiation exposure in the systole can be substantially reduced by a technique called prospective ECG tube current modulation. On the basis of the ECG signal the X-ray tube current is switched to its nominal value during the diastole phase and is reduced significantly during the systole phase of the heart, respectively. This technique is most effective in patients with low heart rates. If the heart rate is lower that 60 beats/min the radiation exposure will be reduced by approximately 50% [1].

Patient Preparation

In 16-MDCT scanners with 420-ms gantry rotation an optimized partial view scan last about 210 ms. Excellent diagnostic image quality with this exposure time can be achieved in patients with low heart rates (40–60 beats/min) [2]. The use of beta-blocker may become necessary for patient preparation aiming at a heart rate of 60 beats/min or less.

To consider beta-blocker for patient preparation, contraindications (bronchial asthma, AV block, severe congestive heart failure, aortic stenosis, etc.) have to be ruled out, and informed consent must be obtained from the patient. In case the heart rate of a patient is significantly above 60 beats/min, 50 to 200 mg of Metoprololtartrat can be administered orally 30–90 min prior to the investigation. Alternatively, 5 to 20 mg of Metoprololtartrat divided in four doses can be administered intravenously [3] immediately prior to scanning. Monitoring of vital functions, heart rate and blood pressure, is essential during this approach. The positive effect of beta-blocker on MDCT scanning is fourfold: better patient compliance, less radiation exposure and cardiac motion artefacts and higher vascular enhancement.

Contrast Application

A timely accurate and homogenous vascular lumen enhancement is essential for full diagnostic capability of coronary MDCT angiography studies. Higher contrast enhancement is superior to identify small vessels in MDCT. However, coronary atherosclerosis is commonly associated with calcifications that may interfere with dense contrast material and hinders the assessment of the residual lumen. A contrast medium flow rate of 1 g/s iodine by peripheral venous injection in an antecubital vein will result in an enhancement of approximately 250–300 HU, that allows for delineation of intermediate (91 ± 21 HU) as well as high dense plaques (419 ± 194 HU) [4].
The circulation time can be determined by a test bolus of 5 g iodine injected with a flow rate of 1 g/s iodine and followed by a saline chaser bolus. A series of scans is acquired at the level of the ascending aorta every other second. The arrival time of the test bolus can be determined by taking the delay time between start of the contrast injection and peak enhancement of the ascending aorta into account.

An additional delay time is required to allow the contrast media to reach the left ventricular system and the coronary arteries. In our current experience another 6 s should be added to the peak enhancement of the test bolus to allow for complete enhancement of the left ventricular system in 16 MDCT. The contrast media has to be injected for the duration of the scan and the delay time, and therefore has to be maintained for 26 s. The sequential injection of contrast media and saline allows for selective enhancement of the left ventricular system with a washout of contrast in the right ventricular system. In general, the use of a dual high-power injector has been found to be mandatory to keep the contrast bolus compact [5], to reduce the total amount of contrast media [6] and to allow for a central venous enhancement profile by a peripheral venous injection [7].

Alternatively, beginning of the CT scan can be triggered automatically by the arrival of the contrast bolus. A prescan is taken at the level of the aortic root and a region of interest is selected in the ascending aorta. When contrast injection starts, repeated scanning at the same level is performed every second. If the density in the ascending aorta reaches 100 HU, a countdown begins until the acquisition starts. Immediately before the CT scan acquisition the patient is instructed to hold his breath. A delay time of 8 s has to be added in 16-MDCT to allow for timely adequate contrast enhancement.

MDCT Scanning

For retrospective ECG gating with MDCT, the pitch factor (detector collimation/table feed per gantry rotation) must not exceed 0.3 to allow for scanning the heart at any heart rate higher than 40 beats/min. In a 16-detector row CT with 0.75-slice collimation, currently 12 channels are used at a gantry rotation time of 420 ms. Tube current is set to 500 effective mAs and acquisition time is 20 s.

Retrospective ECG gating reconstruction always begins with a careful analysis of the ECG trace recorded with the helical scan. The image reconstruction interval is best placed between the T and the P wave of the ECG corresponding to the mid-diastole interval. The point of time for the least coronary motion may be different for every coronary artery. Least-motion artefacts may result on retrospective reconstruction of the RCA, LAD and LCX at 50, 55 and 60% of the RR-interval. Individual adaptation of the point of time for reconstruction seems to further improve image quality [2]. However, the lower the heart rate the easier it is to find the best interval for all three major branches of the coronary artery tree. Images are reconstructed with spatial in-plane resolution of 0.6 x 0.6 mm. The slice thickness and reconstruction increment is 1 with 0.5 mm in 16-MDCT.

The patient room time is approximately 15 min and image reconstruction and postprocessing can be performed within approximately 10 min. Because coronary CT angiography (CTA) is performed with thin slices and low image noise, the radiation dose with tube current modulation is significantly higher (~5 mSv) than for calcium screening. However, the radiation of a CTA investigation is comparable that applied during a diagnostic coronary catheter procedure.

Assessment of Coronary Atherosclerosis

Coronary calcifications can easily be assessed even without contrast media and represent an advanced stage of atherosclerosis. As different stages of coronary atherosclerosis may be present simultaneously, calcifications may also be associated with more early stages of coronary atherosclerosis. The entire extent of coronary atherosclerosis, however, will be underestimated by assessing coronary calcifications alone [8]. With contrast enhancement calcified as well as non-calcified lesions can be completely assessed by MDCT simultaneously.

Cardiac catheter seems to be not suited to assess the entire extent of coronary atherosclerosis completely. Histological and intravascular ultrasound (IVUS) studies have shown that high atherosclerotic plaque burden can be found even in the absence of high-grade coronary stenoses on conventional coronary angiography. From the clinical standpoint, the correlation between acute cardiac events and high-grade coronary artery stenoses is only poor. Recently, it has been reported that 68% of the patients who received coronary angiography by incidence prior to their acute cardiac event did not show any significant coronary artery stenoses [9]. In early stages of CAD, the coronary arteries may undergo a process of positive remodelling that compensates for the coronary wall thickening and keeps the inner lumen of the vessel comparatively unchanged [10]. The pathomechanism of this phenomenon is still unknown, but the underlying type of coro-

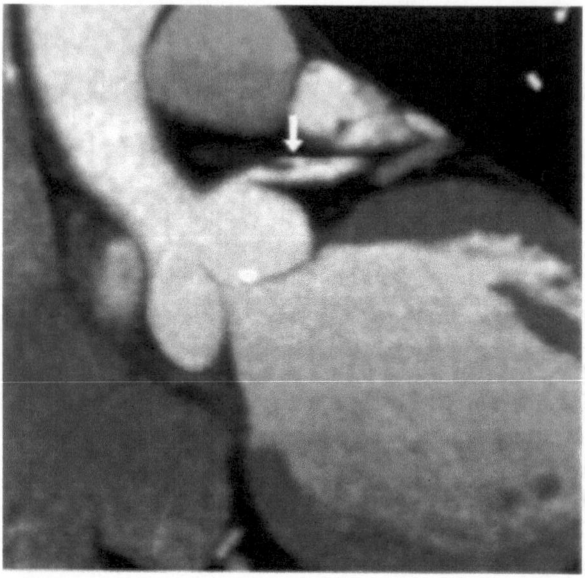

Fig. 1. Fibrocalcified plaque in the left main coronary artery of an asymptomatic 57-year-old male patient. The plaque is well defined and has a homogenous density of approximately 100 HU. At the base of the plaque a calcification can be seen (*arrow*)

nary artery disease may be a fibrous cap atheroma with accumulation of cholesterol. In the case of inflammatory processes, the fibrous cap of an atheroma may become thinned, putting the plaque on risk for rupture and consecutive thrombosis [11].

The current gold standard to assess coronary atherosclerosis in vivo is IVUS. Comparing IVUS with MDCT, Schroeder et al. [12] reported that coronary lesions classified as soft, intermediate and dense as determined by IVUS correspond to plaque with a density of 14 ± 26 HU, 91 ± 21 HU and 419 ± 194 HU in MDCT, respectively.

It seems that different histological stages of atherosclerosis are present with different morphological pattern in MDCT. In heart specimen studies it turned out that HU densities of non-calcified plaques seem to depend on the ratio between lipid and fibrous tissue and may increase from atheroma (~50-HU) and fibroatheroma to fibrotic (~90-HU) lesions. Moreover, fibrotic lesions are commonly associated with calcifications, indicating a progressive stiffness of coronary lesions with high HU densities. Fibrocalcified lesions (Fig. 1) may more often be found in patients with chronic stable angia whereas low-density plaque may be associated more frequently in patients with acute unstable angina. As we have observed in coronary arteries of patients with acute symptoms, coronary thrombi (Fig. 2) present as very low-density (~20-HU) and inhomogeneous plaques [13] (Table 1).

Commonly, spotty calcified lesions may be found in MDCT angiography studies that may be associated with only minor wall changes in conventional coronary angiography [14]. However, it is known that such calcified nodules may also be the source of unheralded plaque rupture and consequent thrombosis (Fig. 3) and may in very rare cases lead to sudden coronary death [11].

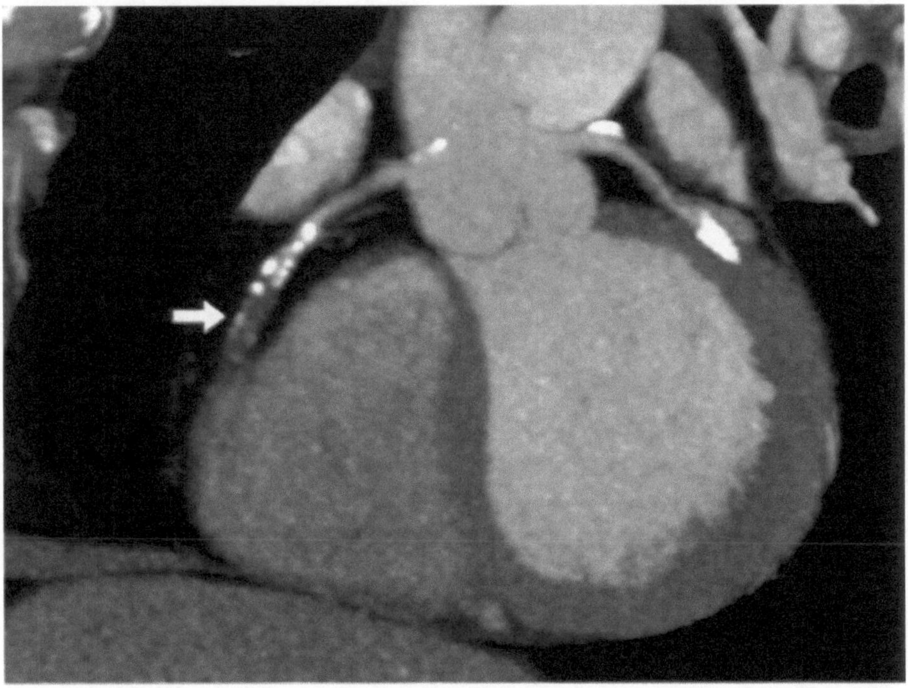

Fig. 2. 48-year-old patient with thrombotic occlusion of the right coronary artery (*arrow*). The density of the inhomogenous plaque is approximately 40 HU. Fresh coronary thrombi may have low density whereas with further organization, coronary thrombi may fibrose and HU densities may increase

Even in contrast-enhanced studies, coronary calcifications can easily be detected and quantified because the density of calcium (>350 HU) is greater than the density of the contrast media in the coronary artery lumen (250–300 HU) [15].

Table 1. Coronary artery plaque entities and morphological appearance in MDCT

Plaque entity	AHA type	Calcification	Density	Shape	Remodelling	Symptoms possible
Atheroma	IV	No	~50 HU	Smooth	Positive	None
Fibroatheroma	Va	No	~70-HU	Smooth	Positive/negativ	None
Fibrotic lesion	Vc	No	~90 HU	Smooth	Positive/negativ	None
Fibrocalcified plaque	Vb	Yes	~90 HU or absent	Smooth	Negative	Chronic stable angina
Thrombus	VI	No	~20 HU	Irregular	High-grade stenosis or occlusion	Acute unstable angina

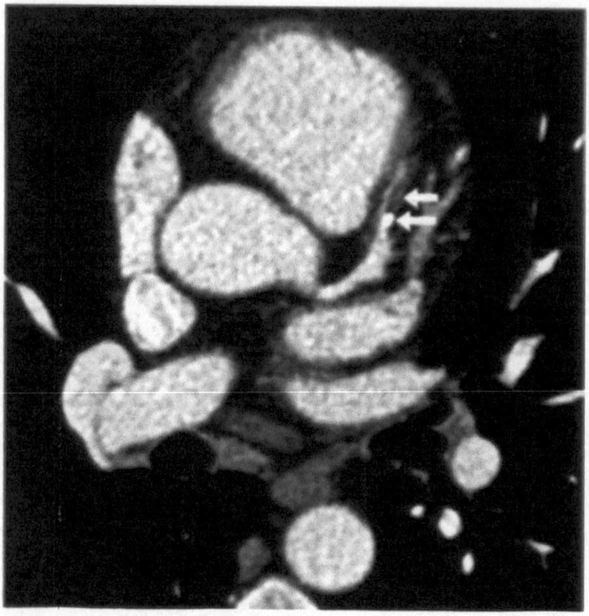

Fig. 3. Symptomatic patient with a calcified nodule (*arrow*) in the left anterior descending coronary artery. The symptoms may be caused by an appositional thrombus behind the calcification

However, because of partial volume effects it is much more difficult to quantify non-calcified plaques. The optimal quantification algorithm for atherosclerosis determined by MDCT is still under development.

In patients with extensive coronary calcifications, non-calcified plaques are uncommon, most likely because the »blooming« artefact prevents assessment. For this reason and because the coronary artery stenosis cannot be reliably assessed [14], contrast-enhanced MDCT is currently not recommended in patients presenting with diffuse calcifications (>100 mg CaHA or Agatston Score >500).

Conclusion

The newest generation MDCT scanners now allow for consistently good image quality when regular sinus rhythm is present and the heart rate is in the range between 40 and 60 beats/min. Extensive calcifications may hinder the detection of coronary stenosis and non-calcified atherosclerotic plaque. The high negative predictive value of CTA may justify the investigation of symptomatic patients with low to moderate pretest probability of CAD [16] to exclude a coronary macro-angiopathy and to avoid unnecessary cardiac catheter procedures. Morphological criteria allow for differentiation of different atherosclerotic plaque entities. The predictive value of atherosclerotic lesions for cardiac events is currently unknown and requires further long-term studies.

References

1. Jakobs TF, Becker CR, Ohnesorge B et al. (2002) Multislice helical CT of the heart with retrospective ECG gating: reduction of radiation exposure by ECG-controlled tube current modulation. Eur Radiol 12:1081–6
2. Hong C, Becker CR, Huber A et al. (2001) ECG-gated reconstructed multi-detector row CT coronary angiography: effect of varying trigger delay on image quality. Radiology 220:712–7
3. Ryan T, Anderson J, Antman E et al. (1996) ACC/AHA guidelines for the management of patients with acute myocardial infarction. A report of the American College of Cardiology/American Heart Association Task Force on Practice Guidelines (Committee on Management of Acute Myocardial Infarction). J Am Coll Cardiol 28:1328–1428
4. Schroeder S, Kopp AF, Baumbach A et al. (2001) Noninvasive detection and evaluation of atherosclerotic coronary plaques with multislice computed tomography. J Am Coll Cardiol 37:1430–5
5. Hopper KD, Mosher TJ, Kasales CJ, Ten Have TR, Tully DA, Weaver JS (1997) Thoracic spiral CT: delivery of contrast material pushed with injectable saline solution in a power injector. Radiology 205:269–71
6. Haage P, Schmitz-Rode T, Hubner D, Piroth W, Gunther RW (2000) Reduction of contrast material dose and artefacts by a saline flush using a double power injector in helical CT of the thorax. AJR Am J Roentgenol 174:1049–53
7. Hittmair K, Fleischmann D (2001) Accuracy of predicting and controlling time-dependent aortic enhancement from a test bolus injection. J Comput Assist Tomogr 25:287–94
8. Wexler L, Brundage B, Crouse J et al. (1996) Coronary artery calcification: pathophysiology, epidemiology, imaging methods, and clinical implications. A statement for health professionals from the American Heart Association. Circulation 94:1175–92
9. Ziada K, Kapadia S, Tuzcu E, Nissen S (1999) The current status of intravascular ultrasound imaging. Current Problems in Cardiology 24:541–566
10. Glagov S, Weisenberg E, Zarins C, Stankunavicius R, Kolettis G (1987) Compensatory enlargement of human atherosclerotic coronary arteries. N Engl J Med 316:1371–1375
11. Virmani R, Kolodgie FD, Burke AP, Frab A, Schwartz SM (2000) Lessons from sudden coronary death. A comprehensive morphological classification scheme for atherosclerotic lesions. Arterioscler Thromb Vasc Biol 20:1262–1275
12. Schroeder S, Kopp A, Baumbach A et al. (2001) Noninvasive detection and evalutation of atherosclerotic coronary plaque with multislice computed tomography. J Am Coll Cardiol 37:1430–1435
13. Becker CR, Knez A, Ohnesorge B, Schoepf UJ, Reiser MF (2000) Imaging of noncalcified coronary plaques using helical CT with retrospective ECG gating. AJR Am J Roentgenol 175:423–4
14. Kajinami K, Seki H, Takekoshi N, Mabuchi H (1997) Coronary calcification and coronary atherosclerosis: site-by-site comparative morphologic study of electron beam-computed tomography and coronary angiography. J Am Coll Cardiol 29:1549–56
15. Hong C, Becker C, Schoepf UJ, Ohnesorge B, Bruening R, Reiser M (2002) Absolute quantification of coronary artery calcium in non-enhanced and contrast enhanced multidetector-row CT studies. Radiology 223:474–480
16. Nieman K, Cademartiri F, Lemos PA, Raaijmakers R, Pattynama PM, de Feyter PJ (2002) Reliable noninvasive coronary angiography with fast submillimeter multislice spiral computed tomography. Circulation 106:2051–4

VI Screening

16 Coronary Artery Disease: Role of Coronary Artery Calcium Detection

R. FISCHBACH, D. MAINTZ

Coronary Heart Disease

Coronary heart disease (CHD) remains the major cause of mortality and morbidity in the industrialized nations [1]. CHD typically manifests in middle-aged and older, predominantly male, individuals. Approximately 50% of patients with acute myocardial infarction die within the first month of the event [2]. At least 25% of persons with sudden coronary death or non-fatal myocardial infarction have no prior symptoms. Therefore, the identification of asymptomatic persons with subclinical disease who are at a high risk of developing a future coronary event and who could potentially benefit from preventive efforts is of major economical and clinical importance. Moderately effective preventive treatment is available: lipid lowering with HMG CoA reductase inhibitors (statins) or antiplatelet therapy (aspirin) have both resulted in decreased incidence rates of coronary events [3, 4].

According to the Air Force/Texas Coronary Atherosclerosis Prevention Study (AFCAPS/TexCAPS), only 37% of acute events can potentially be prevented using lipid-lowering therapy as primary prevention in individuals with average cholesterol levels [5]. Therefore, risk assessment tools or screening tests are required that will identify asymptomatic individuals at high risk of hard coronary events to target therapy efficiently.

The risk of developing CHD depends on a wide range of environmental and biochemical factors, many of which have been identified in prospective epidemiological studies. Among these well-recognized risk factors are tobacco smoking, high LDL cholesterol levels, low HDL cholesterol, diabetes mellitus, arterial hypertension and family history of premature myocardial infarction (Table 1). These

Table 1. Risk factors for developing coronary heart disease

Causal risk factors	Predisposing risk factors	Conditional risk factors
Hypercholesterolemia	BMI > 30 kg/m³	Triglycerides
Arterial hypertension	Sedentary life style	Lipoprotein (a)
Cigarette smoking	Family history of premature myocardial infarction	Homocystein
Diabetes mellitus	Male gender	Fibrinogen
	Metabolic syndrome	Plasminogen acitvator inhibitor
	Social factors	C-reactive protein

and other risk factors interact in a complex way, making a simple risk assessment in the individual patient complicated. However, algorithms derived from large prospective epidemiological studies like the Framingham Study [6, 7] in the United States and the Prospective Cardiovascular Münster (PROCAM) Study [8] in Europe can be used to calculate a person's risk of CHD. A person is said to be at increased risk if his or her absolute risk of suffering a future myocardial event within the next 10 years exceeds 20%. Calculation of an individual's CHD risk is possible by using either scoring systems and risk charts or computer-assisted algorithms. The Framingham risk score is available at *http://www.nhlbi.nih.gov/guidelines/cholesterol/atglance.pdf*. The PROCAM risk algorithm can be accessed interactively on the Internet at: *http://www.chd-taskforce.com.*

Using traditional risk assessment, subpopulations at a significantly increased global risk of CHD can be identified with a high level of exactness. Epidemiological studies have shown that in many individuals without clinically apparent symptoms the risk of developing a future myocardial infarction may equal or even exceed that of persons with a history of coronary heart disease [8]. However, it remains questionable whether the presence of subclinical manifestations of atherosclerosis in these presymptomatic patients can be diagnosed with sufficient certainty based on traditional risk factors alone. In this context, it is noteworthy that a considerable number of subjects at low to intermediate risk may have unexpected events.

Coronary Artery Calcification and CAD

Coronary artery calcification is a well-recognized marker of coronary artery disease (CAD) [9] and can develop before clinical manifestation of atherosclerotic disease. Although calcification is found more frequently in advanced lesions, it may also occur in the lesions that are seen as early as the second decade of life. Calcium accumulation reflects an active process which involves mechanisms similar to bone formation. Calcification probably reflects healing of plaque rupture and intraplaque haemorrhage as well as a response to inflammation in the plaque. The extent of coronary calcification is correlated with the total coronary plaque burden [10, 11], but it is not known if the amount of calcium reflects the amount of total plaque over time or after therapeutic intervention.

Coronary Artery Calcification and Angiographic Stenosis

Reports on the potential for imaging coronary calcifications began early with the papers of Tannenbaum [12] and Agatston et al. [13]. In their study, Agatston et al. demonstrated that EBCT was much more sensitive than fluoroscopy in detecting coronary calcifications and that patients with symptomatic CHD displayed higher calcium scores than asymptomatic subjects (see Fig. 1). Several other investigators reported accuracies for predicting angiographic stenoses that are comparable with those of exercise testing. Table 2 lists the sensitivities and specificities of CT coronary calcium scans for predicting angiographic stenoses. The sensiti-

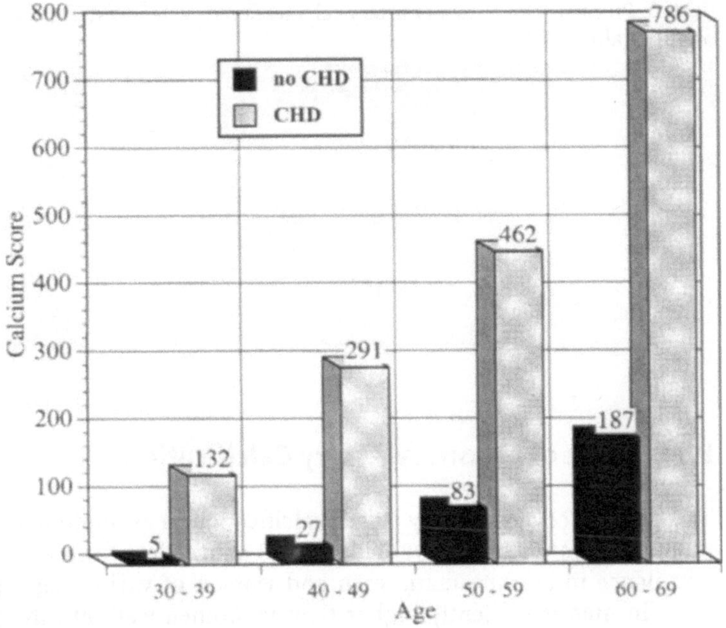

Fig. 1. Comparison of mean absolute calcium scores in 475 symptomatic patients without and 109 patients with a diagnosis of coronary heart disease. The calcium score increases with patient age and there is a significant difference between patients with and without CHD

vity for detecting obstructive CAD ranges between 85 and 100%, while the specificity remains low between 39 and 76%. This gives a positive coronary calcium scan a high negative predictive value for ruling out but a low predictive value for identifying stenoses. Coronary calcium scans can be used in the differential diagnosis of symptomatic patients with atypical chest pain [9]. It has to be kept in mind, however, that even though a negative CT scan result for calcium does imply a low likelihood of significant luminal obstruction, the presence of atherosclerotic plaque cannot be excluded. In this context, it has to be stressed that culprit plaque in sudden coronary death may contain only little calcium [14].

Table 2. Relationship of coronary calcium and obstructive coronary artery disease in coronary angiography

Reference	No. of patients	Age (years)	Sensitivity (%)	Specificity (%)	Positive predictive value (%)	Negative predictive value (%)
Breen et al. [28]	100	47	100	47	62	100
Fallavollita et al. [29]	106	44	85	45	66	70
Devries et al. [30]	140	58	97	41	55	94
Rumberger et al. [31]	139	51	99	62	57	97
Budoff et al. [32]	710	56	95	44	72	84
Haberl et al. [233]	1764	56	99	39	57	97

Table 3. Prevalence of coronary artery calcification detected by CT in asymptomatic men and women. (after [15])

Age	Asymptomatic Men (%)	Asymptomatic Women (%)
– 29	11	6
30–39	21	11
40–49	44	23
50–59	72	35
60–69	85	67
70–79	94	89
80–89	100	100

Prevalence of Coronary Artery Calcification

The prevalence of coronary artery calcification in asymptomatic as well as symptomatic persons is well studied. Table 3 shows data from an early study of the prevalence in asymptomatic men and women of various ages [15]. The prevalence in men is evidently higher than in women well into the postmenopausal period and it is obvious that the prevalence is age-dependent. Several investigators[16–18] have since reported coronary calcium scores in large asymptomatic populations (see Fig. 2). The calcium score distributions published for asymptomatic mainly white American populations can be used to classify patients com-

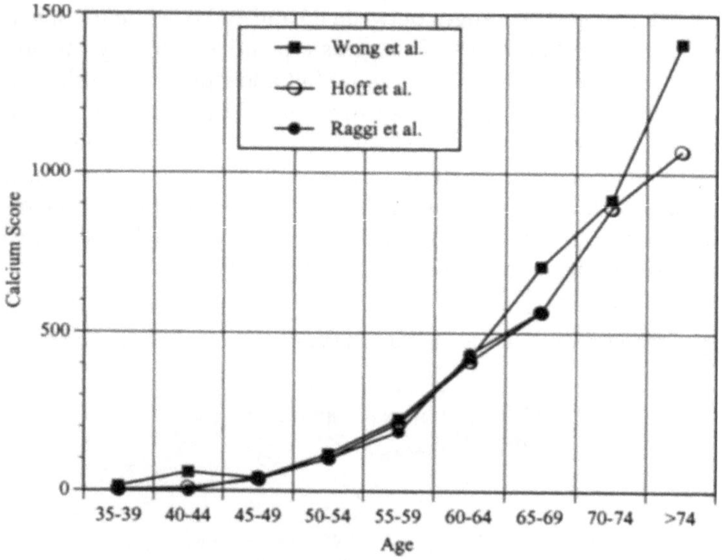

Fig. 2. Age- and gender-adjusted 75th percentile of coronary artery calcium in asymptomatic male patient populations reported by Raggi et al. [18], Hoff et al. [17] and Wong et al. [16]. All investigators found a remarkable increase of calcium scores with age. The reported 75th percentile calcium score is quite similar in the different groups

pared with the expected norm. All investigators report a steep increase in coronary calcium with age. The 75th percentile ranges between 101 and 116 for males between 50 and 55 and 410 and 434 for males between 60 and 65. Interestingly, the absolute calcium scores are quite similar in the different US American populations studied.

Calcium Detection and Predicting Events

Screening for a disease is appropriate if the test used is accurate, effective treatment is available and the costs of screening and treatment remain reasonable. The use of non-invasive measurement of coronary artery calcification as a screening test for coronary atherosclerosis has aroused remarkable interest in recent years and has generated much controversy. Coronary calcium detection by CT makes the assumption that direct demonstration of atherosclerotic vessel wall involvement in asymptomatic populations with increased CHD risk is helpful to identify as well as stratify individuals at risk.

To evaluate a possible benefit from CT calcium screening, we first should realize that the main purpose of CAD screening is classification of asymptomatic persons as likely or not likely to have CAD. Early diagnosis of cases with subclinical CAD ought to reduce morbidity and mortality from the specific disease among the population screened, because screening leads to a course of action proven to save lives. If a significant reduction of morbidity and mortality cannot be achieved by CT screening, it cannot be deemed effective. Therefore, we need to prove that calcium screening of the entire adult population, or even a subpopulation, leads to effective preventive therapy.

Computed tomography is very sensitive for the detection of high-density calcium deposits, and EBCT or MDCT have been successfully used to identify calcified coronary artery plaque [19–21]. From the results of coronary calcium measurements by CT, a future myocardial event can be predicted with sensitivities reaching as high as 89% [22, 23]. Though there is a clear relationship between absolute calcium scores and the severity of CAD, coronary events have been shown to occur even in patients with little or no coronary calcifications. This indicates that the ability to predict a future myocardial event on the basis of an absolute calcium score may be limited.

A meta-analysis regarding the literature on using CT calcium to predict future events in asymptomatic adults was carried out by O'Malley et al. [24]. Their results show that the relative risk of calcification for a myocardial infarct or CAD-related death varies from 1 to 22 with a weighted mean of 4.2. Thus, the predictive value of coronary calcium for new cardiac events remains to be determined. It also remains to be shown that the calcium score predicts coronary disease events better than conventional risk-factor analysis.

While the absolute calcium score has a wide variation in asymptomatic individuals with an increased cardiac event risk, a calcium score in the upper age- and gender-adjusted quartile seems to identify subjects at risk better (see Table 4) than an increased absolute calcium score. A prospective study in 632 asymptomatic subjects showed that approximately two thirds of the observed events

Table 4. Coronary calcium scores and risk of myocardial events according to Raggi et al. [18]. In 632 asymptomatic persons 8 fatal and 19 non-fatal myocardial infarcts were observed. The use of adjusted calcium quartiles discriminates better between risk statuses than the use of an absolute calcium score

	Absolute calcium scores			
	0	1–99	100–400	> 400
Patients	292	219	74	47
Annual event rate	0.11	2.1	4.1	4.8
	Age- and gender-adjusted calcium score quartile			
	1st	2nd	3rd	4th
Patients	351		100	181
Annual event rate	0.2	0.2	1.4	4.5

occurred in patients with mild to moderate amounts of coronary artery calcium (calcium scores below 400) [18]. Subjects with massive calcifications (calcium scores > 400) represented 7% of the population scanned and accounted for 22% of all events. On the other hand, 70% of the events observed (19 of 27) occurred in 181 subjects with a calcium score above the 75th percentile.

On the basis of the investigations in asymptomatic persons, some would argue that the demonstration of coronary artery calcium, which means the presence of subclinical CAD, should shift an asymptomatic patient from a primary to a secondary prevention category [25]. Even though this seems logical, it has not been proven that a positive or increased calcium score is equivalent to a prior myocardial infarction. Even if an increased calcium score put a person at increased risk, as several investigations imply, one cannot be sure that any benefit would be reached by therapeutic intervention.

Three prospective epidemiological trials under way will examine this issue. One part of the Prospective Army Coronary Calcium (PACC) study [26] is a prospective cohort study of 2000 participants followed for at least 5 years to establish the relation between coronary calcification and cardiovascular events in an unselected, »low-risk« Army population. The Multi Ethnic Study of Atherosclerosis (MESA) will use a cohort of 6500 American adults who will undergo CT scanning and will be followed for coronary events for 7 years.

Another population-based, prospective cohort study was begun in Germany in 2000. The RECALL (Risk Factors, Evaluation of Coronary Calcium and Lifestyle) study is designed to define the relative risk associated with EBCT-derived coronary calcium score for myocardial infarction and cardiac death in 4200 males and females aged 45 to 75 years in an unselected urban population from the large, heavily industrialized Ruhr area [27].

Conclusion

Since atherogenesis is a dynamic process, which represents the result of a lifelong exposure of an individual to a variety of predisposing factors, manifestations of subclinical coronary artery disease, as indicated by a positive CT calcium scan, may point to individuals with an increased future cardiac risk. Demonstration of coronary artery calcification may thus be of value in improving risk stratification of asymptomatic persons with moderate to increased global coronary heart risk. There is no formal proof that coronary heart disease risk can be reduced in patients with elevated coronary calcium scores. Neither is there a consensus who should undergo CT scanning and on how to use the results of calcium scoring for risk-factor management or therapeutic decisions.

Due to this lack of data, there is no indication for a population-based CT screening of asymptomatic adults. A clinical examination including history, blood pressure measurement and lipoproteins should always be used to assess a person's coronary event risk based on traditional risk factors. In persons with a low risk, further studies should be discouraged. In groups with intermediate or increased risk, calcium scanning may be of value, but long-term prospective studies that will eventually determine the indications for such an examination are not completed.

References

1. American Heart Association (2001) 2002 Heart and stroke statistical update. American Heart Association, Dallas, Texas
2. Chambless L, Keil U, Dobson A, Mahonen M, Kuulasmaa K, Rajakangas AM, Lowel H, Tunstall-Pedoe H (1997) Population versus clinical view of case fatality from acute coronary heart disease: results from the WHO MONICA Project 1985–1990. Multinational MONItoring of Trends and Determinants in CArdiovascular Disease. Circulation 96:3849–3859
3. Antiplatelet Trialists' Collaboration (1994) Collaborative overview of randomized trials of antiplatelet therapy. I: Prevention of death, myocardial infarction, and stroke by prolonged antiplatelet therapy in various categories of patients. Br Med J 308:81–106
4. Shepherd J, Cobbe S, Ford I, Isles C, Lorimer A, MacFarlane P, McKillop J, Packard C (1995) West of Scotland Coronary Prevention Study Group. Prevention of coronary heart disease with pravastatin in men with hypercholesterolemia. N Engl J Med 333:1301–1307
5. Downs J, Clearfield M, Weis S, Withney E, Shapiro D, Beere P, Langendorfer A, Stein E, Kruyer W, Gotto AJ (1998) Primary prevention of acute coronary events with lovastatin in men and women with average cholesterol levels: results of the AFCAPS/TexCAPS research. JAMA 279:1615–1622
6. Anderson K, Wilson P, Odell P, Kannel W (1991) An updated coronary risk profile – a statement for health professionals. Circulation 83:356–362
7. Wilson PW, D'Agostino RB, Levy D, Belanger AM, Silbershatz H, Kannel WB (1998) Prediction of coronary heart disease using risk-factor categories. Circulation 97:1837–1847.
8. Assmann G, Cullen P, Schulte H (2002) Simple scoring scheme for calculating the risk of acute coronary events based on the 10-year follow-up of the prospective cardiovascular Munster (PROCAM) study. Circulation 105:310–315.
9. Wexler L, Brundage B, Crouse J, Detrano R, Fuster V, Maddahi J, Rumberger J, Stanford W, White R, Taubert K (1996) Coronary artery calcification: pathophysiology, epidemiology, imaging methods, and clinical implications. A statement for health professionals from the American Heart Association. Circulation 94:1175–1192

10. Rumberger JA, Simons DB, Fitzpatrick LA, Sheedy PF, Schwartz RS (1995) Coronary artery calcium area by electron-beam computed tomography and coronary atherosclerotic plaque area. A histopathologic correlative study. Circulation 92:2157–2162
11. Sangiori G, Rumberger J, Severson A, Edwards W, Gregoire J, Fitzpatrick L, Schwartz R (1998) Arterial calcification and not lumen stenosis is correlated with atherosclerotic plaque burden in humans: a histologic study of 723 coronary artery segments using nondecalcifying methodology. J Am Coll Cardiol 31:126–133
12. Tannenbaum S, Kondos G, Veselik K, Prendergast M, Brundage B, Chomka E (1989) Detection of calcific depositis in coronary arteries by ultrafast computed tomography. J Am Coll Cardiol 15:827–832
13. Agatston A, Janowitz W, Hildner F, Zusmer N, Viamonte M, Detrano R (1990) Quantification of coronary artery calcium using ultrafast computed tomography. J Am Coll Cardiol 15:827–832
14. Taylor AJ, Burke AP, O'Malley PG, Farb A, Malcom GT, Smialek J, Virmani R (2000) A comparison of the Framingham risk index, coronary artery calcification, and culprit plaque morphology in sudden cardiac death. Circulation 101:1243–1248
15. Janowitz WR, Agatston AS, Kaplan G, Viamonte M, Jr. (1993) Differences in prevalence and extent of coronary artery calcium detected by ultrafast computed tomography in asymptomatic men and women. Am J Cardiol 72:247–254
16. Wong ND, Budoff MJ, Pio J, Detrano RC (2002) Coronary calcium and cardiovascular event risk: evaluation by age- and sex-specific quartiles. Am Heart J 143:456–459.
17. Hoff JA, Chomka EV, Krainik AJ, Daviglus M, Rich S, Kondos GT (2001) Age and gender distributions of coronary artery calcium detected by electron beam tomography in 35 246 adults. Am J Cardiol 87:1335–1339.
18. Raggi P, Callister TQ, Cooil B, He ZX, Lippolis NJ, Russo DJ, Zelinger A, Mahmarian JJ (2000) Identification of patients at increased risk of first unheralded acute myocardial infarction by electron-beam-computed tomography. Circulation 101:850–855
19. Detrano RC, Wong ND, Doherty TM, Shavelle RM, Tang W, Ginzton LE, Budoff MJ, Narahara KA (1999) Coronary calcium does not accurately predict near-term future coronary events in high-risk adults. Circulation 99:2633–2638
20. Arad Y, Spadaro LA, Goodman K, Newstein D, Guerci AD (2000) Prediction of coronary events with electron beam-computed tomography. J Am Coll Cardiol 36:1253–1260.
21. Becker CR, Kleffel T, Crispin A, Knez A, Young J, Schoepf UJ, Haberl R, Reiser MF (2001) Coronary artery calcium measurement: agreement of multirow detector and electron-beam CT. AJR Am J Roentgenol 176:1295–1298.
22. Arad Y, Spadaro LA, Goodman K, Lledo-Perez A, Sherman S, Lerner G, Guerci AD (1996) Predictive value of electron beam computed tomography of the coronary arteries. 19-month follow-up of 1173 asymptomatic subjects. Circulation 93:1951–1953
23. Wong ND, Hsu JC, Detrano RC, Diamond G, Eisenberg H, Gardin JM (2000) Coronary artery calcium evaluation by electron-beam computed tomography and its relation to new cardiovascular events. Am J Cardiol 86:495–498.
24. O'Malley PG, Taylor AJ, Jackson JL, Doherty TM, Detrano RC (2000) Prognostic value of coronary electron-beam computed tomography for coronary heart disease events in asymptomatic populations. Am J Cardiol 85:945–948
25. Hecht HS (2001) Impact of plaque imaging by electron-beam tomography on the treatment of dyslipidemias. Am J Cardiol 88:406–408
26. O'Malley PG, Taylor AJ, Gibbons RV, Feuerstein IM, Jones DL, Vernalis M, Brazaitis M (1999) Rationale and design of the Prospective Army Coronary Calcium (PACC) study: utility of electron-beam computed tomography as a screening test for coronary artery disease and as an intervention for risk factor modification among young, asymptomatic, active-duty United States Army Personnel. Am Heart J 137:932–941
27. Schmermund A, Möhlenkamp S, Stang A, Grönemeyer D, Seibel R, Hirche H, Mann K, Siffert W, Lauterbach K, Siegrist J, Jockel KH, Erbel R (2002) Assessment of clinically silent atherosclerotic disease and established and novel risk factors for predicting myocardial infarction and cardiac death in healthy middle-aged subjects: rationale and design of the

Heinz Nixdorf RECALL Study. Risk factors, evaluation of coronary calcium and lifestyle. Am Heart J 144:212–218.
28. Breen J, Sheedy P, Schwartz R, Stanson A, Kaufmann R, Moll P, Rumberger J (1992) Coronary artery calcification detected with ultrafast CT as an indication of coronary artery disease. Radiology 185:435–439
29. Fallavollita JA, Brody AS, Bunnell IL, Kumar K, Canty JM, Jr. (1994) Fast computed tomography detection of coronary calcification in the diagnosis of coronary artery disease. Comparison with angiography in patients < 50 years old. Circulation 89:285–290
30. Devries S, Wolfkiel C, Shah V, Chomka E, Rich S (1995) Reproducibility of the measurement of coronary calcium with ultrafast computed tomography. Am J Cardiol 75:973–975
31. Rumberger J, Sheedy P, III, Breen J (1995) Coronary calcium, as determined by electron beam computed tomography, and coronary disease on arteriogram: effect of patient's sex on diagnosis. Circulation 91:1363–1367
32. Budoff MJ, Georgiou D, Brody A, Agatston AS, Kennedy J, Wolfkiel C, Stanford W, Shields P, Lewis RJ, Janowitz WR, Rich S, Brundage BH (1996) Ultrafast computed tomography as a diagnostic modality in the detection of coronary artery disease: a multicenter study. Circulation 93:898–904
33. Haberl R, Becker A, Leber A, Knez A, Becker C, Lang C, Bruning R, Reiser M, Steinbeck G (2001) Correlation of coronary calcification and angiographically documented stenoses in patients with suspected coronary artery disease: results of 1764 patients. J Am Coll Cardiol 37:451–457.

17 Lung Cancer Detection and Characterization: Challenges and Solutions

D. P. NAIDICH

Introduction

The challenge of early detection and characterization of lung cancer represents a persistent clinical problem reflecting the dire nature of this malignancy. In the United States alone, nearly 175 000 new cases are diagnosed yearly, of which only 20–25% will be amenable to potential cure, with 5-year survival remaining less than 15% [10]. Although the use of routine chest radiography for screening has proved ineffective [19], recent technical developments have focused attention on the potential for CT screening, especially the detection of small peripheral lung tumors [12, 31]. These include: increasing availability of multidetector CT (MDCT) scanners with as many as 10 to 16 detector rows; advanced image-processing workstations capable of sophisticated image processing, including automatic nodule segmentation and volume assessment; and the use of computer-assisted diagnosis (CAD) for image analysis. While improving our ability to detect small peripheral lesions, not surprisingly, these technological developments provide us with new challenges and the opportunity to develop innovative solutions.

Lung Nodule Detection

Although CT is well documented to be superior to plain chest radiography for detecting pulmonary nodules, small lesions remain difficult to identify, especially using single detector CT scanners [1]. In a recent study of 5418 CT examinations in 1443 smokers, 7 of 22 lung cancers were retrospectively identifiable [15]. In a similar study reported by Henschke et al., 22 of 63 newly identified nodules could be identified retrospectively [12].

Factors affecting nodule detection have been well documented and include: technical parameters; variability in the morphologic appearance of small nodules; and inter- and intraobserver variability.

Technical factors that have been shown to affect nodule detection include slice thickness, reconstruction interval, pitch and dose, as well as differences in the methods of viewing. While it has been shown that use of thicker sections, larger reconstruction intervals, and pitch decrease nodule conspicuity, especially using single-detector CT scanners, dose appears to be of only minimal importance [9, 28].

Morphologic features that determine nodule conspicuity include size, density, contour, and location. Of these, the most important is size: predictably, smaller lesions, in particular those less than 5 mm in size, prove hardest to detect [15, 28]. Nodules adjacent to blood vessels, as well as those lying near the pulmonary hila, diaphragms, or even airways, also limit conspicuity [35]. Nodule density is another key determinant, with small ground-glass or subsolid nodules particularly difficult to identify.

Observer variability also plays an important role in assessing the accuracy of nodule detection [25]. In a recent study of 23 patients with 286 nodules between 2 and 40 mm in size evaluated by two readers, only 103 of 286 nodules were identified by both [36].

One response to these challenges is the use of MDCT scanners allowing use of a wider range of image-reconstruction techniques. While single-detector (SDCT) scanners allow volumetric data acquisition, increasing the pitch to allow greater anatomic coverage results in broadening the slice profile with a resulting decrease in nodule conspicuity, even when overlapping reconstructions are used. With multidetector scanners, it is now possible to routinely scan through the entire thorax in a single breath hold using 1-mm collimation: this allows both prospective and retrospective reconstruction of thick and thin high-resolution images without the need to rescan patients [16]. Equally important, volumetric acquisition of high-resolution datasets (comprising as many as 600 to 1000 1- to 1.25-mm images) allows a range of reconstruction options in addition to routine cine imaging including high-quality multiplanar reconstructions (MPRs), volumetric renderings and, in particular, overlapping maximum-intensity projections (MIPs). In a recent study of 122 nodules in 25 patients (3–9 mm in size) evaluated by five separate reviewers, Gruden et al. compared cine viewing of routine axial 3.75-mm sections reconstructed every 3 mm with 100-mm-thick MIPs reconstructed every 8 mm [11]. While between 20 and 39% of nodules were missed on axial images, only 9 to 18% were missed using overlapping MIPS ($p <$ 0.001). Maximum projection images proved of particular value in identifying central perihilar nodules, with 33–61% missed viewing axial images versus only 10–31% using MIPs.

Lung Nodule Characterization

While differentiating benign from malignant nodules remains problematic, recent improvements in morphologic assessment, contrast-enhanced densitometry, and accurate assessment of nodule growth over time has allowed improved assessment.

Morphologic Evaluation

Unfortunately, to date, most radiographic and CT signs have proved insufficiently predictive to provide reliable clinical management in individual cases. Noteworthy exceptions include the CT halo sign, indicative of fungal infection in immunocompromised patients [8], the feeding-vessel sign characteristic of metastatic disease in patients with known extrathoracic malignancies [20], and the presence of pseudocavitation within peripheral adenocarcinomas [22]. In the correct clinical setting, these signs may be sufficiently specific to warrant empiric therapy.

Recently, following the introduction of high-resolution, low-dose multidetector CT screening, the significance of previously overlooked lung nodules now requires clarification. This includes tiny nodules less than 5 mm in size, and the finding of small, well-defined ground glass nodules.

Size

Most tiny lesions in the lung are benign, especially when incidentally discovered by low-dose screening, usually representing either small noncalcified granulomas or intrapulmonary lymph nodes [6, 40]. As recently documented by Henschke et al. [13], of a total of 29 cancers identified in the initial low dose Early Lung Cancer Diagnosis Action Program (ELCAP) prevalence study, only one proved to be less than 5 mm in size, while 20% measured between 6 and 10 mm, 45% were between 11 and 20 mm, and 80% were greater than 20 mm in size. Similarly, of 2832 noncalcified nodules identified in 1049 individuals followed with low-dose CT screening at the Mayo Clinic over 2 years, among 35 CT-detected cancers only three measured 5 mm in size, with one additional 2-mm-small cell carcinoma identified [31]. These findings suggest that nodules less than 5 mm in size identified on screening studies may be safely followed. As recently reported by Quaterman et al. [27] in their retrospective review of 84 patients with surgically documented stage I and II non-small cell lung cancers between 1989 and 1999, no significant effect of delay on overall survival was found, with the mean preoperative interval measuring 82 days with a disease-specific 5-year survival of 63%. Further evidence suggesting that »benign« neglect of small nodules may be indicated comes from a retrospective study of 510 patients with T1N0M0 lesions in which no statistical relationship between survival and tumor size could be shown [26].

The Subsolid Nodule

With the introduction of MDCT scanners, there has been a remarkable transformation in our understanding of the nature and significance of focal subsolid pulmonary nodules (Fig. 1). In particular, characterizing lesions as ground glass or subsolid is proving to be an accurate means of defining nodules as belonging to the histologic spectrum of adenocarcinoma, as well as an accurate predictor of prognosis [21, 33]. In particular, there is close correspondence between the spectrum of CT findings (including both pure ground glass and mixed ground glass/solid nodules) and the Noguchi classification of peripheral adenocarcinomas, with pure ground glass nodules more likely representing either atypical adenomatous hyperplasia when less than 5 mm in size and bronchoalveolar cell carcinoma (BAC) with predominant lepidic growth when larger and solid components more likely reflecting the presence of invasive adenocarcinoma [2].

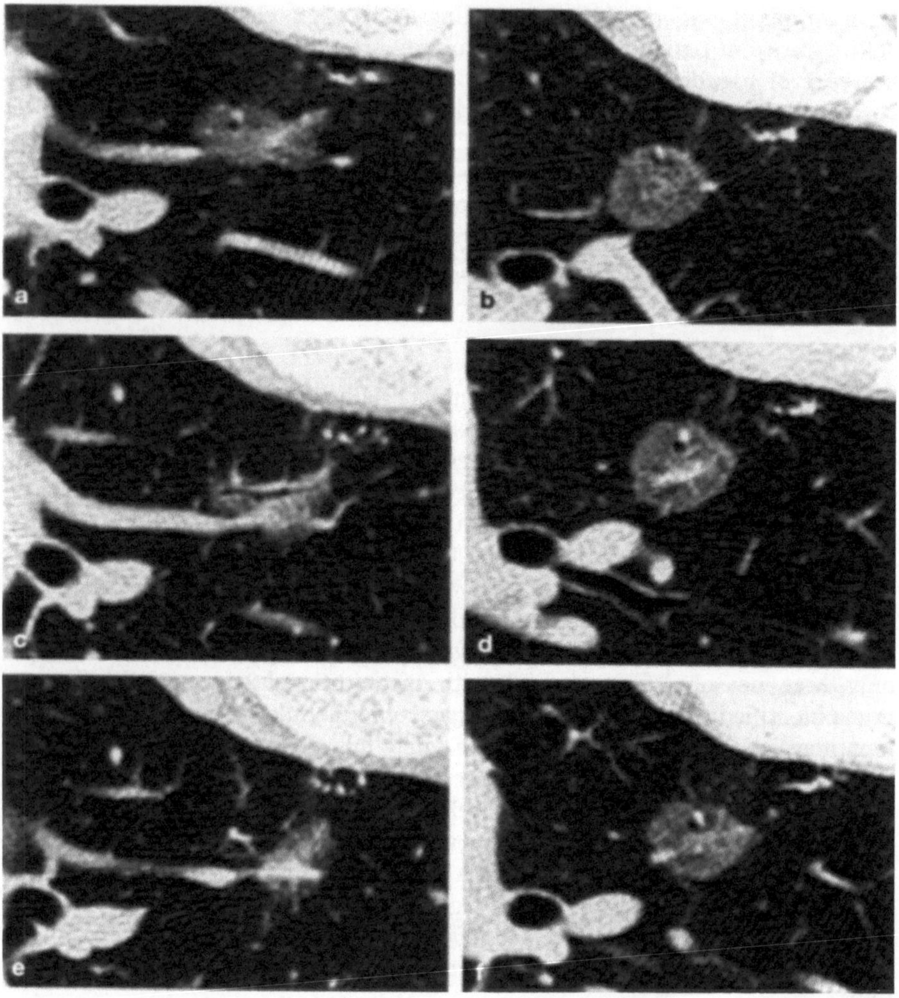

Fig. 1a–f. Bronchoalveolar cell carcinoma. Sequential 1 mm target reconstructed images through the medial aspect of the right lower lobe show the characteristic appearance of a well defined bronchoalveolar cell carcinoma (surgically proved). Note that with the exception of a crossing vessel there are no solid components identifiable. This appearance has been shown to correlate with improved prognosis.

Rarely identified prior to the introduction of low-dose screening, it is now apparent that localized subsolid nodules are commonplace, especially among smokers. As documented by Henschke et al., of 233 nodules initially detected by prevalence CT screening using single-detector CT scanner 44 (19%) proved to be subsolid [13]. More importantly, the finding of a subsolid nodule in this population proved a better indicator of likely neoplasia than solid nodules, with 15 (34%) of 44 proving malignant versus only 7% of solid nodules ($p = 0.000001$).

Not surprisingly, all represented either BAC or adenocarcinomas ($p = 0.0001$). Also not surprisingly, it has been shown that there is good correlation between the extent of ground glass density in subsolid nodules and prognosis [14].

Growth Assessment

In the setting of a nonspecific morphologic appearance and the absence of histologic verification, differentiation between benign and malignant nodules requires assessing the presence of growth. Measurement of growth typically is expressed in terms of tumor volume doubling time (VDT). Measurement of VDT assumes that nodules are essentially spherical: once nodule diameters are converted to volumes, VDT can then be calculated if the time difference (t), initial volume ($V0$), and volume at time t (V_t) is known [39]. Typically, VDTs for lung cancer range between 20 and 400 days, in distinction to benign nodules with volume-doubling times of either less than 20 days, or greater than 400 days, as occurs in patients with hamartomas or granulomas.

As a consequence of the large number of small, otherwise nonspecific, nodules now routinely identified following introduction of MDCT scanners, considerable attention has focused on developing reliable methods for assessing the growth of small nodules [39].

Unfortunately, accurate assessment of growth rates in small lung nodules, especially those less than 5 mm in size, is often problematic, particularly when reliance is placed solely on the use of bidimensional perpendicular measurements [32]. This is because a nodule doubles in volume when its diameter increases by only by one fourth. A 3-mm nodule, therefore, doubles in volume when it reaches 3.8 mm in diameter: not surprisingly, in routine clinical practice it is difficult to reach this degree of accuracy even with use of electronic calipers [36]. This becomes even more problematic for slower-growing malignancies with doubling times in the range of 800 days, such as typically occurs in patients with small localized bronchoalveolar cell carcinomas [2, 38].

For these reasons, recent attention has focused on obtaining automated segmentation and volume assessment of nodules [39]. While accurate and reproducible assessment of the volume of small nodules is dependent on methodology [17, 18], this approach represents a clear improvement over standard bidminensional cross-sectional measurements. Currently, most manufacturers have developed commmercially available software for stand-alone workstations to allow automated segmentation and volume assessment of lung nodules, making this approach likely to replace routine measurements in the near future [24, 25].

Clinical Management

As previously emphasized, the introduction of multidetector CT scanners has resulted in an exponential growth in the number of small nodules identified, even on routine CT studies. Although to date a number of algorithms have been proposed which have in common a focus on the need for close monitoring of small incidentally identified nodules [12, 23, 30], these have in common a growing realization that conservative clinical management is most often appropriate. Given that the vast majority of small nodules less than 5 mm in size are most likely benign, and with increasingly accurate methods for assessing even subtle growth, in most cases it remains only to determine an appropriate time interval for follow-up assessment. While management of solid nodules remains controversial, it is increasingly clear that semisolid nodules do not require as aggressive a follow up. Suzuki et al., for example, in a retrospective study of 69 lung cancers with a large (greater than 50%) ground glass component showed that 47 (68%) were BACs while 22 (32%) were minimally invasive adenocarcinomas, none demonstrating lymphatic invasion or nodal metastases [29]. Based on these data, these authors have proposed that subsolid nodules that show no interval growth over 3 months may either be conservatively managed by continued observation or successfully managed with only limited surgical resection. Similarly, Wang et al., in a study of cancer growth rates in patients identified by low-dose CT screening, concluded that lesions less than 5 mm in size require only yearly follow-up CT exams [34].

In our experience, ground glass nodules less than 5 mm in size need be assessed only yearly, provided there is no history of prior malignancy. While larger ground glass nodules (between 5 and 10 mm in size) should initially be followed at 6-month intervals for at least 1 year, solid nodules between 3 and 8 mm in size require reevaluation in 3 months. Solid nodules greater than 8–10 mm, especially if irregular or spiculated, may alternatively be evaluated using either nodule enhancement following intravenous contrast administration, PET scanning or biopsy, as warranted.

Future Directions: Computer Assisted Detection (CAD)

Considerable interest has recently focused on the use of computer assistance in detecting and characterizing lung nodules [3–5, 7, 17, 37].

In a recent study of 38 low-dose CT scans using 10-mm section thickness, for example, including 50 nodules not prospectively identified by readers, 31 of which proved to be malignant, CAD detected 80% of the nodules including 78% of cancers missed due to detection errors, and 93% of lesions missed due to interpretive errors, providing an overall sensitivity of 84% [5]. Novak et al. [25], in a study of ten consecutive low-dose screening studies obtained with a 4-row multidetector CT scanner using 1-mm collimators, compared 7-mm-thick sections evaluated by three experienced chest radiologists to CAD interpretation using contiguous 1-mm-sections, and showed that while only 8 (31%) of 26 nodules were detected by all three readers (1.4 to 2.1 nodules per patient), CAD identified a total of 3.2 nodules per patient representing an increase in sensitivity of between 114 and 207%. As expected, most of these additional nodules proved to be less than 4 mm in size or centrally located.

Although still in its infancy, it may be anticipated that CAD will play a crucial role in evaluating patients with suspected pulmonary nodules, especially in conjunction with advanced image-processing techniques already available, including the use of automated nodule segmentation and volume assessment as well as computer identification of nodule growth over time. Coupled with sophisticated data mining techniques, these advances promise to revolutionize CT interpretation.

References

1. Ambrogi V, Paci M, Pompeo E et al. (2000) Transxiphoid video assisted pulmonary metastatectomy. Relevance of helical CT for occult lesions. Ann Thorac Surg 70:1847–1852
2. Aoki T, Nakaata H, Watanabe Hea (2000) Evolution of peripheral lung adenocarcinomas: CT findings correlated with histology and tumor doubling times. AJR 174:763–768
3. Armato SG, Giger ML, MacMahon H (2001) Automated detection of lung nodules in CT scans: preliminary results. Medical Physics 28:1552–1561
4. Armato SG, Giger ML, Moran CJ et al. (1999) Computerized detection of pulmonary nodules on CT scans. Radiographics 19:1303–1311
5. Armato SG, Li F, Giger ML et al. (2002) Lung cancer: performance of automated lung nodule detection applied to cancers mssed in a CT screening program. Radiology 225
6. Bankoff MS, McEniff NJ, Bhadelia RA et al. (1996) Prevalence of pathologically proven intrapulmonary lymph nodes and their appearance on CT. AJR 167:629–630
7. Brown MS, McNitt-Gray MF, Goldin JGea (2001) Patient-specific models for lung nodule detection and surveillance in CT images. IEEE Trans Med Imaging 20:1242–1250
8. Gaeta M, Blandino A, Scribano E et al. (1999) Computed tomography halo sign in pulmonary nodules: frequency and diagnostic value. J Thorac Imag 14:109–113
9. Gartenschlager M, Schweden F, Gast K et al. (1998) Pulmonary nodules: detection with low-dose vs conventional-dose spiral CT. European Radiol 8:609–614
10. Greenlee RT, Murray T, Bolden S et al. (2000) Cancer statistics, 2000. CA Cancer J Clin 50:7–33
11. Gruden JF, Ouanounou S, Tigges Sea (2002) Incremental benefit of maximum-intensity-projection images on observer detection of small pulmonary nodules revealed by multidetector CT. AJR 179:149–157
12. Henschke CI, Naidich DP, Yankelevitz DFea (2001) Early lung cancer action project: initial findings on repeat screeings. Cancer 1:1533–1159
13. Henschke CI, Yankelevitz DF, Mirtcheva RMea (2002) CT screening for lung cancer: frequency and significance of part-solid and nonsolid nodules. AJR 178:1053–1057
14. Higashiyama M (1999) Ann Thorac Surg 68
15. Kakinuma R, Ohmatsu H, Kaneko Mea (1999) Detection failures in spiral CT screening for lung cancer: analysis of CT findings. Radiology 212:61–66
16. Klingenbeck-Regn K, Schaller S, Flohr Tea (1999) Subsecond multi-slice computed tomography: basics and applications. Eur J Radiol 31:110–124
17. Ko EJ, Betke M: Chest CT (2001) automated nodule detection and assessment of change over time: preliminary experience. Radiology 218:267–273
18. Ko JP, Rusinek H, Jacobs E et al. (2003) Volume measurement of small pulmonary nodules on chest CT: a phantom study. Radiology Accepted for publication
19. Marcus PM, Bergstralh EJ, Fagerstrom RMea (2000) Lung cancer mortality in the Mayo Lung Project: impact of extended follow-up. J Natl Cancer Inst 92:1308–1316
20. Milne ENC, Zerhouni EA (1987) Blood supply of pulmonary metastases. J Thorac Imag 2:15–23
21. Nakata M, Saeki H, Takata I et al. (2002) Focal ground-glass opacity detected by low-dose helical CT. Chest 121:1464–1467
22. Nambu A, Miyata K, Ozawa K et al. (2002) Air-containing space in lung adenocarcinoma: hgh-resolution computed tomography findings. J Comput Assist Tomogr 26:1026–1031
23. Nawa T, Nakagawa K, Kusano Sea (2002) Lung cancer screening using low dose spiral CT. Chest 122:15–20

24. Novak CL, Naidich DP, Fan L et al. (2001) Improving radiologist' confidence of interpreting low-dose multi-slice lung CT screening studies using an interactive CAD system. Radiology 224pp
25. Novak CL, Qian J, Fan JP et al. (2002) Inter-observer variations on interpretation of multi-slice CT lung cancer screening studies, and the implications for computer-aided diagnosis. In: Medical imaging 2002: image perception, observer performance, and technology assessment. pp 68–79
26. Patz Jr. EF (2000) Correlation of tumor size. Chest 117
27. Quarterman RL, McMillan A, Ratcliffe MB et al. (2003) Effect of preoperative delay on prognosis for patients with early stage non-small cell lung cancer. J Thorac Cardiovasc Surg 125:108–114
28. Rusinek H, Naidich DP, McGuinness G et al. (1998) Pulmonary nodule detection: low-dose versus conventional CT. Radiology 209:243–249
29. Suzuki K, Asamura H, Kusumoto M et al. (2002) »Early« peripheral lung cancer: Prognostic significance of ground glass opacity on thin-section computed tomographic scan. Ann Thorac Surg 74:1635–1639
30. Swensen SJ, Jett JR, Sloan JA et al. (2002) Screening for lung cancer with low-dose spiral computed tomography. Am J Respir Critical Care Med 165:508–513
31. Swensen SJ, Jettt JR, Hartman TE et al. (2003) Lung cancer screening with CT: Mayo Clinic experience. Radiology 226:756–761
32. Therrasse P, Arbuck SG, Eisenhauer EAea (2000) New guidelines to evaluate the response to treatment in solid tumors. European Organization for Research and Treatment of Cancer, National Cancer Institute of the United States, National Cancer Institute of Canada. J Natl Cancer Inst 92:205–216
33. Travis WD (2002) Pathology of lung cancer. Clinics Chest Med 23:65+
34. Wang JC, Sone S, Li Fea (2000) Rapidly growing small peripheral lung cancers detectged by screening TC: correlation between radiological appearance and pathological features. Br J Radiol 73:930–937
35. White CS, Romney BM, Mason AC et al. (1996) Primary carcinoma of the lung overlooked at CT: analysis of findings in 14 patients. Radiology 199:109–115
36. Wormanns D, Diederich S, Lentschig MGea (2000) Spiral CT of pulmonary nodules: inter-observer variation in assessment of lesion size. Eur Radiol 10:710–713
37. Wormanns D, Fiebich M, Saidi Mea (2002) Automatic detection of pulmonary nodules at spiral CT: clinical application of a computer-aided diagnosis system. Eur Radiol 12:1052–1057
38. Yankelevitz DF, Henschke C (1997) Does 2-year stability imply that pulmonary nodules are benign? AJR 168:325–328
39. Yankelevitz DF, Reeves AP, Kostis WJ (2000) Small pulmonary nodules; volumetrically determined growth rates based on CT evaluation. Radiology 217:251–256
40. Yokomise H, Mizuno H, Ike O et al. (1998) Importance of intrapulmonary lymph nodes in the differential diagnosis of small pulmonary nodular shadows. Chest 113:703–706

18 Techniques and Interpretation of Multislice CT Colonography

M. MACARI

Introduction

Virtual colonoscopy is an evolving non-invasive imaging technique allowing detection of colorectal polyps and cancers. Currently, most centers utilize computed tomography (CT) for image acquisition [1]. In Europe and several centers in the United States, some investigators are acquiring virtual colonoscopy data using MR imaging [2]. A potential advantage of MR imaging is lack of exposure to ionizing radiation. However, using CT to acquire virtual colonoscopy data, the radiation dose to the patient can be substantially lowered when compared to routine abdominal and pelvic CT related to the high tissue contrast between the insufflated colonic gas and the wall of the colon [3]. In either case, utilizing either CT or MR, certain fundamental aspects of the procedure have emerged since the first report of virtual colonoscopy appeared in the literature in 1994 [4].

Patient Preparation and Data Acquisition for Virtual Colonoscopy

Bowel Preparation

Virtual colonoscopy continues to evolve in an attempt to increase the diagnostic performance of the examination. Regarding patient preparation, it is desirable to perform virtual colonoscopy in patients with »clean« colons [1, 3, 5–9]. Currently, the biggest limitation of virtual colonoscopy is bowel preparation. Like all other techniques that attempt to image and visualize the colon surface, the colon needs to be cleansed of residual fecal material. At New York University, commercial preparation kits are used as bowel preparation. The instructions are easy for the patient to follow and the kits are inexpensive. The two commercial preparation kits that we utilize are the 24-h Fleet 1 Preparation (Fleet Pharmaceuticals, Lynchburg, VA) or the LoSo Preparation (EZ-EM, Westbury, NY). However, these preparations do on occasion leave more fecal residue than a typical electrolyte preparation or a double dose, that is, two 45-ml doses of phospho-soda. In our experience, approximately 5% of patients who undergo bowel preparation with these commercial kits will have a poor preparation, limiting interpretation.

Given this limitation, the idea of fecal and fluid tagging for virtual colonoscopy is currently being evaluated [10, 11]. Fecal tagging can be performed without bowel cleansing [10] or with bowel cleansing [10, 11, 12]. Fecal tagging without bowel cleansing relies on having the patient ingest small amounts of iodine or dilute barium with low fat and fiber diets beginning several days prior to the examination. When the CT examination is performed, residual fecal material will appear in high attenuation.

Colonic Distension

Once the colon has been prepared, the examination is ready to be performed. It should be noted that different institutions utilize different CT techniques. At our institution, data acquisition is performed entirely by a trained technologist or a nurse [3]. A radiologist is not on-site. Obviously, an experienced technologist or nurse is required, but after adequate training the examination can be performed in this manner, thus minimizing radiologist time commitment to data acquisition.

Immediately prior to the examination, the patient evacuates any residual fluid from the rectum. Therefore, easy access to a close bathroom is essential. For colonic insufflation, either room air or carbon dioxide (CO_2) can be used. The use of room air is easy, clean, and inexpensive. Proponents of CO_2 argue that because it is readily absorbed from the colon it causes less cramping after the procedure than room air insufflation. In our experience, CO_2 is associated with less delayed discomfort. While cramping may be a problem in some patients after room air insufflation, most find the examination to be quick and minimally uncomfortable.

A small rubber catheter is used to insufflate the colon with a hand-held bulb syringe. This catheter is much smaller than a barium enema tip and a balloon is not used. Patients do not feel this catheter being inserted. Patients are encouraged to keep the gas in. Approximately 40 puffs with a hand-held bulb syringe is sufficient to distend the colon. However, we do not use a set strict number of insufflations, since the length of an individual colon is variable. Also, if the ileocecal valve is incompetent, more gas will be required for optimal distension. We do not use a bowel relaxant (Glucagon) for CT colonography [7]. After insufflation, the catheter is left in the rectum and a single scout CT image is obtained in the supine position to verify adequate bowel distension. If adequate bowel distension is present, the CT examination is performed. If adequate bowel distension is not achieved, additional air is insufflated into the rectum. Following air insufflation, CTC is performed first in the supine position in a cephalo-caudad direction encompassing the entire colon and rectum. The patient is then placed in the prone position. Several additional puffs of air are then administered. Following a second scout localizing image, the process is repeated over the same z-axis range [3]. While one study found improved detection of polyps after the administration of IV contrast material, we do not utilize IV contrast [15].

Data Acquisition

The single most important factor in the improvement of the performance of virtual colonoscopy has been the development and installation of multidetector row spiral CT scanners. These scanners allow between 4 and 16 slices to be obtained in a single rotation of the X-ray tube [3, 13–16]. The advantages of these scanners are that they allow large volumes of data to be scanned with very thin sections in a single breath-hold. As a result, motion artifact from respiration and peristalsis is decreased or eliminated. Moreover, interpretation is not limited to evaluation with axial images only. Using improved computer workstations, coronal, sagital, and endoluminal images can all be obtained from the single axial acquisition, thus facilitating differentiation of polyps, bulbous folds and residual fecal material [3]. At NYU, we utilize a 4 x 1-mm slice detector configuration, 120 kV, 0.5 s gantry rotation and effective 50 mAs. This enables the entire colon to be covered within a 30-s breath-hold. CT images are reconstructed as 1.25-mm-thick sections with a 1-mm reconstruction interval. The examination is networked to a workstation where data interpretation can proceed. Some investigators are now utilizing an ultralow dose of 20 effective mAs. However, this limits evaluation of extracolonic findings.

Data Interpretation Techniques

Currently, many sophisticated computer workstations are available to interpret virtual colonoscopy examinations. These workstations allow fast processing of the data as well as an interactive ability to evaluate an abnormality in multiple projections including axial, coronal, and sagital multiplanar reformations as well as endoluminal views. There is some controversy regarding whether virtual colonoscopy examinations should be interpreted using a primary two-dimensional or three-dimensional viewing technique.

Most investigators agree that a primary axial 2-D review is sufficient, with the use of coronal and endoluminal imaging for problem solving. Using these techniques, the colon can be evaluated in approximately 5–15 min by an experienced reader. It is important to remember that whether one uses 2-D or 3-D as the primary review technique, both must be available to accurately differentiate folds, polyps, and residual fecal material.

When interpreting CT colonography data, a number of filling defects may be encountered in the colon. These include polyps, irregular and bulbous folds, and residual fecal material. Using thin-section multislice CTC, most of these lesions can be differentiated from each other [3] (Figs. 1–4). Clearly, the sensitivity of CTC for colorectal polyp detection is directly related to polyp size [3]. There is controversy regarding what should be considered a clinically significant colorectal polyp. Most small polyps are mucosal elevations, hyperplastic polyps, of diminutive tubular adenomas with no or very little clinical significance. Indeed, Bond [17] points out that most small polyps are clinically unimportant because they are tubular adenomas that will never develop the additional genetic alterations to cause malignant degeneration [13]. The suggestion that we shift our attention away from finding and removing all diminutive polyps and toward strategies that allow reliable detection of the less common, but more dangerous, advanced adenomas has been proposed [17].

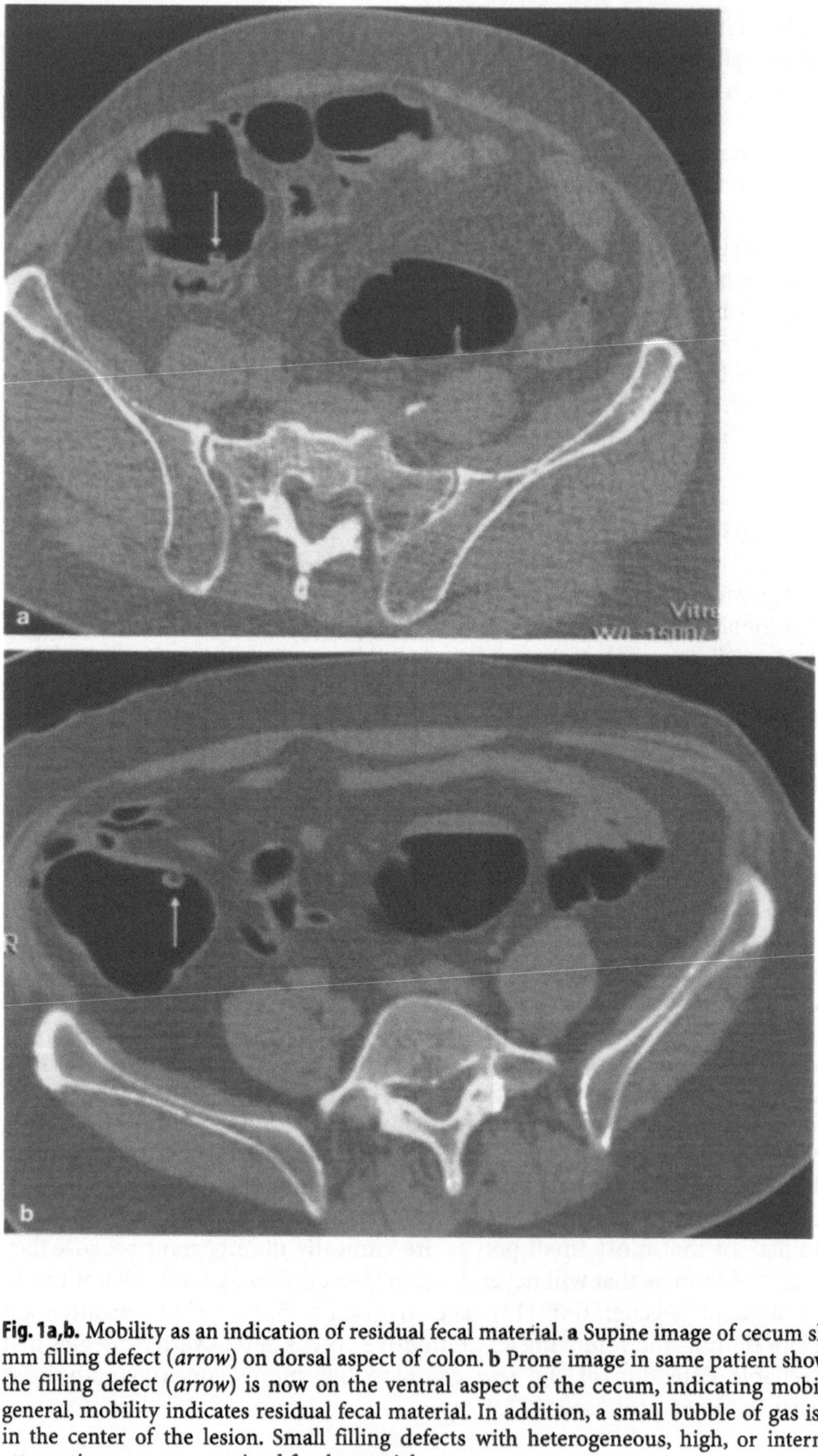

Fig. 1a,b. Mobility as an indication of residual fecal material. **a** Supine image of cecum shows 6 mm filling defect (*arrow*) on dorsal aspect of colon. **b** Prone image in same patient shows that the filling defect (*arrow*) is now on the ventral aspect of the cecum, indicating mobility. In general, mobility indicates residual fecal material. In addition, a small bubble of gas is noted in the center of the lesion. Small filling defects with heterogeneous, high, or internal gas attenuation represent retained fecal material

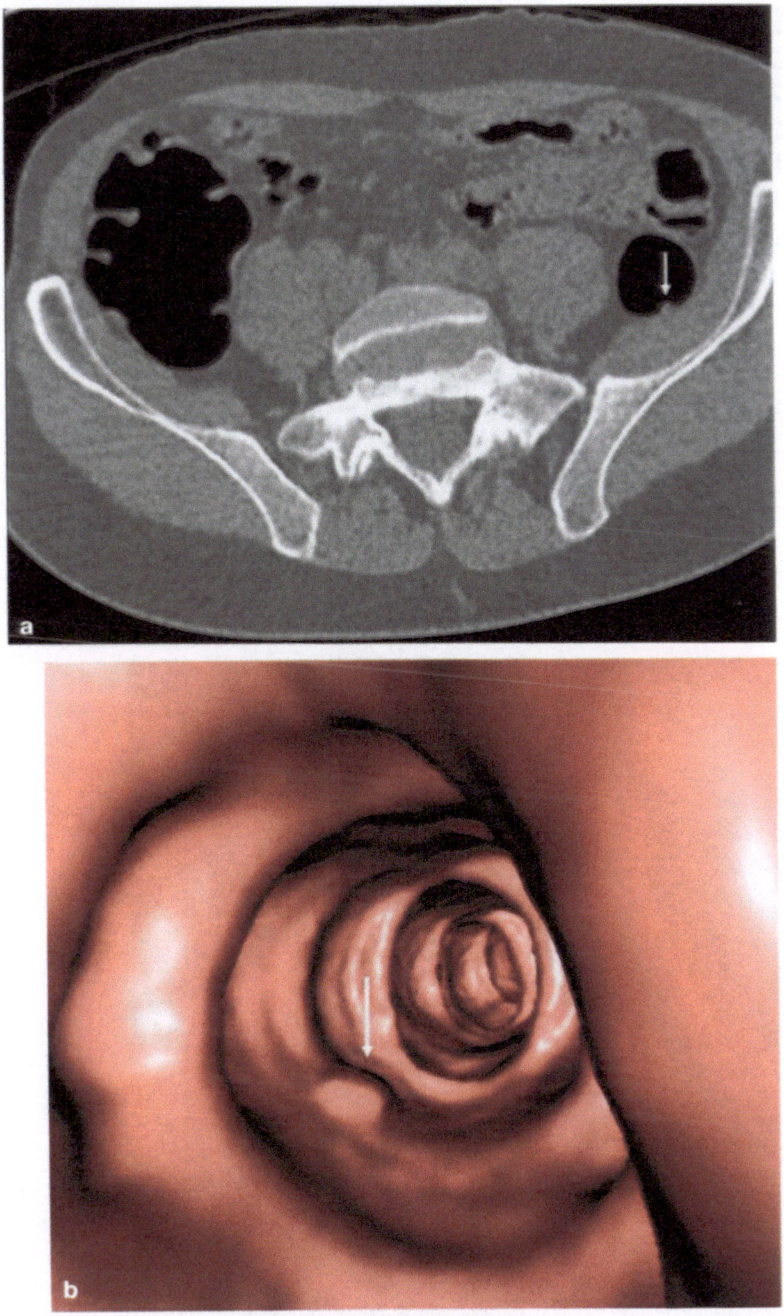

Fig. 2a,b. Small filling defect in descending colon with homogeneous attenuation. **a** Axial prone image show 5 mm filling defect (*arrow*) in the descending colon, which is on non-dependent surface. **b** Endoluminal image confirms small polypoid lesion. At colonoscopy a 5-mm tubular adenoma was found

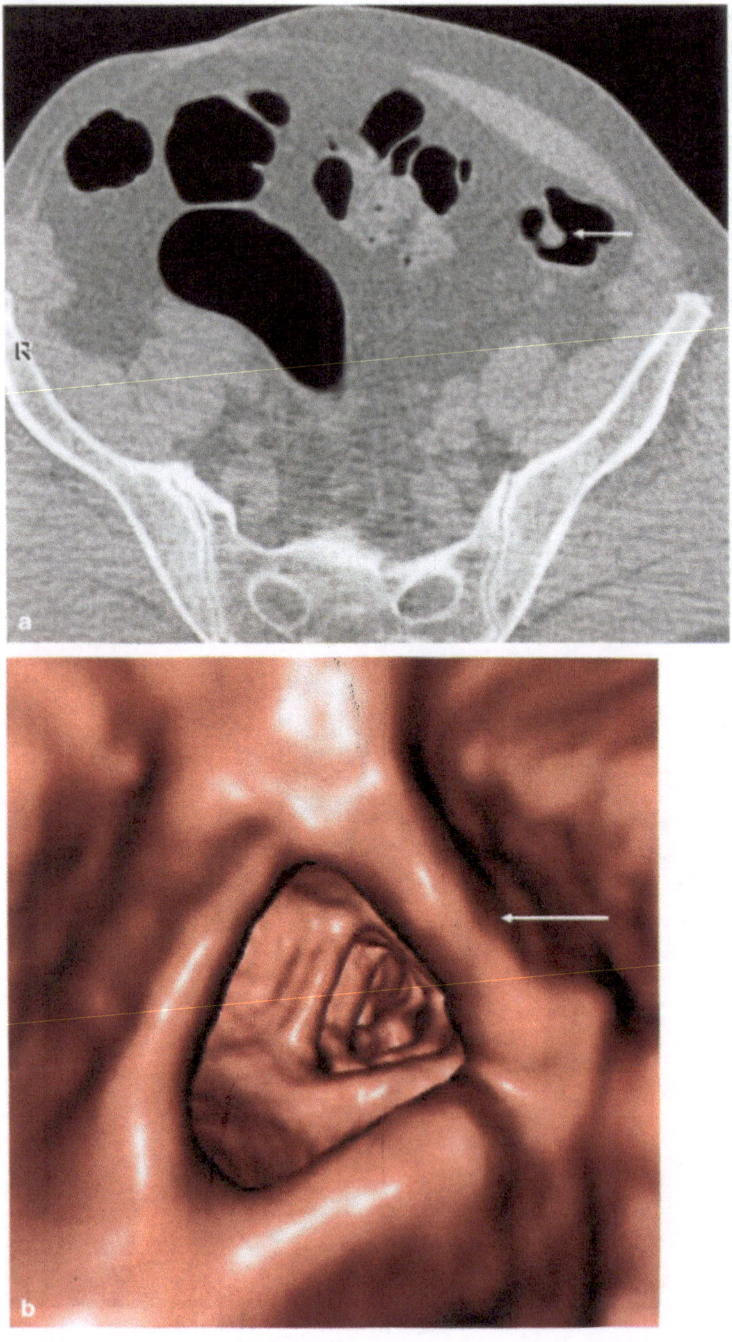

Fig. 3a,b. Use of endoluminal imaging to differentiate bulbous fold from polyo. **a** Axial CT image shows pedunculated filling defect in descending colon (*arrow*). **b** Endoluminal image shows the filling defect actually represents interhaustral fold (*arrow*)

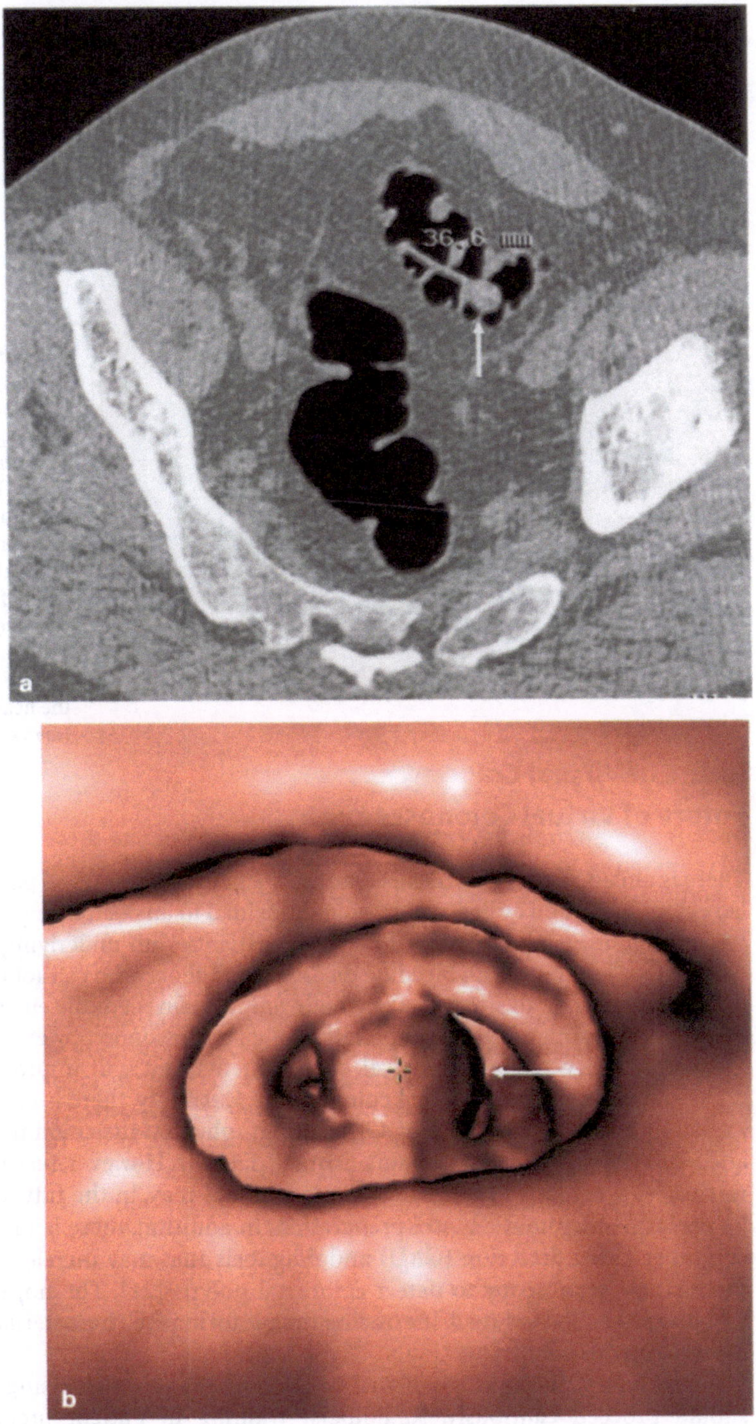

Fig. 4a, b

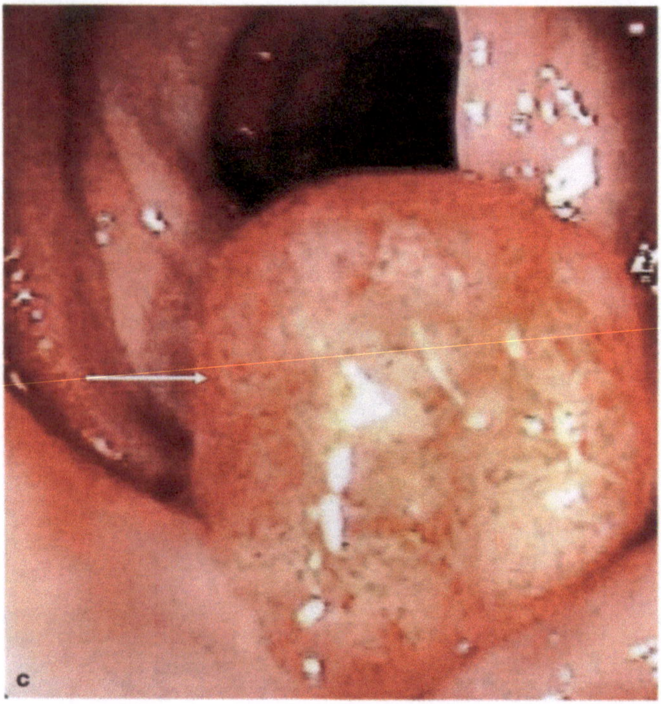

Fig. 4a–c. Pedunculated polyp on stalk. **a** Axial CT image shows polyp on stalk in sigmoid colon (*arrow*). The head and stalk together measure 36.6 mm. **b** Endoluminal image shows head of polyp (*arrow*). **c** Conventional colonoscopy shows similar morphology of the head of the polyp (*arrow*)

Future of Virtual Colonoscopy

There is already a role for virtual colonoscopy in evaluating those patients with failed colonoscopy and evaluating the colon proximal to an obstructing lesion [18–20]. In addition, it may be the test of choice in patients with underlying medical problems as well as those with bleeding disorders and those who cannot undergo sedation. It is important to stress that currently only certain medical centers have expertise in the performance and interpretation of virtual colonoscopy examinations.

There are several technological developments that will improve the performance characteristics of virtual colonoscopy. Currently, there is consensus in the radiology community regarding CT colonography that the colon needs to be cleaned and well distended to obtain adequate datasets. However, research into optimizing fecal tagging with subtraction techniques may, in the future, allow CT to be performed without a bowel preparation. In addition, there is much interest in computer-aided detection (CAD) and diagnosis that may increase the ability of the virtual colonoscopy to detect colorectal polyps [21]. The hope is that CAD will be used as second read, increasing the performance characteristics of virtual colonoscopy in polyp detection.

In summary, the future of virtual colonoscopy is very promising. However, we should proceed cautiously. Radiologist training in patient preparation, data acquisition, and perhaps most importantly, data interpretation is necessary if virtual colonoscopy will ever be able to be used in the general radiology community.

References

1. Johnson CD, Dachman AH (2000) CT colonography: the next colon screening examination. Radiology 216:331–341
2. Morrin MM, Hochman MG, Farrell RJ et al. (2001) MR colonography using colonic distension with air as the contrast material. AJR 176:144–146
3. Macari M, Bini EJ, Xue X et al. (2002) Colorectal neoplasms: prospective comparison of thin-section low-dose multi-detector row CT colonography and conventional colonoscopy for detection. Radiology 224: 383–392
4. Vining DJ, Gelfand DW, Bechtold et al. (1994) Technical feasibility of colon imaging with helical CT and virtual reality (abstr). AJR 162:194
5. Fletcher JG, Johnson CD, Welch TJ et al. (2000) Optimization of CT colonography technique: prospective trial in 180 patients. Radiology 216:704–711
6. Chen SC, Lu DSK, Hecht JR, Ladell BM (1999) CT colonography: value of scanning in both the supine and prone positions. AJR 172:595–600
7. Yee J, Hung RK, Akekar GA, Wall SD (1999) The usefulness of glucagon hydrochloride for colonic distension. AJR 173:169–172
8. Yee J, Akerkar GA, Hung RK, Steinauer-Gebauer AM, Wall SD, McQuaid KR (2001) Colorectal neoplasia: performance characteristics of CT colonography for detection in 300 patients. Radiology 219:685–692
9. Macari M, Pedrosa I, Lavelle M et al. (2001) Effect of different bowel preparations on residual fluid at CT colonography. Radiology 218:274–277
10. Callstrom MR, Johnson CD, Fletcher JG et al. (2001) CT colonography without cathartic preparation: feasibility study. Radiology 219: 693–698
11. Lefere PA, Gryspeerdt SS, Dewyspelaere J, Baekelandt M, Van Holsbeeck BG (2002) Dietary fecal tagging as a cleansing method before CT colonography: initial results-polyp detection and patient acceptance. Radiology 224:393–403
12. Rex D (2000) Virtual colonoscopy: time for some tough questions for radiologists and gastroenterologists. Endoscopy 32:260–263
13. McCollough CH, Zink FE (1999) Performance evaluation of a multi-slice CT system. Med Phys 26:2223–2230
14. Hara AK, Johnson CD, McCarty RL, Welch TJ, McCollough CH, Harmsen WS (2001) CT colonography: single versus multi-detector row imaging. Radiology 219:461–465
15. Morrin M, Farrell RJ, Kruskal JB et al. (2000) Utility of intravenously administered contrast material at CT colonography. Radiology 217:765–771
16. Hara AK, Johnson CD, Reed JE et al. (1997) Reducing data size and radiation dose for CT colonography. AJR 168:1181–1184
17. Bond JH (1999) Virtual colonoscopy—promising, but not ready for widespread use. NEJM 341:1540–1542
18. Macari M, Megibow AJ, Berman P, Milano A, Dicker M (1999) CT colonography in patients with failed colonoscopy. AJR 173:561–564
19. Morrin MM, Kruskal JB, Farrell RJ et al. (1999) Endoluminal CT colonography after incomplete endoscopic colonoscopy. AJR 172:913–918
20. Fenlon HM, McAneny DB, Nunes DP, Clarke PD, Ferrucci JT (1999) Occlusive colon carcinoma: virtual colonoscopy in the preoperative evaluation of the proximal colon. Radiology 210:423–428
21. Summers RM, Johnson CD, Pusanik LM et al. (2001) Automated polyp detection at CT colonography: feasibility assessment in a human population. Radiology 219:51–59

Subject Index